HYPNOTIC TECHNIQUES FOR INCREASING SELF-ESTEEM

EDITED BY R. A. STEFFENHAGEN, Ph.D.

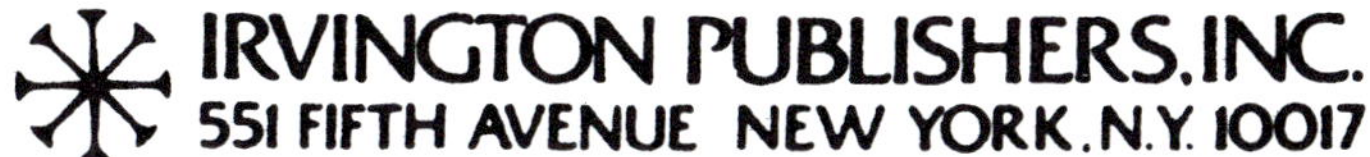

IRVINGTON PUBLISHERS, INC.
551 FIFTH AVENUE NEW YORK, N.Y. 10017

Library of Congress Cataloging in Publication Data

Main entry under title:

Hypnotic techniques for increasing self-esteem.

Bibliography: p.
1. Psychology, Pathological. 2. Deviant behavior.
3. Self-respect. 4. Hypnotism—Therapeutic use.
I. Steffenhagen, R. A.
RC454.4.H96   616.89   82-6551
ISBN 0-8290-0775-X   AACR2

Printed in the United States of America

LIST OF CONTRIBUTORS

BIOGRAPHICAL NOTES ON THE CONTRIBUTORS

NICHOLAS L. DANIGELIS — University of Vermont. Nicholas L. Danigelis Received his Ph.D. from Indiana University, has taught at the University of Wisconsin and is now Associate Professor at the University of Vermont. Dr. Danigelis has published articles on minority politics and suicide and is an expert in the study of Durkehim's contribution to suicide theory.

JULIA R. FLYNN — Julia R. Flynn is a graduate of the University of Vermont. She majored in sociology and is planning to begin graduate work in medical sociology.

RUBEN FOURNIER — Ruben Fournier is a graduate of the University of Vermont and is pursuing an advanced degree at the Massachusetts School of Pharmacy. He was a psychology major and a close associate of the author.

JOSEPH HARRY ASSOCIATE PROFESSOR — Northern Illinois Univeristy. Joseph Harry received his Ph.D. from the University of Oregon and has taught at Oregon, Wayne State University, College of Idaho and is now Associate Professor at Northern Illinois University. He is an authority in the area of deviance, is author of the *Social Organization of Gay Males* and author and co-author of numerous articles. Dr. Harry is one of the leading young sociologists to deal with homosexuality from a theoretical and empirical perspective.

H. GILMAN McCANN — University of Vermont. H. Gilman McCann is an Associate Professor at the University of Vermont. He has his Ph.D. from Princeton with a specialty in the sociology of science, methodology and deviance. He is author of *Chemistry Transformed: The Paradigmatic Shift From Phlogiston to Oxygen* and articles on deviance. He has been the recipient of honors at Allegheny and Princeton. He has taught at Princeton, University of California at Santa Cruz, and New Mexico.

J. MICHAEL MCKNIGHT — University of Vermont. J. Michael McKnight received his Ph.D. from McMaster University. He is an Assistant Professor in the Department of Religion at the University of Vermont. He has published articles on the history of religions and has a special interest in the interaction of eastern and western religious traditions in contemporary society.

GAIL GLEASON MILGRAM — Rutgers University Gail Gleason Milgram received her Ed.D. from Rutgers University in administration and supervision. She is Associate Professor at Rutgers and the author of nine books dealing mostly with alcohol among youth. She has published numerous articles and conducted many workshops on alcoholism. Without question Dr. Milgram is one of the leading authorities on teenage drinking. She is Director of Education, Center of Alcohol Studies Rutgers.

WALTER O'CONNELL — Glass Ark. Walter O'Connell is a Diplomate in Psychology and was Director of Glass Ark in Texas. He is a past president of the American Adlerian Society and is on the editorial board of the Journal of Individual Psychology, Voices, The Individual Psychologist and Catholic Psychological Record. Dr. O'Connell has published over 200 articles and books and is highly respected in his field. He has developed Natural High Therapy as a technique for building self-esteem.

R. A. STEFFENHAGEN — University of Vermont. R. A. Steffenhagen is a clinical sociologist who studied under Marvin K. Opler, Professor of Social Psychiatry in the Department of Psychiatry at the State University of New York at Buffalo. He is now Professor at the University of Vermont. He has pursued research in deviance (drug abuse) since 1968 and has published articles on Drug Abuse in such journals as: International Journal of Social Psychiatry, Journal of Alcohol and Drug Education, Drug Forum, Journal of Drug Education, Journal of Individual Psychology, etc. He has been involved in drug counseling since 1968 and a practicing hypnotherapist since 1975. Out of his interests in research and practice he has developed a self-esteem theory of deviance based upon an Adlerian model and developed a hypnotherapeutic technique based upon the theory of deviance; an attempt to bring theory and practice together. He is a member of the American Society of Clinical Hypnosis, International Society of Hypnosis, professional member of the International Society for Professional Hypnotism, American Sociological Association and American Psychological Association. Dr. Steffenhagen is listed in American Men of Science and Men of Achievement.

MARK RAINVILLE — Mark Rainville is a graduate of the University of Vermont. He majored in sociology and is planning to go to graduate school in counseling.

ACKNOWLEDGEMENTS

Of the twelve chapters in this book all are original material written for this book. Chapter one has/will also appear in the *Journal of Alcohol and Drug Education* by permission of Irvington Publishers. A case history has been added to each deviance chapter to show how self-esteem hypnotherapy can be utilized to deal with deviance. The approach has been to build self-esteem and not work with the sympton — the result being the disappearance of the symptom.

I am indebted to my contributors for their excellent contributions to this text. I am indebted to my mentor Marvin K. Opler who inspired me to pursue research in social psychiatry and Heinz Ansbacher whose tutelage in Adlerian Psychology has revived my interest in theory development.

FOREWORD

William James and Alfred Adler were pioneers in recognizing the importance of self-esteem as a motivator of human behavior. This focus on a dimension of personality, rather than on sexual drive, as the basis of motivation, was largely responsible for Adler's break with Freud. While Freudian theory has tended to dominate the intellectual climate through the first half of the 20th century, the brilliant insights of Alfred Adler have lain dormant. Within the past decade, Adler's greatest contribution, the role of self-esteem as the prime motivator of behavior, has begun to have greater impact on social-psychological research and to influence the *Weltanschauung* of the West. One needs merely to peruse the annotated bibliography presented at the end of this volume to realize that self-esteem is being related to a myriad of behaviors — e.g., work, equality, sex, god images, school, achievement, and sex role stereotypes, to mention just a few of the areas capturing the interest of the researcher.

The references to self-esteem in the literature today are twofold: they are theoretical, such as in Ernest Becker's *Birth and Death of Meaning*, and they are empirical as evidenced by the research cited in the bibliography. Academicians tend to pursue both theoretical empirical avenues in their quest for knowledge. Theory should provide the guidelines for research and research should support theory. As Goethe put it:

"Jeder wandle fur sich und wisse nichtsvan dem andern
Wandelen nur beide gerad, finden sich beide gewiss."

or,

"Each should travel his own path, knowing nothing of the other;
If both travel as they should, they will certainly find each other."

Too often, this is not the case in academia; theorists and empiricists frequently travel their own paths, but they do not find each other.

The present volume explores both theoretical and emprical articulations of a theory of self-esteem as a framework for the study of deviant behavior. Part I, comprising the first three chapters, provides a theoretical-philosophical orientation to the relationship between self-esteem and deviance and illustrates the use of hypnotherapy as a technique for the emelioration of deviance through the building of self-esteem. In Chapter 1, "Hypnosis and Alcoholism: A

Theoretical Perspective," the author points out that hypnotherapy is not a therapeutic modality in its own right, but rather, a process which can be used to enhance a therapeutic perspective. The concept was developed by the author as the result of two research interests, hypnosis and deviance. Chapter 2, "Hypnosis in Building Self- esteem," elaborates the use of a special hypnotherapeutic technique for building self-esteem using hypnosis, and places particular emphasis on enhancing self-esteem through attention to the spiritual component of the self. This theme is continued in Chapter III, "Self-esteem and Hypnosis: A Transcendental Perspective," in which Dr. McKnight discusses self-esteem and hypnosis in relation to eastern religious philosophy.

Part II, a more detailed presentation of the development of a self- esteem theory of deviance, includes an operational definition of self-esteem and a discussion of how self-esteem develops within the individual. In Chapter IV, Dr. Steffenhagen relates the theory of self-esteem to empirical research on the personality of drug users and abusers, and in Chapter 5, "Self-esteem: A Model," Steffenhagen and Fournier more fully discuss the specific nature of self-esteem as a personality component. Chapter 6, "Self-esteem and Social Structure," offers a perspective on the source and development of self-esteem, taking into consideration its physical, psychological and social manifestations.

Parts III and IV explore the relationship between self-esteem theory and other theoretical and empirical approaches to the study of specific deviant behaviors. Part III comprises chapters on anorexia nervosa, youthful suicide, and deviance theory and, in each case, the possibilities, for integrating self-esteem theory with other theoretical perspectives are illustrated. Such integrations, as discussed by Steffenhagen and Flynn, Danigelis, and McCann, may result in models of deviant behavior which would facilitate treatment and broaden the scope of current research.

In contrast to the chapters in Part III, which emphasize a theoretical perspective, those in Part IV, focusing on the deviant behaviors of teenage drinking, heroin addiction, and homosexuality, illustrate a decidely empirical orientation. Milgram provides data on teenage drinking patterns, focusing on studies which include self-esteem, alienation and related concepts. O'Connell contributes a socio-empirical discussion of the organizational and bureaucratic obstacles to the building of self- esteem in a large treatment center. Finally, Harry's chapter on self- esteem and effeminacy in gay males explores the relationships among psychological well-being, social processes, and male homosexuality.

The present volume is intended to illustrate the utility of self-esteem theory in the understanding of deviant behavior, as well as to suggest a diversity of potential applications of a model informed by this theoretical perspective. The interdisciplinary nature of the text reflects the many paths that have already been taken; however, it is hoped that it also suggests many points along the way at which travelers may "certainly find each other."

CONTENTS

R. A. Steffenhagen Ph.D
Department of Sociology
University of Vermont

1

HYPNOSIS IN THE TREATMENT OF ALCOHOLISM: A THEORETICAL PERSPECTIVE

There are many different approaches to the treatment of alcoholism, most of which have been borrowed from human service disciplines. Most of these approaches, however, explain alcoholism using either a moral deficit model or a disease model, the latter being the most accepted model today.

Alcoholism

Alcoholism is viewed medically as an addiction, that is, as a physical dependence as opposed to drugs which only produce psychological dependencies. The English physicians, for example were the first to see heroin as a drug which is required to feel normal; once a person is addicted (physically) the body requires the drug and the individual experiences physical pain and discomfort if s/he is deprived of it. Alcohol is a chemical substance which quickly leads to psychological dependence and then physical addiction; the individual needs it if he is going to feel relatively comfortable. Morever, alcohol is a psychoactive agent as powerful as many more notorious drugs, and is similar in its effects to the sedative-hypnotic compounds. Central nervous system depressants are addictive; thus, valium, librium and the barbituates exaggerate the depression induced by alcohol. Alcohol addiction and dependency *can be* so easily transferred to prescription drugs, because its effect is similar to the sedative hypnotic drugs.

Models

In the late 1800's and early 1900's, alcoholics were viewed as morally deficient in character; they were defined as moral degencrates. The main approach to treatment was religious, since morality was the concern of the clergy; alcoholics were viewed as lacking strength and willpower.

The medical model, on the other hand, treats alcoholism as a disease, taking treatment out of the hands of the clergy and placing it in the realm of the physicians. To what avail? Disease means dis-ease, impling (a.) lack of health in the broader sense, or (b.) physical infection in the narrower sense, which then determines the type of treatment modality. The "lack of health" concept places treatment in the realm of psychology while the "infection" notion suggests medical treatment. Medical intervention rarely goes beyond detoxification and general health maintenance, which in itself does not even alleviate the symptoms. Without a theoretical prospective, a *Leitlinie*, placing treatment in the hands of the psychiatrist is also nonproductive, since the treatment would lack direction.

Theories

Theories of drug abuse have developed from the various social, medical, and biological sciences and they have been characterized in many ways. One of the more exhaustive categorizations is that of Lettieri et. al., (1980) who quantified 43 current separate theoretical perspectives on drug abuse. These have been divided into disciplinary foci including psychiatry, psychology general, psychology learning, social psychology, sociology, criminology, biology, genetics, biomedical sciences, neurosciences, and others. As can be seen, a majority of these theories come from the social sciences which transfers treatment from the medical to the socio-psychological realm.

Although we are still operating within the medical model, the bulk of the treatment is social. It is ironic that when physicians attempt to treat alcoholism chemotherapeutically, the success lies within a shift of dependency. Alcoholics may easily transfer their alcohol dependency addiction to a prescription drug dependency usually barbituates and valium etc., and possibly even a dual alcohol-barbituate dependency. The latter condition frequently leads to purposeful or accidental suicide since the two substances have the synergetic effect of potentiating each other. This is easily substantiated by the fact that alcohol in combination accounts for the largest number of deaths from substance abuse: 2,530 in 1976-77, with heroin/morphine following at 1,680. Moreover, heroin addicts are rarely purists and most are gross multiple abusers whose deaths result from drugs in combination. The third highest death rate is from darvon (1,090) and the fourth highest death rate results from valium, the most widely consumed drug, a drug having the greatest number of prescriptions (57,084,000) with 880 deaths. These data* are important because valium is often prescribed by physicians for patients suffering from the anxiety and depression which often accompanies alcohol abuse. Yet these drugs do not treat the problem; at most, they are geared to symptom relief. Given these circumstances, it is safe to say that medical intervention is practically useless in treating alcoholism, although possibly necessary during detoxification; there is no real effect in terms of rehabilitation or cure.

Rehabilitation

Rehabilitation refers to the treatment of a medical or social ill whereby the person is returned to 'normal' functioning but is not cured of the malady. An example of rehabilitation is the treatment of a chronic illness in which the person is brought back to normal or next-to-normal functioning, although the illness is still prevalent, e.g., pulmonary tuberculosis in the past. In this case the per-

---

*Data reported by NIDA (national estimates) The U.S. Journal of Drug and Alcohol Dependence: April 1978 p.s.

son does not become 'free' of the illness which ultimately remains in the lungs but through the treatment process the Koch bacillus is brought into an inactive state; the lungs, through rest, are able to form calcium 'walls' around the bacillus pockets so that the bacillus are no longer destructive to the lung tissue. However, if the person engaged in too much exertion, the encapsulated pockets may break thus reinfecting the patient with his/her own bacillus. Rehabilitation, then, does not mean complete cure, but functional in a normative sense of behavior. Schizophrenia is another chronic illness which is not cured but (ideally) brought into a state of remission. In Breuler's time, schizophrenia had a poor prognosis: one third recovered, one third vacilated up and down and one third continued unvariably downhill. Today, with the use of thorazine, many of the latter third have been deinstitutionalized and lead marginally normal lives. However, if the medication is withdrawn the patient usually reverts back to a nonfunctional state. Even in the medical model, then, chemotherapy may only rehabilitate but not cure.

Cure
When we speak of cures, we typically refer to the idea of being healed, getting well, restoring to health, making one well. How then do these concepts differ from rehabilitation? In the case of the T.B. patient we might say that he/she is now well, may leave the hospital and go to work. By this we mean that the patient is restored to health, the illness removed or destroyed and the patient is now in a state of health similar to his/her previous condition. The bacillus is removed or destroyed; rehabilitation on the other hand is a state of being healed with restriction, or a conditional state of health.

We see that rehabilitation and cure are different concepts which imply a different state of being. To relate this to alcoholism we may look at the experience of alcoholics anonymous. First of all, AA uses a rehabilitation paradigm. They never assume cure, but view alcoholism as a chronic incapacitating illness-once an alcoholic always an alcoholic. Nevertheless, AA has the highest success rate of any treatment modality; in fact, it is the only truly successful treatment of which we are aware. Alcoholism is often referred to as the revolving door illness. The same clients come through the same treatment centers over and over again with many or most of the facilities boasting of a 5-10% 'recovery rate', a proportion which has been suggested as the recovery rate without any systematic intervention. Using this information, AA follows the medical model since it suggests we look at the alcoholic as a sick individual in need of help. AA further assumes that the alcoholic will never be able to drink again and thus works toward total abstinence from alcohol. Their program is further built upon a total support system, a group support system and therefore, while AA utilizes a medical model as a basic assumption, the thrust is spiritual.

Hypnosis
Hypnosis, although identified with Anton Mesmer's work of 1776, was not given legitimacy until James Braid published his book Neurypnology in 1843. Braid's work served to remove the occult 'flavor' connected to Mesmer's work

and make the use of the hypnotic technique a respectable part of the medical profession. Mesmer's work was called animal magnetism while Braid coined the term hypnosis, which came from neurypnology (nervous sleep).

Before the development of chemical anesthetics other than alcohol, hypnosis was popular in England and India for the purpose of anesthetizing surgical patients and, one might suggest, with great success. When chemical anesthetics became available, the use of hypnosis diminished because of its variability and time consuming characteristics. Hypnosis then became identified with stage entertainment; it acquired an occult flavor and lost respectability. It is only within the past decade that hypnosis has been revitalized, studied and legitimated within the medical profession.

Theories

Although there are various theories of hypnosis a dominant prospective has not yet developed, thus contributing to the confusion and lack of trust. Surrounding the procedure further, because of popular interest in hypnosis as a technique for dealing with smoking and other habit control, coupled with lack of legislative regualtions, a form of pop art is developing in which incompetent or marginally trained practitioners are prevading the field. The membership of the International Society of Hypnosis and the American Society of Clinical Hypnosis, two noteworthy groups, are taking a strong stand against the teaching of hypnosis to technicians, police officers, and others, who lack a broader based expertise in therapy. Hypnosis as a technique is not safe or dangerous, but in the hands of the unskilled or insensitive therapist however it can have untoward effects.

For years, hypnosis was defined in terms of suggestion and the ability of the subject to respond to such suggestion. Of late, hypnotists have become increasingly aware of the importance of trance level, and consquently, much of the variability of reported results are now being attributed to differences in level of trance. Many key researchers are developing techniques for measuring these levels, e.g., the Harvard and Stanford scales. Baudouin (1920), however, proposed that the degree of the hypnotic trance is a function of the suggestibiligy of the subject, thus his incorporating suggestibility and trance levels. Similarly Hilgard (1965), considers the trance level to be a function of the individual; hypnotic susceptibility is a stable personality characteristic and thus there are no major differences in the ability of hypnotists, since the technique and subject properties are crucial in this regard. Steffenhagen (1979), on the other hand, suggested that the function of charisma may be more important than the trance per se, belief in the hypnotist.

Hilgard's (1965) theory of hypnosis views hypnosis as an altered state of consciousness involving physiological mechanisms. It is more than heightened suggestibility. In the hypnotic state, it is the unconscious which accepts the suggestions thus differing from other theories which assume suggestibility to be part of the conscious mind. Under hypnosis, people have an enhanced capacity for receptivity.

Sarbin and Coe (1969) used an interactionist approach in explaining hypnosis. They subscribed to a role theory model and explain hypnosis as a special form of role playing - not mere pretense but an actual role enactment. In role playing, from a dramaturgical perspective we find both the technical and method acting form of role playing, the latter form explaining why some subjects are more susceptible. While this theory has more of an empirical foundation than Hilgard's, it fails to account for the use of hypnosis as an anesthetic in surgery.

T. X. Barber (1969), another leading authority on hypnosis, takes the position that there is no psychological condition called hypnosis but rather deals with the phenomenon as suggestibility. He describes the process in the framework of task motivational instruction in which the subject feels a moral pressure to conform to the demands of the hypnotist or trainer. Although this is a reasonably acceptable theory psychologically, it also fails to account for pain reduction; it can account for pain control, but not reduction.

Hypnosis is a process, not a therapy; it is a process or technique which can be utilized in therapy. Freud developed a therapeutic technique called psychoanalysis for dealing with mental patients. He also developed an interest in hypnosis and studied under several leading experts. If our data are correct, he saw hypnosis as a valuable technique in therapy, but since he was not adept in its use, he developed psychoanalysis in its place. The notion of hypnoanalysis is again surfacing. We now have a new periodical, the *Journal of Medical Hypnoanalysis*. Hypnosis is also being used by behaviorists as part of behavior modification programs. It is now evident that although there are theories of hypnosis (an attempt to explain a behavioral process or condition), hypnosis is not itself a theory or a therapy, but can be used successfully as an adjunct to existing therapies.

From the rather limited number of studies focusing upon the use of hypnosis in the treatment of alcoholism, we see that there is no common denominator or theme presented by the various researchers. See footnotes. Some strongly recommend the use of hypnosis in the treatment of alcoholism and suggest lasting effect. Others (e.g., Wendt, 1970) say there is no effective treatment of alcoholism including hypnosis. Some refer to the use of hypnotherapy, hypnosis, autohypnosis, the use of hypnosis in aversion therapy, covert conditioning, relaxation therapy, etc. It is clear, then, that there is no common theme presented and that the basic assumptions underlying the use of hypnosis are not specified. Nevertheless, Byers (1975) makes (four) 4 basic assumptions about hypnosis: (a.) all hypnosis is self-hypnosis; (b.) 80-90% of the population are hypnotizable; (c.) a common benefit of hypnosis is relaxation; and (d.) hypnosis is functionally a non-chemical tranquilizer. His first assumption is not consistent with hypnosis theory per se but a position. Assumption b is non-specific and c and d are reasonably accepted non-specific effects of hypnosis which cannot account for why hypnosis should be effective.

Lack of Consistency in Theory and Practice

So far, we have briefly sketched the history, theory and treatment of alcoholism and the history, theory, and the use of hypnosis in therapy. What has become increasingly evident is that there is no consistent or accepted theory of alcoholism and no consistent and accepted theory of hypnosis. Hynotherapy is itself a misleading construct, in that what is really meant, is that the hypnotic technique (the process) is used in or as part of an existing therapeutic modality but this is never made clear.

The purpose of this chapter is, as the title denotes, the presentation of the use of hypnosis in the treatment of alcoholism. Before we can constructively present a valid typology we need to present a coherent theory of alcoholism and then tailor a therapeutic technique to the theory - theory should be the *Leitlinie* for the therapy. Are many therapists less than effective because they lack a coherent theoretical focus?

A Theoretical Model of Alcoholism

The author (an Adlerian) has been working on a theory of drug abuse for the last six years and has developed a theory of deviance which includes drug abuse and alcoholism - a self-esteem theory of deviance. To be effective a drug abuse theory must be able to explain non-use, use, and abuse or it has limited applicability; further, separate theories for drug and alcohol abuse, sex differences, age differences, etc., become questionable.

In order to explain drug abuse, we find a need for a theoretical perspective which can also explain normal behavior. Theories which only explain abnormal behavior are relatively useless since abnormal or deviant acts are cultural constructs: behavior which is deviant in one culture, context or time frame may be normal, if not even desirable, in another context, e.g. marijuana use which, although legally deviant, has become an accepted norm on most college campuses today. A Vermont authority has commented that if you drink more than once a week you are into incipient alcoholism, a statement I would totally disagree with; the ritualistic use of wine among the Jews did not lead to alcoholism.

The self-esteem theory of deviance is derived from the broader Adlerian theory of behavior. It assumes that all behavior is a striving for success (superiority) and a diminution of inferiority - the dialectical process. For Hegel, every phenomenon has its own opposite tendency suggesting a theory of unity of opposites, a vital aspect of the Adlerian model. One cannot resolve conflict since life is dynamic, constantly in flux, in change, and change is itself conflict, new opposed to the old, superiority opposed to inferiority. The goal is not the resolution of the conflict, but the balance achieved in which the opposing forces find a functional unity and the individual perceives himself or herself neither as inferior, the starting point of action, nor superior, the goal. An excess of definitions at either pole leads to low self-esteem since inferiority leaves one feeling inadequate and an excess of superiority leaves one without goals which itself is inaction - the opposite of life.

Man is born inferior, physically, mentally and socially. He strives for superiority, and hence a decrease in inferiority. When this striving is inadequate, it leaves one with low self-esteem, and compensatory mechanisms for coping are necessary. Compensation is not, as Freud thought, an ego protecting mechanism, but a mechanism for protecting a fragile self-esteem and these mechanisms are frequently viewed as deviances e.g. drug abuse, occult membership, compulsive eating or dieting, delinquency, promiscuity, etc. Sometimes the behavior is not directed outward but inward and then the result is not viewed as deviant but as illness, either physical or mental.

All behavior is goal-directed; the ultimate goal is to build self- esteem and the achievement of lower goals help us to tackle the higher goals. When we fail to set goals, we stagnate; when we set them too high ("God-like"), we cannot achieve them and our self-esteem is threatened. We are then likely to resort to compensatory behavior to protect the little which is left. Alcohol serves such a purpose: it covers up guilt, anxiety, depression, melancolia, anger, etc., and also offers one an excuse for failure: "If it weren't for the alcohol, I would have succeeded."

One doesn't become an alcoholic in a vacuum. Drinking does not lead to alcoholism, but drinking and low self-esteem provide the fertile environment in which it is nurtured. We know that alcoholics tend to come from homes in which alcoholism is a problem. This leads to the development of theories which explain alcoholism in terms of socialization, role modeling, etc. The difficulty with such theories is that they fail to explain use and cannot explain exceptions. If familiarity and role modeling were the answer, then the number of estimated alcoholics should increase geometrically. Self-esteem theory provides an explanation for non-use, use, and abuse, as discussed in chapter IV.

If the self-esteem theory of deviance is viable, then therapy should focus upon building self-esteem and not on the symptom-alcoholism. Most alcoholics know why they drink and therapy directed at making these factors known to the client are useless. Some time ago, a beautiful young lady who we will call Ms. X came to me and told me she was drinking too much and becoming concerned. She commented on the fact that she couldn't go out socially without first having several shots of alcohol and then she would also drink more than she wanted to at the party. She knew why she drank - she felt insecure, and uncomfortable socially - she didn't like herself. If you cannot like yourself, how can you ever like someone else; before you can love someone else, you must first be able to love yourself. Ms. X was 21 years old and came from an upper middle class family. She was the second of two children, an older brother receiving much of the attention of the family. They were Jewish and the push and emphasis upon an education was largely directed towards the brother. The daughter was sent to a high status college, but little was said about her choice of a career, the tacit assumption being that she would marry and that her education would only be of value to her socially. As was stated, she was strikingly beautiful and certainly had no difficulty eliciting male response (while women may have been envious). She was also very intelligent and could easily develop a successful career for herself, if that were what she wanted. Why then the need to drink for fortification? She had very low self-esteem, felt inadequate and didn't like herself. Within the familial and college peer group, alcohol was an accepted social commodity - a milieu fertile for the development of problem drinking. She had everything going for her and yet the most important factor was missing; good self-esteem. We will return to Ms. X later.

Alcohol researchers more frequently focus upon the lower SES range when discussing the problem and therapy. They stress the restrictive milieu, the cultural deprivation etc. - the polar opposite of Ms. X and yet both result from low self-esteem. If therapy is to be effective, it must focus upon building self-esteem. Walter O'Connell has developed a therapeutic model he terms Natural High Therapy; John Henderson has developed a technique called Developmental Rehabilitation Therapy; while the author has pursued Self-esteem Hypnotherapy all directed at building self-esteem. These therapies have been successful in the treatment of alcohol and drug abuse. If therapy is to be directed at building self- esteem, then a model of self-esteem is important to provide the *Leitlinie* for the therapeutic process. In this way the process can be tailored towards the specific needs of the problem.

The Problem

Although hypnosis may be an effective tool in the treatment of alcoholism, the literature does not accurately reflect the success rate of the process. Given the paucity of coherent theories of alcoholism and hypnosis, there is no wonder that therapeutic models lack credibility. If therapy is to be effective, it must be based on a coherent credible theory. Hypnosis itself should be used as a tool molded to the needs of that theoretical orientation.

Moreover, within this context, it becomes evident why hypnosis has not become a more important technique in the treatment of alcoholism and further why all existing therapies have such a dismal success rate. In order for therapy to be effective it needs (a.) a coherent theory, (b.) a clarification of its key concepts, and (c.) a therapy directed by the theory. When these requirements are met, the potential of hypnosis is great. From a theoretical point of view then, in the case of Self-esteem Hypnotherapy we have (a.) the self-esteem theory of deviance, (b.) a model of self-esteem and (c.) a hypnotherapeautic process geared to building self-esteem. In fact, the author recommends the use of hypnosis and has had success in the treatment of alcoholism and problem drinking. Ms. X had three sessions of Self-esteem Hypnotherapy, after which, she felt good; her self-esteem had increased dramatically and the need for alcohol, as a crutch, was gone. She had moved from an introverted, insecure person to an outgoing person who was able to assert herself at home and in company.

Conclusion

What has been proposed is that there are two deficiencies in the determination of the effectiveness of hypnosis in the treatment of alcoholism: (a.) there isn't a consistent and coherent theory of alcoholism and, (b.) there isn't a consistent therapeutic model.

Self-esteem theory provides a consistent and coherent theory of drug abuse, of which alcoholism is only one type. Since, alcohol addiction can be transferred to other drug addictions (e.g. barbituates) an adequate theory must be more comprehensive than a theory is of alcoholism. If the efficacy of hypnosis as a treatment modality is to be determined, it must be used within the framework of a consistent theory.

Further, if the treatment modality focuses upon rehabilitation, then rehabilitation will become the logical denouement of successful therapy. On the other hand, if cure is the goal, then the resultant condition should be cure. The model presented here offers cure as the goal.

Theory and practice should develop together so that each can strengthen the other.

Footnotes

1   Langen, D. (1967), Lassoff S. (1970), Redlick, F.C. and Freeman, D.T. (1966), Smith-Moorhouse, P.M. (1969) and Von Dedenroth, T.E.A (1965) have all commented on the success of hypnotherapy with individual alcoholics. Beahrs and Hill (1971) report success with a group interaction approach for alcholics in which the subjects are in hypnotic trances during the sessions.

2   Byers (1975) uses hypnosis for relaxation as part of alcholism treatment. While no positive conclusions are presented, the study suggests that the use of self-hypnosis in relaxation therapy can be beneficial. Relaxation therapy was cited as effective by the Colorado State Hospital in the treatment of alcoholism.

3   Cautela (1975) uses covert conditioning in behavior modification of phobias, alcoholism etc. and comments on the use of hypnosis in this type of conditioning.

4   Van Pelts (1975) argues that many behavior problems, e.g. alcoholism, migraine, panic attacks etc., are the result of accidental self-hypnosis and are reactions to the intense emotional experiences accompanying the procedure. He suggests that hypnosis can then be used to re-educate these patients; seven cases are presented as support for the theory.

5   Seguin (1974) describes the value of folklore, herbs, aversion therapy, hypnosis, etc. in the treatment of patients. He comments on the treatment of chronic alcoholism by nature healers and suggests we incorporate the use of folklore techniques in modern pyschiatry.

6   Paterson (1974) notes that auto-hypnosis has been used in English prisons for the treatment of alcoholism and drug addiction; three case histories are presented.

7   Dunn (1972) describes the use of aversion therapy in drug rehabilitation. A conditioning process is used which causes the patient to vomit when alcohol is ingested. The total therapy includes the use of an emetic, possibly a mild electro-shock, relaxation training and hypnotherapy.

8   Grannone (1971) presents data on 40 alcoholics who were treated with hypnotherapy for alcoholism in an Italian clinic. Forty percent of the patients continued hypnotherapy after discharge and were considered successful one year later.

9   Wendt (1970) suggests that therapy of alcoholics is difficult because there are no physical or personality types which characterize the alcoholic. He discusses different psychotherapeutic techniques used in the treatment of alcoholism, including hypnosis and dismisses these as having no lasting ef-

fect, which seems generally to be the state of the *art* at the moment.

10 Field (1969) compared a group of alcoholics with a group of college students to determine whether they differed in level of trance. Both groups were similar in trance depth but the alcoholics seemed to show more impulsive enthusiasm and conscious awareness. He mentions that personality or organicity might be the answer although other researchers would contend that in this respect they do not differ from the normal population.

11 Fox (1967) suggests that for any treatment of alcoholism to be effective a multidisiplinary, approach is necessary with hypnosis as a possible component.

REFERENCES

Barber, T. X. *Hypnosis: A Scientific Approach*. New York:Van Nostrand, Reinholt Co., 1969.

Baudouin, C. *Suggestion and autosuggestion*. Norwood Additions Reprint, 1920.

Beahrs, J.O. and M.M. Hill, Treatment of alcoholism by group interaction psycho-therapy under hypnosis. *American Journal of Clinical Hypnosis*, 1971, *14* (1)

Braid, James *Neurypnology*. London: J. Churchill, 1843.

Byers, A.P. Training and use of Technicians in the Treatment of alcoholism with hypnosis. *American Journal of Clinical Hypnosis*, 1976, *18*, 90-93.

Cautela, J.R. The use of covert conditioning in hypnotherapy. *International-Journal of Clinical & Experimental Hypnosis*. 1975, *23*, 15-27.

Dunn, B. A new comprehensive, intense care program for the treatment of alcoholism. *Psychosomatics*. 1972, *13*, 397-400.

Field, P.B. Experiences of alcoholics during hypnosis. *American Journal of Clinical Hypnosis*. 1969, *12*, 86-90.

Fox, R. A multidisciplinary approach to the treatment of alcoholism. *American Journal of Psyciatry*. 1967, *123*, 769-778.

Granone, F. Hypnotism in the treatment of chronic alcoholism. *Journal of the American Institute of Hypnosis*. 1971, *12*, 32-40.

Henederson, J. Unpublished work on developmental rehabilitation therapy.

Hilgard, E.R. *Hypnotic Susceptability*. New York: Harcourt, Brace & World, 1965.

Langen, D. Modern hypnotic treatment of various forms of addiction in particular alcoholism. *British Journal of Addictions*, 1967, *62*, 77-81.

Lassoff, S. Evaluating group hypnosis with alcoholic patients. Personal communication study completed at Agnew State Hospital, 1970.

Lettieri, D.T. Sayers, M. and Pearson, H.W. eds. *Theories on Drug Abuse: Selected Contemporary Perspectives*. National Institute on Drug Abuse Research Monograph 30. DHHS Pub. No. (ADM) 80-967. Washington, D.C.: Supt. of Docs. U.S. Gov't. Print. Off. 1980.

Mesmer, Franz Anton Doctoral dissertation on the influence of the Planets on the Human Body.

O'Connell, W.E. *Super Natural Highs*. New York. North American Graphics Inc. 1979.

Paterson, A.S. Hypothesis as an adjunct to the treatment of alcoholics and drug addicts. *International Journal of Offender Therapy & Comparative Criminology*. 1974, *18* 40-45.

Redlich, F.C. and Freeman, D.T. *Theory of Practice of Psyciatry*. New York Basic Books, 1966, p. 762.

Sarbin, T. and Coe, W. *Hypnosis: A Social and Psychological Analysis of Influence Comminication*. New York: Van Nostrand, Reinholt Co., 1969.

Sequin, A. What folklore psychotherapy can teach us. *Psychotherapy and Psychosomatics*. 1974, *24*, 293-302.

Smith-Moorhouse, P.M. Hypnosis in the treatment of alcoholism. *British Journal of Addictions*, 1969, *64-*, 47-55.

Steffenhagen, R.A. An Adlerian approach toward a self-esteem theory of deviance: a drug abuse model. *Journal of Alcohol & Drug Education*. 1978, *24*, 1-13.

Steffenhagen, R.A. Hypnosis and charisma. *Journal of the Society for Professional Hypnosis*, 1979, *8*, 14-16.

Van Pelt, S.J. Not merely a treatment, more a way of life. *Journal of the American Institute of Hypnosis*, 1975, *16*, 44-45.

Von Dedenroth, T.E.A. Some newer ideas and concepts of alcoholism and the use of hypnosis. *British Journal of Medical Hypnosis*, 1965, *16* 27.

Wendt, H. Principle questions of psychotherapy of alcoholics. *Psychiatrie, Neurologie and Medizinische Psychologie*. 1970, *22*, 365-369.

R. A. Steffenhagen Ph.D
Department of Sociology
University of Vermont

2

HYPNOSIS IN BUILDING SELF-ESTEEM

Since, Decartes, we have been left with the mind-body dichotomy in philosophy and psychology. Western philosophy and science have all focused upon the body and its components when explaining human behavior. Simplistically, we have in behaviorism a stimulus-response theory which says that the organisms behavior is the result of external stimuli. The body is translated in terms of its components and, in terms of human behavior specifically, the brain is then seen as the analog of a computer-mechanistic theory.

Theodore Roszak, in *Unfinished Animal* (1975), has commented on what he calls the upside-down nature of culture in modern society. He has shown how myth, magic and mystery have become perverted in terms of their true meaning and in terms of their integrating qualities of culture, vis-a-vis personality. Man, who's Weltanchauung was built around myth, magic and mystery was able to develop an identity with which he is comfortable. How can modern man who has perverted each one of these qualities develop a meaningful identity when his place in the universe can only be seen in terms of his physical body? The body, as a physical unit (including the brain), houses the mind, that ethereal spiritual entity which science has not been able to explore, discover, test for, etc. In the process of idealizing the physical, man has changed myth to history, magic to reason, and mystery to technology. This creates an inverted or profane triangle with and earthly orientation. (p. 159).

Sociologists have long spoken about religious vs. secular cultures and in recent times have so taken for granted the secularization of the world that little time and effort have been spent upon the religious *Weltanschauung* which has previously been the focal point of the *Weltansicht* of the individual. Roszak comments that the sacred theme is buried beneath the profane (p. 57). We might further point out that Karl Marx, a "profound" atheist, had merely supplemented the secular nature of culture "science" for religion in his personal philosophical development. The difficulty with a trascendant reality is of course that it is not amenable to present day scientific measurement, but this does not mean that the spiritual element of man is unimportant. Weber (1947), has stressed the importance of the *verstehen* approach to studying man. Science has defined man as the analog of the machine and now as an analog of the com-

13

puter. Any theory of behavior which excludes the ethereal quality of man, the mind, the spiritual component which gives man a *Weltansicht* in which he develops a unified identity is an approach which ultimately must end in disaster. Many writers have seen the present period as a return to the sacred. If there is a hope for modern man, it is not in science, but rather in a spiritual reintegration. This theme is well developed by Theodore Roszak who suggests, in *Unfinished Animal,* that modern man is suffering from spiritual malnutrition, has been cheated by progress to make do with trivial or even demonic substitutes for the unifying theme inherent in true myth, magic and mystery (p. 179). Any *Weltanschauung* which fails to integrate the spiritual with the physical is doomed to failure. The spiritual is there, whether the individual is aware of it or not, albeit starved.

Therapists frequently comment on the importance of building self- esteem. It if frequently felt that there is nothing which succeeds like success and that nothing increases one's self-esteem quicker than positive reinforcement. To a degree, this is true, but success by itself insures no one of personality integration. We find innumerable examples of extremely successful people, by our usual standards, who commit suicide, become drug addicts, become alcoholics, or who resort to other forms of deviance as self-esteem protecting mechanisms. If success builds self-esteem, then how can one explain our "successful deviants"? It is because success is only one aspect in the process of building self-esteem. Success does not produce the unified, cohesive, integration of the personality. Success has positive reinforcement value, just as failure leads to poor self-concept. Success can only be translated by the individual in terms of his own perceptions and apperceptions. Although acquired through the socialization process, it is still in part removed from the culture vis-a-vis the mind. Success, encouragement, and support are the triad of factors for building self-esteem on this level. Equally important, however, is the transcendent or spiritual. We need to build self-esteem on both levels. When we have only the first (material), we are subject to the winds of adversity but when the spiritual is developed, our triangle cannot be tipped and we can then cope with adversity.

Gurdjieff's approach in therapy was not to bring to consciousness the causes of neurosis but to awaken the higher levels of the mind, thus therapy could be used on the essentially well person as a means of awakening the mind and promoting growth. He felt that most people never became awakened.

Henri Bergson saw the need for the masses to free themselves from this narrow secularism (the sleeping consciousness), to reach a higher reality, if cosmic evolution is to proceed. (For an enlightening discussion of the role of the cosmic evolution, see the works of Pierre Tielhard de Chardin.) This secularism is the imprint of the age of science, where all hope is based upon science rather than the spirit. To give up the role of the spirit is to relegate oneself to the sleeping consciousness. In the words of Soren Kirkegaard (1941 p. 146), "That Despair is the Sickness Unto Death"; he further says that, "Despair is a Sickness in the Spirit." Man is his spirit says Kirkegaard and this simple proposition has been lost. Science thinks that reason can supplant 'magic' but it cannont if man is to move towards the cosmic evolution.

In 1978, a time when youth are supposed to have everything to look forward to, almost 5,000 youths commited suicide. Suicide is the number two cause of death among young people. Can there be any question that despair is the sickness unto death. When the mind, body and spirit are not integrated, we have despair, a sleeping consciousness. The 'evil' in the world today is not a crime of commission but rather a crime of omission - omitting the importance of the spirit in man's cosmic evolution. Scheler was aware that modern man is living a delusion of his own making; i.e., he thinks unconsciously that he knows what is real and for modern man only materialsim is real, whereas in reality, ultimate reality transcends the material to the plane of the spiritual and the sacred.

Self-esteem is not a unidimensional characteristic; it is the core around which the personality revolves. If too much self-esteem is lost, the individual will resort to suicide, or morasmus a mental form of suicide. A fragile self-esteem needs to be protected and frequently is protected through compensatory mechanisms which may take the form of social deviance (physical manifestations) or mental manifestations (as neurosis or psychosis).

Self-esteem exists on three levels: self-concept (mental), self-image (physical), and social concept (cultural or interpersonal). Individuals are not necessarily weak or good in all three areas and treatment itself may need to focus more on one area or another. It has been my experience that when self-esteem hypnotherapy is effective, it will produce improvement in the deficient dimension or dimensions and that these dimensions will not improve equally but differentially as treatment continues.

Hypnosis is a process which can be used to help build self-esteem on both levels, the material and the spiritual. Hypnosis is a process and not a therapy and therefore can be used within various therapeutic modalities.

Definition

Self-esteem hypnotherapy eminates from the Adlerian tradition. It is an attempt to use hypnosis in the building of self-esteem. The theory presented is that self-esteem exists on two levels: the material and the transcendental; for a person to have good self-esteem, he needs both.

William James (1890) defined self-esteem as S. E. - $\frac{\text{SUCCESS}}{\text{PRETENSION}}$ which is an adequate formula for the material component of self-esteem but misses the spiritual. Success, encouragement, and support are necessary but not sufficient for good personality integration. It is fine when everything is going well but, when the winds of adversity strike, the individual lacks the inner strength necessary to cope with the adversity. This may be diagramed as follows:

SELF-ESTEEM

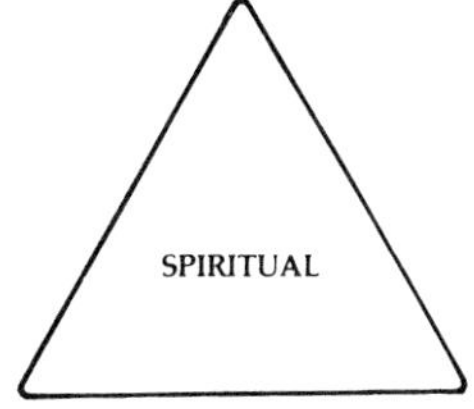

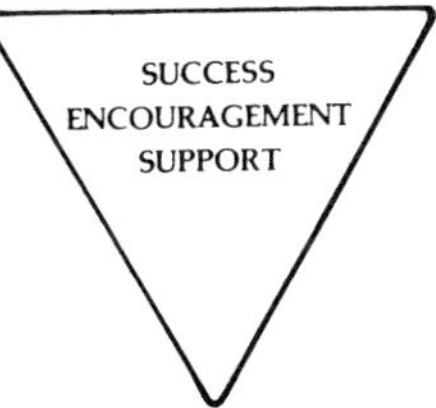

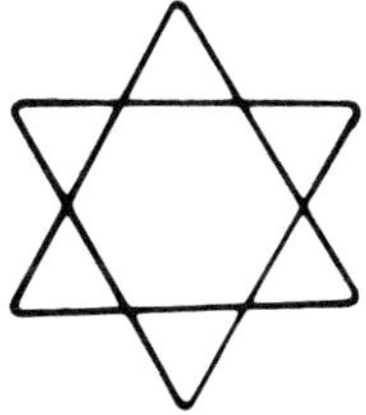

Freud's ego-defense mechanisms are more often self-esteem protecting mechanisms. Forms of deviances are compensatory mechanisms used to cope with or protect a fragile self-esteem. The alcoholic uses alcohol to protect his weakened self-esteem ("If it weren't for the alcohol I would have succeeded"); it provides him with an excuse for his failure to achieve his goals. Only achieved goals are non-constrictive. However, even achieved goals may be inadequate when the individual has created "God-like" goals for himself. When you have to be the "best", nothing is good enough. People frequently spend their energy merely sustaining a fragile self-esteem which keeps them in a neurotic state and prevents them from becoming the productive, creative people they are capable of becoming. The development of inner spiritual strength and self-acceptance while promoting the material manifestation of self-esteem are the goals of self-esteem hypnotherapy.

History

As indicated self-esteem hypnotherapy comes from the Adlerian tradition; when people have good self-esteem they don't need compensatory mechanisms. The goal of the hypnosis is to strengthen the self-esteem, not to focus upon the problem. Many young people today are totally self-centered and, when queried as to what their problem is, respond, "I am not happy" which is like saying "I only want to be perfect."

Ego strength and self-esteem are not the same. One may have good ego strength and yet have low self-esteem. Self-acceptance is crucial to good self-esteem; a good ego does not provide self-acceptance. It is difficult to be happy when one looks in the mirror and cannot accept what s/he sees. Modern culture, vis-a-vis the mass media (T.V., movies, teen and fashion magazines) and advertising have created an all-pervading myth of youth, beauty and virility which is close to Weber's ideal type, a good methodological research tool, but not a reality. However, more and more young people have internalized this myth and then feel cheated, inadequate; others are more handsome or beautiful, more intelligent. Many of the inmates in our prisons are there because of their need to maintain their macho image, which is a poor substitute for true feelings of self-acceptance. Further, they are caught up in Merton's Anomie condition - internalized cultural goals and low perceived means of attainment. The good life is brought before everyone vis-a-vis T.V. The slums are always depicted as repulsive and to be shunned. Need we look any further for causes of deviance on a cultural level? Concomitant with this is the development of low self-esteem and then the development of compensatory mechanisms for coping. Alcoholism is not the problem, but the effect. Self-acceptance must transcend these perceived cultural values or rehabilitative therapeutic techniques will not work.

Out of my self-esteem theory of deviance developed the hypnotic technique for building self-esteem. Hypnosis is a process whereby the unconscious mind is programmed during a state of deep relaxation (See Hilgard, 1965). Hypnotherapy is, in essence, a misnomer since the therapist is using hypnosis as a device to facilitate his theoretical perspective. This is most easily explained using the behavior modification approach to therapy in which hypnosis is used to create the desires or aversions. David Kopay's hypnotist attempted to use hypnosis to implant the idea that he wanted to get married and become heterosexual. He did get married but, it was short-lived and he still preferred sex with a man. David's problem was not being gay (sexual preference) but, the cultural norms and pressures (family and associates who do not see jocks as being gay). In my work, I find that the greatest problem many homosexuals face is not the sexuality but, low self-esteem which frequently accompanies the sexual preference, resulting from the cultural values and pressures.

My approach to therapy is to work on self-esteem and not on the problem presented (e.g., homosexuality, obesity, etc.). The important thing is the self-acceptance. When you feel good about yourself you have the strength and motivation to do something about your problem. It is my experience that I can facilitate weight loss with hypnosis on a short term basis but that the diet program itself does not hold. I explain that I am going to work on self-esteem and that I will use the hypnosis to help get them started but, that the hypnosis is no miracle cure. I explain that when they feel good about themselves they then can make the decision whether they want to put forth the vast amount of energy it will take to lose a lot of weight and maintain it.

Technique

Self-esteem exists on the two levels cited: the material and the transcendental. We will present two models for using hypnosis to strenthen self-esteem.

Model I utilizes any conventional hypnotic induction process and the individual is programmed to feel good about himself outwardly and inwardly.

> Pay close attention to what I am going to say: Everyday in every way I am getting better and better. Everyday in every way I am becoming more self-confident, more self-assured, more positive. I am totally and completely acceptable, just the way I am, 24 hours a day, waking or sleeping. I am becoming more positive; negative thoughts will have no influence over me whatsoever. My body is a holy temple in which my spirit lives; my body is a holy city in which my spirit resides. I am both spiritual and physical. As I become more aware of my own inner power I will become more productive, creative, efficient on the material level; (along with this you may also work on whatever behavior problem needs work, e.g. smoking, eating, etc.).

Model II is the most innovative aspect of self-esteem hypnotherapy. It is a suspension of the ego, a form of dis-association or a cosmic transcendence in which the client loses contact with this reality. Many of my clients who have 'dropped acid' (LSD) have commented on the fact that it is similar to an acid trip but much more pleasant, much smoother. It is interesting that the typically straight individual also doesn't have any difficulty transcending reality; however, he doesn't have the sign posts that the individual who has dropped acid does. The level of trance state doesn't seem to affect the technique although there are a few individuals who don't seem to be able to let go. The hypnotist's instructions are as follows:

> "In our western society we have built up a reality based upon a framework of Newtonian science, ever since Newton, and the concept of gravity, we tend to be

caught in a reality dealing with *up and down.* — I count you down into a deeper state of relaxation, I bring you out by counting up from one to five. Now we are going to deal with the Eastern concept of *out and in, in and out* and in a moment I shall begin to speak German, at that point your consciousness will be allowed to go out, out to a different reality, a different dimension, a different existence, it will remain out as long as I continue to speak German and as soon as I speak the first word of English it will return back to this reality, this existence. I shall remain as your guide on this plane of existence, I shall be your psychic guide, it is *Perfectly* safe, you can explore as much or as little as you want, you are free to roam as far or stay as close as you desire and then when you return — you will bring back a greater source of energy or power - a spiritual strength to help you in this reality."

Now I speak German for approximately 10 minutes (I frequently read from a German novel) or as long as you wish to let the individual out. I use the German because I can read it with little or no difficulty and most of my clients don't know German. It must be a language unkown to the client or s/he will not disassociate. For those few who do know German I use a tape of a Swami chanting in Sanskrit. The reference to being his/her guide is important. The Cashinahua Indians use hallucinogenic drugs and refer to "Have a good trip" and then sit together and have physical contact during the drug induced experience and have no "bad trips". I have had occasion when it was necessary to hold the client's arm in order to establish the security for the technique to work, especially when the client had had a bad drug experience. Not all individuals respond in like manner but, even those who don't seem to "let go" still appear to derive benefit.

The technique allows for a suspension of the ego. The ego keeps us rooted in reality and gives us a sense of security. Many people have such strong egos they resist losing contact (even for brief periods) with our material reality. When the hypnotist starts talking in a foreign language (German,) the client is able to allow his mind to flow freely. It offers a form of disassociation. This form of disassociation is reminiscent of right brain activity. After the experience the subjects have difficulty describing what they saw, felt, etc.-the same difficulty experienced by people who have right and left brain separation and have sensory experiences in the right hemisphere. After these sessions, clients express a greater sense of contentment, well being and self-acceptance. They feel much more in control of their environment, with an increase in their self-esteem, (see client transcripts at the end of the chapter).

Application

This process can only be beneficial and can be used with clients manifesting minor behavioral problems to those of a serious nature. It can be used with any client, including the most skeptical. I would recommend it only be used with people truly seeking help. Further, I have dramatic behavioral changes with as few as two sessions. I have found that my most dramatic successes have been young clients and that as the individual becomes older, s/he is more resistant and more time is required although I have had changes in 40 year olds even when all traditional therapies weren't successful.

Generally, when the technique isn't going to be effective, two or three sessions are sufficient to discern this and then a more traditional approach can be utilized. I have had success with personality disorders, intermittent explosive disorders, anorexia nervosa, homosexuality, depression, poly-drug abuse, alcoholism and others.

References

Roszak, T. *Unfinished Animal: The Aquarian Frontier and the Evolution of Consciousness.* New York: Harper Colophon Books, 1975.

Kierkegarrd, S. *Fear and Trembling and the Sickness unto Death.* New Jersey: Princeton University Press, 1974.

Hilgard, E. R. *Hypnotic Susceptability.* New York: Harcourt, Brace and World, 1965.

Weber, M. *The Theory of Social and Economic Organization.* Trans. by A. M. Henderson and T. Parson, New York: Oxford University Press, 1947.

J. Michael McKnight, Ph.D
Department of Religion
University of Vermont

3

SELF-ESTEEM AND HYPNOSIS:
A TRANSCENDENTAL PERSPECTIVE

> "Ignorance is to take what is
> non-eternal, impure, painful
> and not-self, for what is eternal,
> pure, happy and the atman, or self"
> — *Yoga Sutras II, 5.*

While the effectiveness of hypnotherapy has been demonstrated in numerous studies, the reasons for this effectiveness remain somewhat obscure. It seems that nothing relating to hypnosis or the human mind can be easily explained. This is especially true of the improved level of self-esteem which an individual achieves through hypnotherapy. How can an individual's fundamental self-concept be altered through hypnotic sessions? In order to begin to answer a question such as this, we must be clear on the significance of self-esteem and the process of hypnotherapy. Therefore, the first part of this chapter will be devoted to an analysis of the concept of self-esteem and the second part will discuss the actual process of hypnotherapy. The work of Professor Ronald Stef fenhagen of the University of Vermont will be utilized as the model for the sec ond part. Professor Steffenhagen's success in improving his clients' self-esteem is demonstrated in dozens of case histories. After discussing the key componen of his technique, this chapter will conclude with a few cautious generalizatio about the real source of an individual's self-esteem.

The compound term "self-esteem" presents many difficulties for anyone see ing a basic universally valid definition. The second component of the co pound, "esteem", is relatively clear. It is derived from the Latin word *aestima* "to value, appraise, estimate". "Self-esteem" would therefore denote the val opinion, or respect one places on one's self. Closely following the etymolog origin of "esteem", it may be said that "self- esteem" is one's estimate of his or total value. This value has no direct or casual relationship with one's monet value, but in a society which places great emphasis on economic status an dividual's self-estimate *may* by porprtional to one's income. Fundament however, the value one places on one's existence is derived from an inner viction about personhood. It becomes a question of ultimate concern: "Wh

I? What is the nature of the self which I esteem?, etc."

The real difficulty in defining self-esteem centers on the term "self", a precise word, the very etymology of which is obscure. In common parla the word presents no problems. Everyone seems to know that they have a "se and it is undesirable to become too "selfish". It is understood to be that essenti identity, character or quality of each person. However, beyond this superficial understanding, the notion of "self" is very difficult to define precisely. The quest for a definition of this term rapidly becomes a philosophical enterprise of the most challenging nature. For the purpose of the present discussion of self-esteem, two important aspects of the nature of selfhood should be noted.

In the first place, part of the difficulty in defining "self" is the fact that one is attempting to define an evolutionary process rather than a static entity. We are continuously forming and altering our concepts of self through our choice of action. This makes the "self" more of a verb than a noun, as Buckminister Fuller noted, "an evolutionary function of the universe." The attempt to define "self" as a thing is doomed to failure because it is more akin to an evolutionary process. This characteristic of selfhood is very significant for the present discussion for it underscores the fact that one's self-concept is naturally altered as one goes through life. This alteration may take place in three ways: consciously, unconsciously, or under the guidance of a psycho-therapist. Using a technique such as hypnosis, a psychotherapist may bring about a radical alteration of the individual's self-concept. This point will be discussed at greater length after we examine another aspect of selfhood.

The second aspect of "self" is closely related to the first. As one experiences the self as a process of continous formation, one often perceives that there are definite divisions or levels to the phenomenon of self. These levels have been called by many different names in the long course of philosophy. Frequently, they are designated the "higher" and "lower" selves as in the works of Nietzsche. The higher self is taken to be what is real or true in the individual, while the lower self is considered only conditionally real and ultimately untrue. The perception that man possesses two levels of selfhood or personal identity is both ancient and widespead among diverse cultural systems.

In the *Upanishads*, philosophical texts composed in India as early as the eight century B.C., the two levels of selfhood are characterized as two birds who roost in the same tree.

> Two birds, fast bound companions,
> Clasp close the self-same tree.
> Of these two, the one eats sweet fruit;
> The other looks on without eating.
>
> On the self-same tree a person, sunken,
> Grieves for his impotence, deluded;
> When he sees the other, the Lord, contented,
> And his greatness, he becomes freed from sorrow.

(Mundaka Upanishad III, 1-2
Sourcebook in Indian Philosophy, P.54.)

In this passage, the bird who refrains from eating the sweet fruit of the senses is identified as the higher transcendent self of man, called the *atman*. The authors of the *Upanishads* openly acknowledged the difficulty of defining the *atman*:

> That Self (*atman*) is not this, it is
> not that (*neti neti*). It is unseizable,
> for it cannot be seized; indestructible,
> for it cannot be destroyed; unattached,
> for it does not attach itself; is unbound,
> does not tremble, is not injured . . .
>
> Brhadaranyaka Upanishad,
> IV, V, 15.

According to the Upanishadic philosophers, called vedantins, the whole purpose of life lies in the realization of one's higher self. They perscribe certain methods for achieving correct knowledge: study of sacred texts under a qualified teacher; philosophical reflection on their inner meaning; and meditation. Repeatedly, it is said that the key to unlocking the *atman* is obtained through a condition of mental equanimity.

One of the great affirmations of the *Upanishads* concerns the relationship between the self *(atman)* and the source of all existence *(Brahman)*. This identity is taken to be a fact not a theory: "...it signifies that *moksa* or release does not consist in becoming something. It only means the discovery of what has always been a fact and is compared to the discovery of a treasure which was all along lying hidden under the floor of one's house, but which one had so far failed to find, though passing to and from over it constantly" (Hiriyanna, 1970, p. 75). One of the methods which the ancient Indian sages employed to bring about a realization of this higher identity was the mental repetition of certain "great sayings" (*mahavakya*) such as "That thou art" and "I am Brahman".

It is not necessary to dwell on the Upanishadic material. The essentials of this ancient doctrine are clear: man possesses two dimensions of selfhood, the *ahamkara* or ego and the *atman* which corresponds to the concept of highest self or soul. A radical dichotomy is posited between these selves of the individual. The lower self is characterized by ignorance, sensuality, and evil, while the higher self is eternally free, all-knowing, and one with the cosmos. Reverence and esteem should be directed only to this cosmic self according to the upanishadic seers. When union with this ever-present and unchanging essence occurs, one is liberated from fear and suffering. This union was sought through yoga, meditation and renunciation of ordinary life commitments.

The doctrine of the dichotomous nature of selfhood which permeates the *Upanishads* and other sacred texts of the East is echoed in Western mystical traditions. The terminology and theology varies, but the fundamental idea that man possesses two natures, divine and mortal, remains the same. By a variety of means, mystics throughout the ages have sought to awaken consciousness of the transcendental level of selfhood. One of the most insightful interpreters of mysticism, Evelyn Underhill, speaks of this "hidden self" as the primary agent of mysticism, the only self which can have any communion with the Absolute or transcendental world. Like the Eastern philosophers, Underhill has difficulty in defining the higher self since it is "a self which the circumstances of diurnal life usually keep 'below the threshold of consciousness,'" (Underhill, 1961, p. 67).

The dichotomous self concept appears in a variety of guises in sources as divergent as Gurdjiefian teachings, Jungian psychology, and the contemporary human potential movement. It is not our present purpose to describe all the articulations of this concept, nor will we attempt to judge its ultimate validity. Our purpose is simply to underscore the pervasiveness of this notion of selfhood and then proceed to comment on its possible relevance in a discussion of self-esteem. However, before moving to this discussion it should be noted that many authors, scholars and mystics alike, recognize that the bifurcation of self into the higher/lower, true/false, levels is not an absolute dichotomy. That is, it is a matter of convenience or a heuristic device used to point toward·a more fulfilling life. Commenting on the Jungian distinction between the ego and the Self, Dr. Edward Edinger (1980) notes, "Considering ego and Self as two separate entities is merely a necessary rational device for discussing these things," (p. 6). Although they are ultimately different sides of the same sphere, man's psyche, the ego and the Self function as autonomous centers of psychic being.

The distinction between the polarities of selfhood has been belabored up to this point in order to make one central point: if there are two levels of selves, there are correspondingly two types of self-esteem. The first and most common variety of self-esteem relates to the normal egotistical level of being. This type of self-esteem is aptly described as situational in nature for it is largely dependent on external factors such as physical appearance, social acceptance, economic prosperity, etc... The essential ingredient in maintaining a high level of self-esteem of the situational variety is the praise and approval of one's peer group. This necessary approval forms a protective umbrella which protects the individual's fragile self-image. Yet, as one authority on self-esteem has noted, there are definite disadvantages entailed in deriving one's self- esteem principally from the opinions of others. Ernest Becker (1971) recommends that the individual seek self-esteem on "the highest level of generality" for this level alone gives the individual a feeling of ultimate value in what Becker calls "the cosmic hero system". This is essentially a call for the development of self-esteem relating to man's higher self, the other mysterious pole of the dichotomous self.

As noted above, the type of self-esteem relating to the ego level of consciousness may be designated situational. Conversely, the type of esteem relating to the higher or deeper self is non-situational in nature. In order to distinguish this variety from the first we will use the adjective "cosmic" in the same sense that Becker used the term to characterize the "highest level of generality." Cosmic self-esteem is fundamentally spiritual in nature. Traditionally, individuals enhanced this sense of cosmic value through "religious" activities such as rituals, prayer and meditation. The world's religions provide their followers with all-embracing life-orientations which impart a sense of positive value and meaning to their lives. However, means of enhancing cosmic self-esteem have never been limited to the bounds of organized religion. One means of effecting dramatic change in a person's self-valuation is hypnosis, a technique which is commonly considered to be non-religious. When the individual's diurnal ego-consciousness is lulled to sleep, the hypnotherapist is able to work with the deeper levels of the personality. The results are often astounding.

We owe the word "hypnosis" to Dr. James Braid of Manchester, England who coined it in 1842. Although the word is fairly recent, the phenomenon is ancient. For example, a form of self-hypnosis can be discerned in the meditative exercises of Indian seers: gazing steadily at a fixed point and repetition of a *mantra* until a trancelike state is attained. The aim of these exercises was the realization of a higher level of being (*atman*). In the nineteenth and twentieth centuries, hypnosis has fully entered the world of medical science. Many professionals have acknowledged its effectiveness in curing or alleviating certain maladies. Since any suggestion given to a person during hypnosis has a much greater effect than the same suggestion during normal consciousness, hypnosis can be used to change people's habits and enhance their enjoyment of life. But, can hypnosis be used to alter a person's self-esteem? In order to answer this question in the affirmative, it is necessary to move from generalities to specifics and look at the work of a practicing hypnotherapist.

Professor Ronald Steffenhagen's approach to therapy has been largely influenced by the work of Alfred Alder. Yet, his own work in the sociology of deviance and his knowledge of hypnosis have added a new dimension to Adler's theories of self-esteem. He utilizes the deep hypnotic levels of consciousness to establish or buttress a client's sense of personal value. This revitalized sense of value will in turn help to solve the client's particular problem whether it may be curbing a bad habit or improving academic performance. Self-esteem is the key.

In the hypnotic state the mind is far more receptive and less obstructive than it is in the waking state. The following lines which form a part of Dr. Steffenhagen's basic "script" in a hypnotic session might be rejected automatically by the "normal" self-defeating mind:

> Everyday in every way I am getting better and better; everyday in every way I am becoming more self-confident; everday in every way I am developing a greater self-assurance. My body is a holy temple in which my spirit resides. I am both spiritual and physical. It is my spiritual essence that will help me achieve those things in this life that are beneficial to me and to humanity.

If the subject is truly in a hypnotic condition these statements sink in like rain into dry soil. He or she may not remember them afterwards but they will remain with the person constantly enhancing their sense of value on a subliminal level of consciousness.

A close examination of the lines quoted above reveals that they are directed to "other pole" of the dichotomous self: the spiritual or cosmic essence of the individual. For Dr. Steffenhagen, a positive sense of self-esteem must be based on an interrelationship of the spiritual and material essences of the individual. It means establishing a connection between the levels of selfhood discussed in the first part of this chapter. The consequences of a disconnection between levels include emptiness, despair, meaningless, and an overriding sense of futility. All of these consequences are characteristic of low-self- esteem. High self-esteem, on the other hand, brings about the opposite consequences: meaning, purpose, a sense of value within the cosmos.

The question that is probably in the mind of the reader at this point is: "yes, but... can it really be that simple?" Hypnosis is not a universal panacea. Key elements in its success are the desire on the client's part to change, a willingness to set realizable goals and work to attain them. As John Dewey emphasized, choice of action is pivotal in self-formation. Therefore, Dr. Steffehagen pays close attention to the goal-setting process.

> When goals become unattainable, we see a dimunution in self-esteem because the individual can never feel truly good about himself. He is never capable of attaining anything worthwhile in terms of his own perceptions.

Professor Steffenhagen has also done extensive work with a new hypnotic technique he refers to as Model Two. Like the first model discussed above, Model Two has proven to be very effective in elevating self-esteem. However, the reasons for its effectiveness are more difficult to explain since it entails the use of a language which is incomprehensible to the hypnotized subject, usually archaic German. This tecnique, which Steffenhagen discovered almost by accident in 1978, is utilized in certain cases to achieve an experience akin to spiritual transcendence. The essentials of this advanced technique are given by Professor Steffenhagen as follows:

> In utilizing this technique any hypnotic technique can be used in placing the individual in the hypnagogic state. At this point, one can utilize model one as a preparation for the second model. Then, I say the following: 'In our western society we have built up a reality based on a framework of Newtonian science. We are caught in a gravity-oriented reality of up and down. I count you down into a deeper state of relaxation, and I bring you out by counting up from one to five. Now, we are going to deal with the eastern concept of out and in, in and out. In a moment, I shall begin to speak in a language which you do not understand. At that point, your consciousness will be allowed to go out, out to a different reality, a different dimension. It will remain there as long as I continue to speak German. As soon as I speak the first word of English, it will return to this reality, this dimension, this existence. I shall remain as your guide on this plane of existence. It is perfectly safe. You can explore as much as or as little as you want, you are free to roam as far or stay as close as you desire. When you return you will bring back a greater source of energy, power and spiritual strength from the other dimension to help you in this reality.' Then, I speak old German words and phrases to the individual for five to ten minutes. Finally, the individual is brought back to waking consciousness through the standard technique.

The key factor which separates Model Two from the standard hypnotic technique is the use of German when the subject is in a deep hypnotic state of consciousness. The choice of German as the language medium was natural for Dr. Steffenhagen since he is familiar with this language. However, he notes that any other language, archaic or modern, can be used with equal effectiveness provided that the subject is not conversant in it. The purpose of the incomprehensible monolog in Model Two is to release the subject from any ego involvement in the transaction. Since the rational portion of the psyche cannot comprehend the incoming sounds, it tends to surrender. Normal blocking of self-consciousness in curtailed, and the individual experiences a dimension of freedom which is extraordinary.

After each of these sessions utilizing Model Two, Dr. Steffenhagen taped an interview with the subject. Extracts from these interviews are given below.

> The process was one of floating very deep down into my own physical and mental being, eventually reaching a unified, whole relaxed state of being. At this point, I was no longer conscious of my body or mind . . . just of being.
>
> When suggested to travel outwards, outwards I went — it was and felt like a natural extension — the only place left to go from my relaxed, deep down state of being was to an extended, outward state of experience. I began the travel outwards above my eyes and into my head until I was only aware of darkness. I transcended through my head into a place that was still me but not necessarily the same me that I was in touch with in the downward flow. I saw purple, my favorite color, all around me until eventually I was travelling through a purple tunnel.
>
> I awoke with incredibly mellow, smooth, warm energy flowing in a complete pattern through and around me.
>
> Throughout the first part of the induction during the standard procedure I found myself going a lot deeper than I have ever gone before. I haven't been hypnotized for awhile now. It was a standard count but when you entered into the second part when you started telling me that we would no longer be dealing with the opposition of up and down but with the opposition between in and out. The first thing I remember when that started to happen I started to have experiences like hypnogogic experiences or just before I go to sleep I have quite a bit of flash recurring images but not focusing on anyone thing. I got the feeling I was travelling along a road ah un — two of the things I remember especially was a row of a couple hundred coffee cups with incredibly rounded glistening edges. This was all during the very first part when you were explaining in and out and I was getting at a place-along the road was a fence blocking the path and from then on things got much more abstract. It wasn't a matter anymore of being able to formulate specific images that have reference to objectsin the world that I could say I just started projection patterns of extreme colors — beautiful colors on this fence and the fence itself disappeared and I seemed to be free floating — a weightless feeling something I have never felt before. With the standard procedure I always feel heavy. But, this was very weightless . . . not to have to worry about . . . gravity seemed to play no part in it and I couldn't say I was in a trance — it was something entirely different and if I did project any the colors were extreme especially purple — purple — bright and prominent and I really enjoyed looking at it. I was never sure if I was sitting in a chair and I was never sure where I was in relation to what I was seeing. That was part of it more than anything else which is something in regular hypnotic techniques I always feel as though I am feeling very heavy and in a deep trance but there is always a point of reference for my thoughts, my projections and my fantasies or my dreams or whatever relates to me in a place either answering questions or having a dream but in this case it seemed relatively absent.
>
> What struck me especially was the fact that in the beinning it seemed as though it was a journey rather than a static position. In regular hypnosis you almost feel like a piston. You are in one position. You are constantly moving up or down in

that position in that place whereas in this there are no referential points and movement was always out — a journey kind of thing and once that passed there was no problem. I didn't try to say I am moving this way or that way or worrying about coming up or going down. I just seemed to be part of a continual flow.

The extraordinary inner experiences reported above are corroborated by similar statements by a score of other individuals who have been put through this technique. Almost without exception, they say that they experienced the sensation of leaving their physical body and journeying into limitless space. This is a difficult experience to describe, and many of the reports reveal that the subjects were groping for words to convey and ineffable feeling. A typical example of this groping occurs in this extract: "I don't know what I felt. It wasn't like being high. I didn't have any great insights or visions. I still felt well . . . I just knew I was above it . . . I could have been undereath it. Anyway, I was out of it."

The reports indicate that Model Two is effective in improving self-esteem by giving the individual an immediate awareness of the unbounded spiritual side of the psyche. The standard indicators of self-esteem which are situational and dependent in nature are no longer as meaningful for one who has been opened to the further reaches of the psyche. When asked about self- esteem in a post-session interview, one subject responded as follows:

> It doesn't really matter . . . when I used to think about self-esteem I thought it was just feeling good about yourself — liking yourself. Now when I think of it, it's dumb to have to either like yourself or dislike yourself, because you are just you anyway, whether you like it or not. I never thought of it this way; you don't have to feel better in order to feel good.

By the last comment, the interviewee aptly distinguishes between the two levels of self-esteem, the situational and the spiritual. Previously, he thought that self-esteem must entail doing better at something than other people: being more successful, handsomer, smarter, etc. However, having travelled "outside himself," he realized that self-esteem can be independent of a situational reference. His comment: "There is nothing to compare it to."

The nature of Model Two requires that the hypnotherapist be a competent guide, knowledgeable in the psychic terrain. Dr. Steffenhagen emphasizes this point in the following manner:

> When using this hypnotic technique for bringing the individual in touch with his own spirituality and thereby developing a spiritual foundation for self-esteem, the hypnotist must accept the responsibility for functioning as the guide. He must intuitively know how to deal with each individual situation that might arise.

When properly administered in a suitable hypnotic state, both model one and model two have shown great potential as elevators of self-esteem. Of the two, the success of model one is more comprehensible and explicable. It has long been known that, "any suggestion offered to a person during hypnosis has an exaggerated effect on his mind." Model Two's success is more difficult to explain. Through this innovative technique, individuals can gain a new foundation for a self-esteem which is not contingent on outperforming one's neighbors.

The goal of elevating an individual to a larger sense of self and significance is not a luxury which enhances life for the fortunate few who can achieve it. It is essential if we are to overcome the contemporary sense of alienation and meaninglessness which plague modern man. As Alan Watts (1966) wrote in *The Book (On The Taboo Against Knowing Who You Are)*:

> No one who has been hoaxed into belief that he is nothing but his ego, or nothing but his individual organism, can be chivalrous, let alone a civilized, sensitive, and intelligent member of the cosmos. (p. 126)

Although hypnosis is certainly not the only means of bringing about cosmic self-esteem, perhaps it is the most accessible means available for most people. Because the consequences of low-self-esteem are so disasterous for the individual's psychic and physcial well-being, there is an urgency in making hypnotherapy available to more people, especially disturbed teenagers. We do not possess all the answers in regard to self-esteem and hypnosis. However, with the successes that Dr. Steffenhagen has achieved with his clients there is little doubt about its effectiveness in improving self-esteem.

Chart — Characteristics of Self-esteem levels

SITUATIONAL	COSMIC
Dependent largely on external circumstances	Dependent on inner sources
ego-related	Self-related
secular	spiritual
constant state of flux	permanent
sense of self as a separate entity	sense of unity with Nature
oriented to becoming	oriented to being
consumer	self-sufficient
fearful (esp. of death)	steadfast

REFERENCES

Becker, E. *The Birth and Death of Meaning.* New York: The Free Press, 1971.

Edinger, E. *Ego and Archetype.* New York: Penguin Books, 1980.

Hiriyanna, M. *Outlines of Indian Philosophy.* London: George Allen & Unwain, 1970.

Upanishads. *A Sourcebook in Indian Philosophy.* Ed. by S. Radhakrishar, Princeton, N.J.: Princeton University Press, 1973, p. 54.

Underhill, E. *Mysticism.* New York: E. P. Dutton & Co., 1961.

Watts A. *The Book (On The Taboo Against Knowing Who You Are).* New York: Collier, 1966.

*A reduced version of this chapter appeared in the
Journal of Alcohol and Drug Education Vol. 24, No. 1,
Fall 1978 under the title: "An Adlerian approach toward
a self-esteem theory of deviance: a drug abuse model".*

R. A. Steffenhagen Ph.D

*Department of Sociology
University of Vermont*

4

A SELF-ESTEEM THEORY OF DEVIANCE:
A DRUG ABUSE MODEL

Introduction

While there are many theories of drug dependence, all are inadequate in one important respect: they fail to account for the individual who manifests all of the preconditions for drug abuse but does not abuse drugs. Regardless of the theory — psychogenic, socio-genic, or pharmacological — individuals who are occasional, or social drug users, or individuals who according to all criteria are abuse prone but instead find other solutions are not dealt with.

The purpose of this chapter is to use the problem of drug abuse as a basis for the development of a new theory of deviance. Theories of drug abuse are not alone in their failure to predict the behaviors they attempt to explain — this is a characteristic drawback of most theories of deviance. Some of the more important theories of drug abuse, or addiction, will be examined and their inherent weaknesses will be discussed. The ways in which the new theory remedies deficiencies in each of the older theories will be described.

It is our belief that, to be of value, a theory must be able not only to explain the phenomenon under consideration (in this case, drug addiction) *after the fact*, as most do, but must also be able to make *predictions* about individuals' behavior. Most theories fail miserably in the latter task, primarily because they are parochial in their focus and fail to take into account the relationships among a large number of factors predisposing the individual to a particular form of deviant behavior.

Personality theories of drug abuse categorize abuse-prone individuals but fail to predict which potential drug-abusers will actually become drug-dependent. Socio-dynamic theories concentrate on family patterns and the impact of social deprivation on these patterns, but still fail to account for choice of deviance. These theories fail to predict because they do not take into account the social milieu of the abuse-prone individual. Sociolgical theories of drug abuse, on the other hand, by concentrating upon the social context of deviant behavior, ignore the role of personality and of family background.

The theory proposed here incorporates several perspectives and proposes a single underlying factor in drug abuse. This underlying factor is *self-esteem*. While psychological theories have been unable to account for the fact that widely varying personality types are found within any population of drug abusers and sociological theories have been unable to account for the fact that members of drug abusing subcultures vary widely in their use of drugs, self-esteem theory postulates that the reactions of individuals to their social environment are mediated by a common factor—self-esteem.

Self-esteem theory, developed within the framework of Alfred Adler's Individual Psychology, places self-esteem at the apex of personality, and assumes that individuals of any personality type vary with respect to self- esteem and that self-esteem itself, as well as distincitve styles of coping with the need for or lack of self-esteem, develops in a social context. Self-esteem is seen as the most important psychological variable in the etiology of drug abuse and in the rehabilitative process.

While Adler saw a feeling of inferiority as a common denominator of individuals, he placed a great emphasis upon each individual's unique style of dealing with this feeling. Styles of coping with feelings of inferiority are developed according to each individual's choices concerning his own goals, or life-plan, and cannot be understood apart from the social context in which the individual makes these choices. Furthermore, although this point was not developed by Adler, individuals differ in the degree to which they feel inferior. The variability of feelings of inferiority, or the variability of feelings of self-esteem, affords an excellent opportunity for exploring the relationship between inferiority and individual behavior as well as offering an explanation of deviant behavior.

Inferiority feelings on the part of the individual reflect the extent to which he sees himself as unable to attain his goals. Both psychological (the extent to which the individual, through early experiences, comes to see himself as able to achieve his goals) and sociological (the extent to which the society in which the individual lives offers viable routes for the individual to attain his goals) processes are relevant. Furthermore, the fashion in which an individual chooses to deal with inferiority or with an inability to attain goals is also socially as well as psychologically determined.

In analyzing earlier theories of drug abuse, we have been conscious of the fact that the proponents of each theory begin their research, start their analysis, and interpret their data with a built-in bias which leads them to see exactly what they expect to see. Clausen suggests, in interviewing an addict it is almost impossible not to attribute to him, personality characteristics that your education and ideologies claim must be present (see Lindesmith, 1968). Theorists ask questions that stem from their theoretical bias and then submit the realtionships they find to statistical tests that support their hypotheses. While phenomenologically oriented researchers are criticized for their lack of well-developed hypotheses, prestated hypotheses may cause researchers to miss significant variables.

Self-Esteem

There are many concepts in the literature which deal with the self, including self-concept, self-image, self-esteem, ego-strength, individation-deindividuation, looking-glass self, alienation and identity. We will focus upon the Adlerian concept of self-esteem; the regard we have for ourselves.

Associated with self-esteem are the important Adlerian concepts of inferiority and superiority. The individual who feels inferior has a poor regard for himself, and generally withdraws from meaningful social participation. He tends to see the group as valuing him even less than it in fact does. An individual who sees his social environment as hostile or threatening may respond to it in a hostile manner, provoking further hostility from the group and leading to increased alienation. It is not uncommon for an individual with an inferiority complex to compensate for it by manifesting a superiority complex, causing the group to reject him for his "egotism." Allport (1937) sees compensation as the handmaiden of self-esteem. Compensation, like anxiety, can be valuable to the individual. Anxiety is a key source of motivation for the individual but becomes debilitating when it reaches a neurotic level. Inferiority can play a similar role. In a child, if the feeling of inferiority is not overwhelming, s/he will work toward being socially worthwhile. The child will show concern and true interest in others around him; hence the *correct* compensation for normal inferiority is toward a social adjustment.

For purposes of our theoretical development we will concentrate on the concept of self-esteem and will attempt to explain not only drug abuse, but deviance in general, in terms of a self-esteem theory.

Self-esteem, or self-concept, develops along with the rest of the personality through the socialization process. Its lack can be the byproduct of a pampered-life style or of the polar opposite, a neglected life-style. In the pampered-life style the individual is given everything—he develops no feeling of self-worth through his own accomplishments. When a person has developed his early character in a situation of excessive care and attention; and where an extreme dependency relationship was nurtured, the individual finds every situation unacceptable in which the pampering partner of the relationship is absent.

In juxtaposition to the pampered-life style is the neglected lifestyle. Here the personality is built up in a situation of deprivation and neglect where the child gets no support from within the family. He finds the world hostile and reacts in a hostile manner, promoting the very hostility he perceives in others. In neither case do the individual's own efforts lead to a sense of accomplishment. In the case of the pampered individual, his efforts are irrelevant because he is given everything he needs whether he strives for it or not. In the case of the neglected individual, his needs remain unmet regardless of how much he strives.

It is our main contention that low self-esteem is the key psychodynamic mechanism in deviance. This is presented in the following typology as it relates to drug use.

Self-Esteem	Social Situation	Drug Use Pattern
Low	No pressure to use drugs	non-use
	Pressure to use drugs	abuse
High	No pressure to use drugs	non-use
	Pressure to use drugs	drug use but not abuse

It is our contention that self-esteem becomes the basic psycho-dynamic mechanism underlying behavior—social or anti-social. A person with a low self-esteem may well resort to socio-pathic behavior to raise his self-esteem. Behavior problem children in school are merely attempting to achieve a mistaken goal of success. Dea (1970) concludes that delinquents' self-perceptions are less positive in comparison to non-delinquents and delinquents also believe that the eyes of society view them more negatively.

Any theory of drug abuse which fails to account for the social situation is destined to fail, but to emphasize the social situation to the exclusion of psychological factors is equally useless.

One of the prime difficulties in drug research is that samples typically contain only drug abusers, which at best, may be compared with nonusers. In our research (McAree, Steffenhagen & Zheutlin, 1972), we were able to compare the drug user, the drug abuser, and the non-user on the basis of the Minnesota Multiphasic Personality Inventory (MMPI) Scales. We found that the marijuana user could not be distinguished from the non-user on the clinical scales—he is as normal as the non-user. The gross-multiple drug user, the person who tries or uses a wide variety of drugs, was clearly distinguished from the non-user on all the clinical scales (P .01). But, what does this say? Only that the students who were using a variety of drugs (and probabley with greater frequency than those who used marijuana only) tended to have more emotional problems than the marijuana only and the non-user groups. In a related article, Steffenhagen, Schmidt & McAree (1972) suggested that emotional disturbances in students cause them to use drugs self-medicatively. It has been our position that drug abuse in college is symptomatic of deep seated emotional problems and not the cause of psychic disturbance. We found more emotional disturbance among the gross multiple drug users in college than among the non-users as evidenced by MMPI scale values over 70. Eighty percent of the polydrug users had one or more scale values over 70 as compared to 45 percent of the non-users.

The important point here is that there was no conistent pattern although we found that the gross multiple users showed schizoid (not schizophrenic) patterns. This last finding is consistent with out theoretical development in that, if self-esteem is the key mechanism, we would expect to find varied personality profiles among the abuser group, with low self-esteem being the common denominator. This last point is probably the reason why the personality theorists have failed dismally to produce any substantial inroads into developing an adquate theory of drug abuse. There is no consistent profile of the drug-user and, as we will attempt to show, not even pathology is a necessary requirement for drug abuse.

Self-Esteem and Goal Orientation

Self-esteem has been defined by William James (1890) as $\frac{\text{SUCCESS}}{\text{PRETENTIONS}}$ = self-esteem. This would fit withing the Adlerian framework if pretensions are viewed as what Adler called goal orientations. An individual who has unrealistic goal expectations will not be able to achieve and, thus, his self-esteem will be low. It is important to realize that what may appear as success to an outside observer may not be success for the actor in that goal orientation may be so far beyond reality that the achievement for him is not success but failure. Goal orientations become a very important concept within the framework of self-esteem theory because if one is to explain drug abuse by this approach, it is necessary to understand the actor's goals and not look at success or failure in terms of the researcher's perspective. In this respect Adler (1914) says:

> In the psychological schema there are two approximately fixed points: the low self-estimation of the child who feels inferior, and the over-life-sized goal which may reach high as godlikeness. Between these two points there rest the preparatory attempts, the groping devices and tricks, as well as the finished readiness and habitual attitudes. It is from these that the above mentioned goal, which is actually hidden, may be inferred . . . an increased insecurity feeling in childhood causes a higher and more unalterable goal setting, a striving which goes beyond human measure, and at the same time brings about the best-suited efforts or safeguards for attaining the goal. (p. 145-146)

A good example is an individual setting his goals so high as to make them unattainable. He may get excellent grades in school but his goal becomes to "know" everything there is to know in the course, so when he gets an A it does not give a feeling of satisfaction—he rationalizes it as "The course was easy and I really didn't do the amount of work necessary to really understand the subject in depth." The pampered life style leads to insecurity through being dependent upon others. Adler (1935) comments: that psychological and physical characteristics of the neurotic, z.B. discouragement, hesitation, oversensitivity, need for support etc. are direct evidence that the patient continues to clutch to his early pampered life style which invariably supports the exaggerated goal setting.

Over-life-sized goal orientatation and low self-esteem are as Adler says, two approximately fixed points in the psychological scheme of personality development, and in the attempt to cope with these the person may resort to drug use as a coping mechanism.

Self-Esteem and Life Style

The term "life style" was borrowed by Adler from Max Weber. Originally, Adler used the term "Lebensplan" or life plan and later called it "Lebenstil" (style of life) and finally life style. He defined life style as "the wholeness of his individuality" (Adler, 1912) and further comments that a child, in order to best orient himself environmentally and to attain needs satisfaction, avoid displeasure and gain pleasure, must have formed a guiding line (*Leitlinie*), a guiding image (*Leitbild*), taking into account these expectations.

In a sociological (group) context Weber (1946) comments:

> Styles of life are the conventions passed on by the status groups (occupation and professional). Stylizaton of life originates or is conserved by the status group and reveals certain typical traits of that group. (p. 191)

In essence they are both saying the same thing except one is writing in terms of a guiding principle for individual behavior and the other in terms of a guiding principle for group behavior.

Charles Cooley clearly understood Descartes' dictum, "Cogito Ergo Sum," as the starting point for man's cognitive development, since man can only start with a societal *given*: the language and "life style" of the groups are superimposed upon him through the socialization process. The teleological basis of man's behavior stems from his social class—with the family as mediator—and becomes his "life style," the core around which his personality revolves. The group is logically prior to the individual, the "I" is the result of a relatively advanced stage of consciousness and is subservient to a "we" consciousness (society—the group). See Cooley (1956, p. 181).

Adler (1929) defines: Individual Psychology as the consistent movement toward a goal a plan of life and that in order to avoid confusion it has become style of life. Style of life has become equated with various other terms, such as ego, self or "man's own personality" (Adler, 1931). This is interesting because the term life style is popularly used by the press in similar fashion. Adler (1929) argues that the life style determines behavior, the whole commands the parts. Freud's ego, the administrator of the personality, has a similar function. The ego is the executive of the personality. Every individual represents a unity of personality and creation of that unity. The personality of the child is a prototype of the personality of the immediate group (the *Gemeinschaft*) which is a prototype of the personality of the larger group (the *Gesellschaft*). However, while the individual is like everyone else the individual is also unique—just as each snowflake is different, each individual is different both physically and psychically.

The existentialists see man as a summation of his "choices" or as Tillich says: "Man is his choices." What are these choices? This is just another way of viewing man as a summation of his life style, because it is the life style which provides and permits the choices. In dealing with behavior, social scientists deal with the milieu interior and the milieu exterior. The choices within each are derived from the life sytle of the child as developed through the socialization process.

The uniqueness of the individual is what made Adler choose the name Individual Psychology for his school. The uniqueness and unity of the individual are the ying-yang of the universe. Sociologists have also looked at individual adaptations. Merton (1938), in the development of his theory of anomie, emphasized the role of the congruence or disjunction between the cultural goals and the institutional means: the role of the social order. Adler, on the other hand, emphasized the psychological process, although he never underestimated the importance of the social order, which he called "Social Interest." All behavior has to be seen in light of the individual's efforts to achieve success, to overcome minus situations and achieve plus situations. Adler sees each individual as striving for superiority and sees life as a process of goal striving. In psychology we speak of motivation as goal-directed behavior. There is no behavior which is not ultimately goal-directed. While goals are treated under goal-orientation in the previous sections, the idea of striving for superiority, or goal striving, is particularly important in light of the individual's uniqueness as derived from his life style.

The role of "apperception" is most important in understanding the life style: the world is organized by the individual — life is seen in terms of the individual's "*Weltansicht*," which is created from meanings layered upon the perceptions of the individual's past experiences. A stimulus is interperted not merely in light of its sense experience but in terms of this appreceptive mass, these past perceptions. Ideology may be more important than reality.

In an individual's style of life, his goal is not built upon an objective view of reality, but rather a subjective one. The personality is formed by the individual's perception of social facts and for that reason, people have different realities and mold themselves differently while exposed to the same world of facts.

Generally speaking, culture helps make for constancy of behavior, so that an individual's life style has much in common with everyone elses but because of subjectivity, each individual is also *unique*. Thus while social deprivation in the ghettos may provide the cultural basis for heroin addiction, not all ghetto youth become heroin addicts. In this environment many of the kids, but not all, because of curiosity and peer pressure, try and use heroin; further, while some become "hooked," others are able to kick the habit without help (medical intervention). We have consistency and uniqueness existing simultaneously in the same individual.

In our Adlerian typology we will call such deprivation a neglected life style, and it is certainly important in explaining drug abuse. On the opposite end of the continuum we have the pampered life style, which helps account for such drug abuse as alcohol or poly-drug abuse, which is frequent in the middle class and college environments.

The understanding of the individual's life style and its relation to the social class life style is important in understanding drug abuse. While the individual's life style becomes a guiding image for him, much of "his" guiding image is also part of the guiding principle of the group. A middle class youth with low self-esteem (often manifesting a pampered life style) who has developed unattainable goals will probably move towards counseling or poly- drug abuse, both of which are consistent with the middle class college subculture. On the other hand, a youth from the slums with low self-esteem (generally manifesting a neglected life style) probably will move in the direction of delinquency and/or drugs as a coping mechanism. In attempting to predict the direction behavior will take, it is essential to deal with both individual and group life styles, and the life style concept becomes crucial in developing a theory of drug abuse.

Self-Esteem and The Social Milieu:
Differential Association and the Role of Peer Group Pressure

Under the social milieu we include the role of differential association with the family and the peer group. First, we shall look at the role of differential association and its impact on drug use. One of the theories of deviance which has relevance to self-esteem theory is Sutherland's (1955) Differential Association Theory. Sutherland established nine propositions concerning behavior which would be important in establishing norms for the individual which would then serve as guide-posts for behavior. This theory is based upon learning theory—socialization. The individual is socialized into being a conformist or deviant. Sutherland's original theory is concerned with crime and attempts to explain crime in modern society. In order to make this theory more relevant to our needs, we are substituting deviance for crime, so his first proposition reads: "Deviant behavior is learned."

There is no question as to how important the role of socialization is in molding the personality and consequently in determining the behavior of the recipient. Becker (1956) refers to the role socialization plays in the process of turning on to drugs. The alcohol user is socialized into the use of alcohol—he is taught what to expect and how to consume. The marijuana user is likewise taught how to "smoke" and what a marijuana high is, as Becker (1967) suggests that when someone first uses marijuana, even though it is obvious to others that he/she is 'high', he may not realize he is feeling the drugs effect.

In reference to "pot" smoking, differential association is particularly important because the individual must associate with users if he or she is to be able to obtain a "stash." Not only is there the preference for association with other peers with similar interests, there is the necessity if one is to obtain the marijuana. This theme has been developed in a paper by McCann, Steffenhagen, and Merriam (1976):

> The data showed that youthful experimentation with drugs was the major factor in extensive drug participation, that it results in a high frequency of marijuana use, which in turn leads to other drugs and the selling of various kinds of drugs. We attribute deep involvement in a drug culture or syndrome primarily to self-selection for early experimentation and the resultant development of roles and values conducive to drug use along the lines of differential association theory and to the necessity for the regular user of marijuana to become more deeply involved with other drug users in order to avoid negative legal sanctions. These two factors combine to produce a pattern of a deviant career. (p. 22)

Under this section we have analyzed the role of differential association from the perspective of research data. It is evident that peer group association is an important factor in the socialization process of the individual. The adolescent peer group, as a subculture, may be either an agent of social change or an agent supporting the status-quo. In this capacity it plays a vital role in putting pressure upon youth to conform to the values "it" has established for itself, be they delinquent or non-delinquent (drug use or non-drug use).

In reference to the establishment of core attitudes in the personality, we find the primary group playing the most important role. The family, along with other primary groups (peer group, the next most important), develops basic core attitudes and values from its primary social institutions (see Barnouw, 1973). In this way, according to Kardiner, as cited by Barnouw, the personality thus formed may also exert an influence upon the formation of secondary institutions, e.g., folklore and religious beliefs. The interrelationship between the family and the peer group is a most complex process—who has the greatest influence upon development of core attitudes which will determine the direction of the behavior of the individual?

Related to the theory of excess of definitions favoring deviance or conformity is the role of the psychological support system, which is essential in helping the individual to develop and maintain his self-esteem. Psychological support systems may come from the family, peer group, intimate friend, or counselor, and can help one cope with stress and at times "buck the system" or reject pressure from one of the groups. Not unrelated to this is David Riesman's typology of social character and his emphasis upon modern youth as being other-directed so that the peer group plays a much more important role in socialization than it had in the tradition-or inner-directed person. Here the peer group may provide the excess of definitions, not merely by virtue of time spent with the group (frequency or duration) but because of the importance of the group's opinions to the individual (intensity). One's contemporaries provide the major source of direction for the individual, and modern youth are particularly sensitive to the opinion and values of others. The breakdown of the traditional extended family and an even further attenuation of the nuclear family further this process. Where the elders used to provide the role models for youth in their transition from adolescence into adulthood, youth today are finding the peer culture a substitute for the traditional family and are finding interpersonal support from within the peer group (Flacks, 1971).

Self-Esteem and Social Interest

Paramount to the development of a healthy personality is social interest. Man is a social animal, a symbolic being. Probably one of Aristotle's most important dictums was that man is by nature a social animal, which leads us to a contemporary corollary that the group is logically *prior* to the individual. S. Hecht (1929) comments that the organism does not adapt to the environment but that the environment adapts the organism to itself.

It is through social participation that the individual develops his feelings of inferiority, and it is only through social participation that he can deal with these feelings of inferiority and develop high self-esteem. Man's humanness arises out of social interaction and out of this interaction the self develops. Man is born with biological needs which must be met through social interaction if he is to live, which accounts for the learning process. This learning process takes place in a socio-cultural milieu which leads to the process we call socialization and it is through this process that he develops his personality. The socialization process can only be accounted for in terms of the social group, particularly the primary group which perpetuates and gives uniformity to social action which accounts for cultural patterns.

From the perspective of the Adlerian model, social interest is necessary to mental health. The pampered life style leads to a lack of social interest; self-interest, whereby the actor feels society is his plum to be picked even at his own choosing. This further leads to inferiority feelings because the gratification of his needs comes from other and not from self-accomplishments. He is only able to maintain a functional balance when he has his significant others to provide for the physical and emotional support. Praise is good for the ego and helps the individual to develop self-esteem when it is given for socially useful acts. When praise is given for socially useless acts or only for exemplary behavior, pampering, ($5.00 for an A) he doesn't develop an inner feeling of self-worth and never outgrows these feelings of inferiority or compensates by outwardly manifesting a superiority complex. Good social interest can only develop out of a concern for and an interest in the welfare of others. This other-directedness further needs to be in conjunction with socially useful goals.

Self-Esteem and Deviance

Who will become a drug user or abuser cannot be explained on the basis of self-esteem alone but must be coupled with an understanding of the total social situation and the life style of the individual. We are postulating that an individual with low self-esteem will be a prime target for drug abuse today, because of the widespread prevalence and availability of drugs and because the mass media have so thoroughly dispersed drug information through the population. The following model is presented to help clarify the issues:

Condition	Effect
Low self-esteem	Psychosis
	Delinquency
	Crime
	Drug Abuse
	Occult
	Neurosis
	etc.

The behavior accompanying low self-esteem can be explained by the individual's social situation and life style. Drug abuse and delinquency may go together in the ghetto environment whereas drug abuse may exist independently or with the use of the occult among the college population (see Steffenhagen, 1974): Drug abuse is frequently an expression of a pampered life style. An individual uses drugs to safeguard self-esteem; to shirk responsibilities and blame others for their lack of success without giving up their high goals.

In this same paper the interrelationship between neurosis and the occult was examined. The occult is being used here in its negative sense to refer to the faddish proliferation of secret societies, devil worship, etc. In a study of a newly formed cult, John Lofland (1966) states that the first condition necessary for conversion is that the prospective convert experience a condition of acutely felt tension over a period of time. There is a close relationship between drugs and cult membership, many cult members having had previous drug abuse histories and many cult members dropping out and becoming drug abusers. The relationship is more clearly understood in light of Adler's reference to the role of the exaggerated goal of self-enhancement. Adler indicates that there are two relatively fixed points in this schema, over-life-sized goals which may reach proportions of god-likeness and the low self-esteem of the person who feels inferior. The striving for a goal set beyond all possibility of attainment is in a sense striving for power. The "normal" person with social interest seeks success in accordance with the dictates of reality, whereas the neurotic with the over-life-sized goals may seek success in terms of immediate gratification and little energy output on his part: "I will pray to the devil for immediate power."

We can build a similar case for the close connection between drugs and delinquency, both having a possible basis in inferiority and neurosis. We see that not just drug abuse but deviance in general may be the bulwark of the person with low self-esteem who uses these various techniques (deviance) as coping mechanisms for dealing with inferiority. Just as the drug abuser is distinguished from the normal drug user by deep seated inferiority feelings, the "neurotic" delinquent must be distinguished from the "normal" delinquent whose delinquency is a result of an adverse environment or an excess of definitions for delinquency. As previously stated, it is not uncommon to see individuals engage in more than one type of deviant behavior simultaneously—drugs-occult, drugs-delinquency, drugs-psychosis, or even drugs-occult-delinquency.

In dealing with heroin addiction, Winkler and Rasor (1953) postulated that there are four types of addicts in terms of personality types— the neurotics, psychopaths, psychotics and normals. The normal addict is the person who manifests no abnormal personality characteristic and who uses drugs to relieve pain. It is necessary to elaborate here because one could say the abnormal also uses drugs to relieve pain. However, the normal user seeks the relief of physical pain. The now famous (or infamous) "soldier's disease" of the post Civil War period would be an example of drug addiction of this type. Individuals, because of the physically addicting nature of the drug, became addicted to morphine when they were administered morphine for the control of pain.

Psychological dependence is more difficult to explain than physiological addiction, but is nonetheless one of the most important processes in the analysis of drug abuse in today's culture. This refers to a compulsion to use a drug for its psychologically pleasurable effect. Such drugs include stimulants, tranquilizers, marijuana and psychedelic drugs. The federal government has dropped the distinction between physiological addiction and psychological dependency in favor of the term "dependency producing drugs."

The concept of the poly-drug abuser generally refers to the individual who uses a variety of drugs rather than just one drug. Such use usually involves the psychological dependency producing drugs. It may also include the physical dependency producing drugs, but not to the point of addiction. This category of poly-drug user for the normal is far more difficult to explain than the opiate addict who started for the control of pain.

Becker and Strauss (1956) and others have spoken of the socialization process involved in drug use. Every drug researcher who has studied marijuana use is familiar with the idea that most users enjoy turning on another person and the social camaraderie which emanates from "doing" drugs together. Here is an example of how a normal person can become involved in drug use without having any emotional instability. McAree, Steffenhagen, and Zheutlin (1972) concluded that the gross-multiple drug users showed more emotional pathology thru the non-user, as measured by the MMPI. However, on an individual basis, we had MMPI profiles of gross-multiple drug users who had normal profiles with no scales above 70.

McCann, Steffenhagen and Merriam (1976) were able to show, through the use of a path analysis, that the marijuana user is put into a situation where he is forced to become a part of the deviant subculture in order to pursue a behavior pattern which he finds pleasurable and satisfying. We found that there was strong support for our theory that frequency of drug use is fostered by socialization into the subculture. The path analysis produced the following model: low age at turn-on leads to high frequency of use, which leads to use of other drugs, to selling marijuana and to selling other drugs. While we are not directly concerned with selling at this point, it is part of the total picture of involvement and the key point is that the frequency of marijuana use had a strong positive effect upon the use of other drugs — our gross-multiple use.

As we indicated earlier in our discussion of the conditioning theory, it is possible for a heavy drug use pattern to emerge from the conditioning process itself without pathology. Does this negate our contention that drug abuse is related to low self-esteem? No, because "heavy" drug use is not necessarily abuse. As with physical addiction, abuse may be reflected in the difficulty incurred in abstinence. If someone can become a poly-drug user through this normal entrance into the drug behavior pattern, then how can one distinguish between the person with high and low self-esteem? It will be hypothesized that given drug abuse, the high self-esteem individual will be able to give up his drug abuse behavior in a therapeutic setting; or, as in the case within delinquent gangs, when the group decides a particular drug is no longer "cool," the person with high self-esteem will give it up whereas the person with low self-esteem will not.

Self-Esteem Related to the Existing Theories

Personality theories fail to account for the fact that the choice of deviance is dependent not only upon the pathology (which may not even be necessary) but also upon the life style of the individual. While one would predict that a boy from the slums might easily turn to delinquency as a form of deviance and as a mechanism for coping with feelings of inadequacy, the middle-class college student might turn to drugs. The pathology per se is insufficient; the life style and self-esteem are crucial.

The socio-dynamic theories, concentrating on family patterns and social deprivation, fail to account for the choice of deviance. It is clear that youth from the ghettos do provide more than their share of delinquents, but what of the siblings who do not become delinquent? Also, why does one become a delinquent and another both delinquent and addict? Our theory contends that the pattern of deviance will be determined to a large extent by the social situation, and that the youth with low self- esteem will be the one most likely to become a drug abuser and/or delinquent and be the least amenable to rehabilitation.

The social theories, while concentrating on anomie and the social structure, fail to account for the differential behavior of individuals as do the socio-dynamic theories. Self-esteem and life style will predict who will tend to abuse drugs and who won't. A person who is free of neurotic inhibitions and anxiety may still get into drugs as a result of peer-group pressure and his life style but without developing a dependency relationship. Also, siblings within a single family may react differently as a result of their different personalities or life styles.

The social theories tend to ignore the role of personality in deviance. Self-esteem is important in determining the behavior of individuals within the social structure. An individual with low self-esteem may develop strong dependency needs for drugs while still subscribing to the acceptable means-ends of society. An area of growing concern would be the middle-class, middle-aged woman who resorts to the use of barbituates to cope with boredom in her life. She has internalized all the acceptable means-ends, but this may provide the very basis for her neurosis. A woman of low self-esteem would be a prime target for barbituate addiction, especially since the use of drugs to alter mood is encouraged within our social structure.

Within the framework of the psychological theories the major weakness is a lack of consideration of the importance of the structural elements, but more important to our paradigm is the lack of emphasis upon the life style and upon self-esteem. The role of self-esteem is important in relation to the acquired drive theory in that it is the individuals with low self-esteem who are most prone to find the drug satisfying and to use it to block unpleasant perceptions. The avoidance theory, in similar fashion, is inadequate in understanding the role of self-esteem. Here, too, the individual with low self-esteem will seek drugs to allay unpleasant perceptions of life. The individual's personality will also be crucial since it will most likely be the pampered and/or neglected "child" who will seek relief through mechanisms requiring little effort on their part.

The metabolic theory, even if it were to be grounded in fact, still needs to take into account the personality, life style and social structure to provide an adequate explanation for exceptions. Certainly, one would not assume that a major genetic mutation in the population can account for a serious drug problem today that didn't exist twenty years ago. Such social factors as Zeitgeist, Volkgeist and alienation cannot be ignored: these factors coupled with life style and self-esteem are necessary social-psychological correlates of drug abuse.

Conditioning theory also is inadequate without considering self-esteem and life style. Given a social situation where the individual partakes of drugs due to social pressure, we still need to be able to explain which individuals will move towards dependency and which ones will be able to withstand the habituating nature of the drug. Here again it will be the individuals with low self-esteem who will be most likely to succumb to drug abuse.

The existentialist theory, although promising, still lacks the important mechanics of self-esteem and life style. For example, Greaves (1974) postulates that drug use is automedicative, i.e., the user will use drugs to minimize pain and anxiety, and that such individuals are those who are lacking in pleasurable sensory awareness, who cannot create their own needed euphoria. This explanation is the first step in advancing an adequate theory, but who are the individuals lacking in pleasurable sensory awareness?

Low self-esteem, a feeling of lacking in self-worth, would be the psychodynamic mechanism sufficient to create the situation where the individual is unable to produce his own needed euphoria. The reaction to such a situation depends on the life style. The main difficulty in this position is that it still focuses upon the symptomatic level and not on the dynamic level of self-esteem. How can euphoria be increased? Only by strengthening the individual's self-esteem.

Four Adlerian concepts which are crucial to self-esteem theory are: life style, social milieu, social interest and goal orientation. Life style is seen to be equally important for the different types of abusers, both the pampered life style of the college student and the neglected life style of the ghetto dweller. The social milieu is important because peer pressure and/or lack of a primary group support system may provide the reason for drug use. We have found that curiosity was the primary reason given by college students for experimenting with drugs, and some peer groups certainly promote curiosity. Social interest, or lack thereof, helps explain the drug abuser who is so self-centered that he fails to consider the effects of his behavior on others. Social interest is essential to good mental health.

It is becoming increasingly evident that the MMPI is of little use in attempting to explain the etiology of drug use and abuse. It is merely a measure of emotional stability. The *psychodynamic mechanism underlying* drug abuse is *lack of self-esteem*. Does the subject see himself as adequate, does he feel confident and secure about himself? Self-confidence in an individual is an important psychological dimension in understanding the etiology of drug abuse and in the rehabilitative process. Those lacking in self-esteem must defend themselves against their poor self-image and insecurity. They are likely to be situation- dominated and particularly subject to the erratic fluctuations of their emotional milieu. They will perceive stress differently than will persons with high self-esteem and this perceived stress will have an inordinate effect upon them. Inferiority feelings, a dimension of low self-esteem, will result in compensatory maneuvers — e.g., drug abuse.

Self-esteem, while the basic psychodynamic mechanism underlying deviance (drug abuse), is however, not sufficient to predict who will engage in deviant behavior — an understanding of the individual's life style and goal orientations and social milieu is also needed. Given the psychodynamic mechanisms we also need to understand the input of the social structure. This, then, leads to the following paradigm:* Self-Esteem — Life Style — Personality Traits — Goal Orientation — Primary Group — Social Milien = Behavior where:

> Self-Esteem — High or low
> Life Style — Self-centered vs. contributive
> Personality Traits — Normal or Neurotic
> Goal Orientation — Socially useful vs. useless
> Primary Group — Supportive or unsupportive
> Social Milieu — Friendly or hostile

---

* These are not mutually exclusive categories, since the life style of the parents provide a basis for shaping the prototype of the personality but self-esteem is being posited as the foundation rather than the apex of the personality.

Conclusion

Our theory postulates that the psychodynamic mechanism underlying deviance is low self-esteem. Self-esteem develops in the individual through repeated experiences of mastery, i.e., repeated experiences in which efforts to achieve a goal are met with success. As such, an individual's self-esteem is a reflection both of his level of aspiration and of his self-confidence. A person may be quite competent, but set his goals too high; or a person may have realistic goals, but feel unsure of his ability to achieve them. William James's formula for self- esteem reflects this situation: success/pretensions = self-esteem. The ratio, for the individual, of success to pretensions, is not solely a result of intra-psychic processes. As Merton points out, goals are set and approached in a structural context, and social structures differ in the extent to which they enable individuals to attain valued goals. The American Credo of Success, so aptly described by Merton, creates aspirations for our youth which are fairly universally shared due to mass media. Because of differential access to means for achieving success, however, discrepancies between aspirations (goals) and expectations (adequacy, self-confidence) are inevitable for a large segment of the population. On this issue, Short (1964) suggests that position discontent among boys, (the mean discrepancy between occupational aspirations and expectations) is approximately related to their official delinquent activities. The Negro gang members, who have the greatest police involvement have the greatest discontent with their position. In other words, Short found structurally created discrepancies between individuals' aspirations and expectations reflected in individuals' tendencies to pursue deviant (delinquent) life styles.

As Cloward and Ohlin have pointed out, however, in their book *Delinquency and Opportunity: A Theory of Delinquent Gangs* (1960), low self-esteem, or a sense of being unable to live up to culturally valued goals, does not in itself predict delinquency. Delinquent behaviors are generally learned through interaction with peers who participate in a delinquent peer culture. Not all individuals with low self-esteem encounter such a peer culture. It is certainly true that youth in poor neighborhoods are more likely than youth in more privileged neighborhoods to encounter an organized delinquent subculture, but even then membership in a delinquent sub-group is not automatic for poor youth. Furthermore, individuals whose self-esteem is unimpaired may temporarily engage in delinquent activities in response to peer pressure or other social contingencies.

Even when the achievement of culturally prescribed goals is precluded by an individual's economic disadvantage, low self-esteem is not inevitable. Family structure and early socialization may play an important role in the development of an individual's self-esteem. An individual whose early family experience provided him with opportunities to set realistic goals and to achieve them through his own efforts may carry that perspective with him in later years. On the other hand, an individual who was unable to cope successfully in early life, either due to pampering or to neglect, may continue to see himself as unable to live up to his goals even when he does possess the means for achieving them.

Behavior, then, is a product of several influences, with self-esteem as the underlying psychodynamic mechanism, as seen in the following model: Self-Esteem — Life Style — Personality Traits — Goal Orientation — Primary Group — Social Milieu = Behavior.

Going back to Adler, all behavior is goal-oriented behavior or goal striving, a fact recognized by all psychologists but frequently lost sight of because of differences in conceptual framework. Psychologists point out that to complete the S-R circuit, the individual must be motivated and motivation is defined as an energizing state of the organism which directs it toward a goal. While Adler and comtemporary psychologists are in agreement as to the basis of behavior, Adler placed more emphasis on goal orientation. Because Adler, a humanist, looked for a uniform principle underlying behavior, he avoided the reductionist traps. If we view all behavior as goal striving and note that the individual evaluates himself in terms of his ability to achieve the goals he sees as important, we begin to understand why self-esteem is the psychodynamic mechanism underlying deviance as well as normal behavior. If the individual feels inadequate, he feels insecure and needs to protect his poor self image. This results in feelings of inferiority which are frequently compensated for in behavior. These compensatory behaviors generally create further problems in interpersonal relations and increase inferiority.

Neurosis and psychosis are attempts to compensate for inferiority feelings. Adler noted that everyone has feelings of inferiority, which provides us with a continuum from those with appropriate and useful ways of dealing with inferiority to those whose guiding principles become fictional life-plans and result in accentuated inferiority. Self-esteem, then, is not merely high or low but varies continuously: those with lower self-esteem are more inclined to deal with inferiority inappropriately (deviance) than are those with higher self-esteem.

On the applied level, Adlerian theory also explains why both AA and Synanon are rehabilitative and not curative.* Evidence in the field indicates that ex-drug abusers who leave Synanon have a high recidivism rate and that AA members have a need to continue to attend meetings. In both therapeutic models, the individual is made to abase himself before the group: "I am an alcoholic who has *no* control over himself" or "I am a *no* good Junkie." In each instance an individual who is already low in self-esteem is made to degrade himself still further before the group which then offers group support. Research by Lieberman, Yalom and Miles (1973) suggests that encounter groups are beneficial for some and not others. Sociologists have long been aware of the socializing function of the group—in AA and Synanon the drug-dependent person is socialized to remain drug free only *with* the support system of the group. It is our contention that both of these groups offer group support to the

---

* By "rehabilitative" we mean that the individual is restored to "normal" functioning although the original pathology is still present but not disruptive. As in the case of T.B. or schizophrenia the person may be restored to normal function although he still has the T.B. or schizophrenia but is in remission. By "curative" we mean the individual is restored to normal function as a result of having destroyed the pathology (he had the flu and now is cured).

individual, but that they do little to help him develop his *own* self-esteem. Therefore, when the individual leaves the group and no longer has the group to fall back on, he returns to old self-esteem safeguarding mechanisms, drugs. He remains rehabilitated as long as he has the group support but since his self-esteem has not been increased he is not cured.

REFERENCES

1. Adler, A. *Der nervose charakter*. In Heilen & Bilden, pp. 140-150, 1914.
2. Adler, A. *Uber der nervosen charakter*. (1912). 4th Edition. Munich: Bergmann, 1928.
3. Adler, A. *The Science of Living*, New York: Greenberg, Publishing, Inc., 1929.
4. Adler, A. *What Life Should Mean to You*. Boston: Little, Brown & Co., 1931.
5. Adler, A. *Social Interest* (1933). Trans. by J. Linton and R. Vaughan. New York: Capricorn Books 1964.
6. Adler, A. "Presentation of Nervosis", *Int. In. Indiv. Psychol.* 1 #4 3-12.
7. Allport, Gordon. *Personality: A Psychological Interpretation*. New York: Henry Holt & Co., Inc. 1937.
8. Ansbacher, Heinz L. and Rowena R. Ansbacher. *The Individual Psychology of Alfred Adler*. New York: Harper Torchbooks, 1956.
9. Barnouw, Victor. *Culture and Personality*. Illinois: Dorsey Press, 1973.
10. Becker, H.S. and Anselm Strauss. Careers, Personality, and Adult Socialization. *American Journal of Sociology*. 62: 253-263), November, 1956.
11. Becker, Howard S. History, Culture and Subjective Experience, in *Student Drug Involvement*. Ed. by Charles Hollander. Washington: U.S. National Student Association, 1967.
12. Cloward, Richard A. and Lloyd E. Ohlin. *Delinquency and Opportunity: A Theory of Delinquent Gangs*. New York: The Free Press, 1960.
13. Cooley, C. H. *Social Organization*. Illinois: The Free Press, 1956.
14. Dea, K. L. Concept of Self in Interpersonal Relationships as Perceived by Delinquent and Non-delinquent Youth. Dissertation Abstracts International, Vol. 31 (9-A): 4893, 1970.
15. Flacks, Richard. *Youth and Social Change*. Chicago: Rand McNally (Markham Book), 1971.
16. Greaves, George. Toward an Existential Theory of Drug Dependence. *Journal of Nervous and Mental Disorders*, 159 (4)263-273, 1974.
17. Hecht, S., in Murchison (ed.) *The Foundations of Experimental Physchology*. 1929, p. 268-269.
18. James, W. *Principles of Psychology*, Vol. 1. New York: Henry Holt, 1890.
19. Lieberman, M.A., I.D. Yalom and M. B. Miles. *Encounter Groups: First Facts*. New York: BasicBooks, Inc., 1973.
20. Lindesmith, Alfred R. *Addiction and Opiates*. Chicago: Aldine Publishing Co., 1968.

21. Lofland, John. *Doomsday Cult*. New Jersey: Prentice-Hall, Inc., 1966.
22. McAree, C.P., R. A. Steffenhagen and L. S. Zheutlin. Personality Factors and Patterns of Drug Use in College Students. *American Journal of Psychiatry* 128 (7) 890-892, January 1972.
23. McCann, H. G., R. A. Steffenhagen, and George Merriam. Drug Use: A Model for a Deviant Sub-culture. Prepublication manuscript.
24. Merton, Robert K. Social Structure and Anomie. *American Sociological Review* 3:672-682 (October, 1938).
25. Short, James F. Gang Delinquency and Anomie. in *Anomie and Devient Behavior*. Ed by Marshall B. Clinard, New York: The Free Press, 1964.
26. Steffenhagen, R. A., F. E. Schmidt and C. P. McAree. Emotional Stability and Student Drug Use. *Journal of Drug Education* 1(4), 347-357, December, 1971.
27. Steffenhagen, Ronald A. Drug Abuse and Related Phenomena: An Adlerian Approach. *Journal of Individual Psychology*, Vol. 30, 238-250, November, 1974.
28. Sutherland, Edwin H. *Principles of Criminology*. Philadelphia: J. B. Lippincott, 1947.
29. Weber, Max. *The Theory of Social and Economic Organization*. Trans. by Henderson A. M. and T. Parsons. New York: Oxford University Press, 1947.
30. Weber, Max. *Essays in Sociology*. Trans. and edited by H. H. Gerth and C. W. Mills. New York: Oxford University Press, 1946.
31. Winkler, A. and W. Rasor. Psychiatric Aspects of Drug Addiction. *American Journal of Medicine* 24, 566-570, 1953.

R. A. Steffenhagen Ph.D
Department of Sociology
University of Vermont

and

Ruben Fournier, B. A.

5

SELF-ESTEEM: A MODEL

The conceptualization of and research on self-esteem has been plagued with ambiguities. Self-esteem, self-acceptance, ego-strength, self-regard, individualism, identity, anomia, self-concept, personality integration and other terms are frequently used interchangably. William James (1890) discussed the concept and it has been amply reviewed since (Wylie, 1961-1968, Shaver 1969). Robinson & Shaver (1976) state that despite its popularity the self-esteem concept has no standard theoretical or operational definition. Yet, the theory of self-esteem is more important in understanding human behavior than are any of the theories of personality development. Carl Rogers (1961) for example, has taken the position that the main motive of man is to actualize, maintain and enhance the idea of one's "self", a theme comparable to Maslow's (1950) concept of self actualization.

In the framework of Adler's individual psychology, even suicide, privately committed, is interpreted as self-enhancement; the individual would be too proud to go on in a self-effacing milieu, and would rather die than lose face. Thus, suicide becomes a preservation of his self-esteem. Within the framework of self-esteem, the most important motive force is the preservation of the "self", stronger and more crucial than the drive for physical survival. All human behavior centers around the interpretation and preservation of the "self" or the maintenance of self "esteem".

In contrast, typical therapeutic approaches used today are essentially theories of personality. Freud's psychoanalytic model had for many years overshadowed other important work and it is this context that Alfred Adler's major contribution has been underemphasized by many contemporary psychologists and therapists. In his emphasis upon sexuality, Freud lost sight of the most important motive force in man: the preservation of the self (self-esteem). In fact, the sex drive and sexual energy is frequently used not to fulfill any sexual need, but rather to protect one's self-concept. Rape, for example, may be committed not for sexual release, but as a device to protect a fragile self-esteem. Here then, we see that Adler's major contribution to psychology was not his *Individual Psychology*" but his theory of self-esteem.

The role of self-esteem is crucial to an understanding of human behavior. Personality is developed as a result of the socialization process and is a reflection of the *Kultur*. What is important is not, for example, whether one manifests an oral or anal personality, but rather how *s/he* protects *s/he* self-esteem. In the psychosomatic literature, we find a myriad of references to the role of repression, contained hostility, etc. In the drug literature we see references to the triad of factors present in the etiology of heroin addictions but these do not explain heroin addiction, as shown by the many individuals who manifest this symptomatology, but are not addicted. A more important factor is how the individual protects his self-esteem, which in turn relates to his exterior milieu.

It is the purpose of this chapter to develop a model of self-esteem which is placed solidly within the social context and to frame the Adlerian role of self-esteem in a broader theory of social adjustment which will then provide a basis for explaining the development of deviant behavior. Although behavior is only deviant in a socio-dynamic context, the basis for the deviance is psycho-dynamic. Deviance can only be explained on this macro-micro level. We will attempt to define self-esteem in terms of a model which can then be applied to deviance.

Figure 1

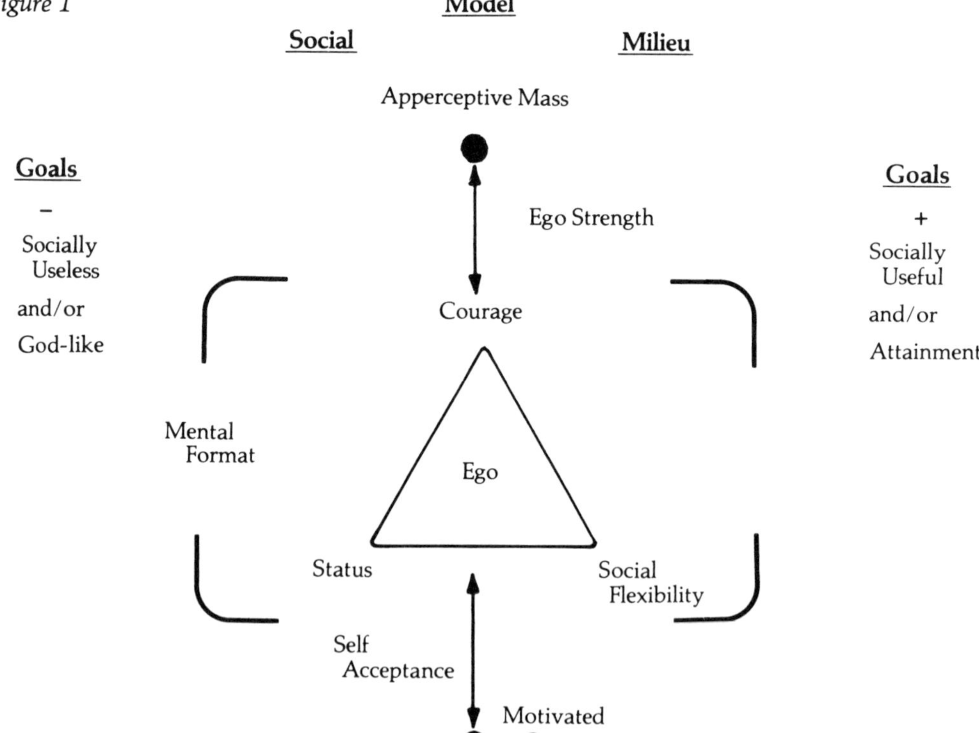

Footnote: Mental format has interesting similarities to Joseph B. Gittler's (1952) diagram of Social Process.

Defining Self-Esteem

It has become evident that nominal definitions applied to self-esteem have not only been inconsistent, but inadequate. We have found self-esteem defined as self-image, ego strength, self-concept, etc. and it is clear that if these terms are interchangeable, they must of necessity reflect the same thing. For the moment, let it suffice to point out that our research has found self-esteem and ego strength as commonly measured to be independent, separate phenomena and not identical as the literature tends to indicate.

Figure 1 presents a model of self-esteem, the components of which are: (1) the apperceptive mass, (2) the mental format, (3) courage, (4) social flexibility, (5) status, (6) social milieu, (7) goals, (8) self-acceptance, (9) ego strength. These concepts are treated at the end of the chapter, but it is necessary to outline them briefly here. The order of consideration is somewhat arbitrary as they are closely interrelated and understanding one involves understanding some or all of the others.

1. *Apperceptive Mass*

The apperceptive mass is the constellation of past perceptions which shape the "mental format". Within the apperceptive mass and the mental format components of the model, there is a basic time reference framework called the *Zeitgeist* which is very important in determining both positive and negative goals, especially within technological cultures.

2. *Mental Format*

The mental format is the interaction of three culturally imposed traits: courage, social flexibility and status which yield a basic orientation towards the reality established by the apperceptive mass.

3. *Courage*

Courage is particularly important in the development of self-esteem. This special quality of holding to one's convictions is an essential element in the development of the individual's perceptions of himself and relates to the guidelines inherent within the apperceptive mass.

4. *Social Flexibility*

Social flexibility becomes important in the development of self-esteem because now, more than ever before, behavioral flexibility is required for survival in an industrialized society built upon rapid social change.

5. *Status*

Modern man is a status bound organism. He evaulates himself in terms of the status ascribed by the group. If he perceives his status as high, he feels good, if he perceives it as low, he feels emotionally destroyed. This is expressed in Liebow's description of the lower calss black male in *Talley's Corner*. We evaluate ourselves in terms of the status we feel we have achieved in the framework of the social milieu.

6. *Social Milieu*

The social milieu determines the feasibility of an individual achieving a goal: (a) From the perspective of the apperceptive mass positive goals are measured in terms of prosperity, economy and interpersonal relationships between the individual and his milieu; (b) In relation to the mental format, goals in the positive direction are revealed to the individual only by way of the apperceptive mass vis-a-vis the social milieu. It should be noted that both positive and negative values are determined strictly by the mental format and by the apperceptive mass which depend on social milieu.

7. Goals

Goals are crucial in the Adlerian development of self-esteem since our evaluations of ourselves frequently depend on the goals that we have or have not achieved. Thus, by setting goals in a god-like manner, the individual is destined to low self-esteem. If he sets his goals too low, their attainment is meaningless and likewise, he is destined to low self-esteem. Realistic goal setting combined with adequate challenge bring about individual satisfaction.

8. Concept of Self-acceptance

Self-acceptance is the ability to relate to oneself realistically within the social milieu. Such self-acceptance can and will only move in the direction of the apperceptive mass. It is the ability to say that I do not have to be better or worse than someone else but this is me, and this is the me I can relate to realistically within interpersonal relationships.

9. Ego Strength

Ego strength may be defind as a realistic orientation to life. The individual who evaluates himself realistically in relationship to the way others view him has high ego strength. (a) It must be understood that the genesis of the ego occurs within the mental format and that which we commonly measure as *ego-strength* is nothing more than the cognitive and intellectual functions (what the individual thinks others think about him) of the individual. (b) The ego is the administrator, the cognitive function of the personality and it is defined in relationship to the mental format and the apperceptive mass. To the degree that the individual evaluates himself appropriately in relationship to the social milieu he has good self ego strength, while to the degree that he is not aware of his true position vis-a-vis the social milieu through the apperceptive mass his ego strength is weak.

Self-esteem is not necessarily related to ego-strength since it is possible to have good ego strength and very low self-esteem. On the basis of the mechanics of motion of the model, it should be pointed out that the mental format when moving towards positive goals leads to high self- esteem. A state of low self-esteem will occur when the mental format moves towards socially useless and/or god-like goals. Man is a forward moving organism and in the state of his movement, the healthy individual will be in line from the self to and through the apperceptive mass. The individual who is oriented toward negative goals or living in the past will be in the state of psychic disequilibrium.

It is possible to have good ego strength and still have low self- esteem. This is the situation when the reality of the mental format is in accord with the apperceptive mass but where the goals are negative. However, the case of low ego strength and high self-esteem may not exist because self-esteem is in large measure dependent upon the reality principle; and in line with the past perceptions of the individual within the social milieu.

Self-image is also not concommitant with self-esteem. We will demonstrate the difference between the two concepts by use of measures demonstrating that self-esteem may be low while ego strength is high. The Brownfain self-concept test which purports to measure self-esteem while consistent with Adlerian principles was used. The difficulty with this test of self-concept, however, is that it actually taps "concept of self". The problem is that tests of this nature are subject to the weakness of 'time boundries' — i.e., they are the reflection of an individual within a specific time frame. Another way of looking at this weakness is that these tests are self-concept tests and that, while the self-concept may be an adequate measure of self-esteem at a given point in time, they are useless as after-measurement tests, because they fail to account for the variable of self-acceptance. Evidence of this contingency is presented here in case histories 1 & 2, which deal with individuals who were clients of the author.

CASE #1: An individual was doing failing work in college due to an automobile accident which caused a permanent ringing in his ears. He lost two years of school while a spinal fusion of a vertebrae in his neck and other therapies were attempted. He came to me for help with studying since the ringing in his ears was preventing concentration. Hypnotherapy was used and he was again able to read and retain. The semester proved quite successful. As a result of the hypnotherapy, there was a major increase in self-esteem which became evident through normal clinical observations. Yet, given the Brownfain at two month intervals, his test scores went up 15 points, which is an indication of lower self-esteem.

CASE #2: The individual was hypnotized for better academic performance and went from a 3.0 to 4.0 GPA. This was followed by a 3.8 and a 4.0. It was also evident from clinical observation in the second case that self-esteem had increased, yet his Brownfain score when up 20 points, indicating a rather dramatic decrease in self-esteem.

I. *Apperceptive Mass*:
   "You see my dear Watson, but you do not perceive". The apperceptive mass is the stored content of past experiences in the nervous system. Thus, what we perceive is interpreted in terms of the past. For example, an aborigine seeing a 1958 Cadillac for the first time would probably call it a double horned monstrous rhinoceros.
   Perception may be defined as: Stimulus (afferent input interpreted by a central mediating process) = *Response*: Under response we are forced to place a question mark because the response becomes directed by the cultural conditioning of the actor. Even in our culture we will find many psychological variations in terms of the unique experiences of the individual. Perception is not influenced merely by the culture per se but also by the learning experiences unique to the individual and also by the subcultural groups within the total configuration. Thus we have ethnic, religious and class variations among others. Kinsey, in his first book, *Sexual Behavior in the Human Male*, (1948), clearly pointed out some of the major variations that human sexual responses may take in terms of class differences within a single cultural framework. He found a difference in

sexual patterns among the three social classes as well as other cultural variations. For example, a lower class male who has higher educational aspirations
will tend to adapt the sexual patterns of the next social class, unconsciously if
not consciously, while being subjected to the value system of his own class. It
is not sufficient to know the ideational content of the culture to understand
the response patterns; equally important is to understand the subcultural
variations.

Perception is not merely dependent upon the individual actor but rather is
the result of the actor in a specific sociocultural milieu. Phenomenology
develops the method of looking at things by means of "epoche" or leaving out
all things which are not relevant for the study, i.e., viewing a single object,
removed as it were, from all other objects. Perception follows a similar procedure by singling out not merely objects but sense data and then placing an
interpretation upon these data. The organism is constantly bombarded by an
array of stimuli which our sense receptors pick up and transmit to the cortex
for interpretation. The old concept of SOR has been proven quite inadequate
in understanding human behavior since it leaves out the concept of motivation, which is crucial in understanding behavior. Motivation may be briefly
defined as a goal-directed drive. Morgan (1966, p. 204) explains motivation in
the form of a cycle:

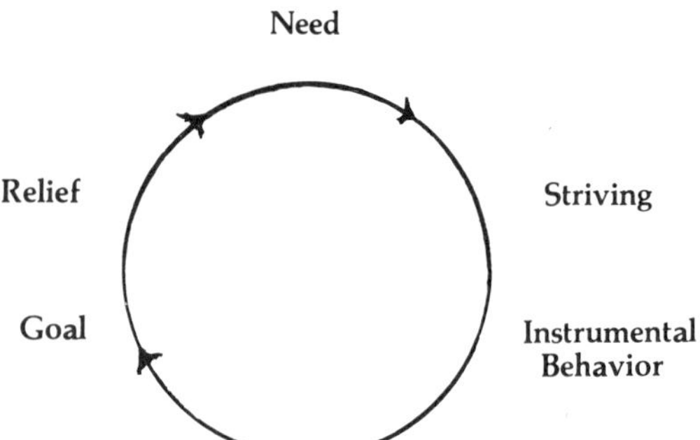

One cannot explain motivation purely on the level of physiologically-derived
needs but must take into account psychogenic or sociogenic needs which are
culturally conditioned. Cross-cultural studies clearly indicate that the specific
psychogenic or sociogenic needs of the individual vary from one culture to
another. Ruth Benedict's (1948) typology of the Appolonian and Dyonesian
groups indicates that particular behavioral patterns of staisfying needs vary in
terms of culture. Although W. I. Thomas's (1951) four basic wishes are probably
universal psychological needs (Response, Recognition, Mastery and Security),
the means of satisfying these basic desires varies from one group to another.

Discussing Mastery, Wallace (1959) suggests that when the Seneca identifies
with one of the masks (representing a legendary figure) and then acts out one of
his infantile roles (modified to conform with the norms and goals) he should
and often does get medical and/or psychological benefit.

Here we see the cathartic effect that the "society of faces" has on the individual by allowing a release of tension and socially acceptable means of venting this without social ostracism. The social change which had taken place in the Iroquois Society by virtue of the impact of the White culture and the reduction of land produced a major change of emphasis in the strategy of the religious psychotherapy. Prior to the cultural invasion (when the culture was an integrated, organized unit), the emphasis had been upon the cathartic aspect, release of tension, of the religious practices. During the succeeding period of dislocation and disorganization there was a shift of emphasis to constriction, repression and control. The former values of bravery, skill at hunting, courage, and self-reliance were no longer realizable under the new socioeconomic structure and placed the individual in a morass of confusion. In view of this, Handsome Lake developed a new philosophy which tended to emphasize values based on self- control, responsibility and order. This view strengthened the superego and constricted the spontaneity of the personality and had a major effect in developing a new organization for the groups.

II. *Ego Strength:*

Ego development is fundamental to all reality orientation and probably for many other functions, as well. Therefore, ego strengh and ego weakness must be viewed in relation to the total maturational stage of ego development. The ego as the executive branch of the personality must produce an effective integration of the id and superego if personality harmony is to prevail. The ego has control over all the cognitive and intellectual functions of personality and comes under the service of the secondary process (realistic thinking). Ego strength goes beyond the relationship of the ego to the id and super ego and includes the ability of the individual to cope with and have mastery over his milieu exterior. A person with a strong ego relates meaningfully to his social milieu. Ego strength may be simply defined, now as a functional reality orientation (an intelligent orientation to life).

For illustrative pruposes, we will focus upon Barron's (1953) ego strength scale as an operational test of ego strength. The scale is composed of 68 items of the MMPI and is designed to prognosticate success in therapy. Working with 33 psychoneurotic patients in an outpatient clinic, Barron (1953) found that the mean of the improved group was 52.7 and of the unemproved group was 29.1—a significant difference beyond the .01 level with a test retest reliability of .72.

The psychological homogeneities in the test as specified by Barron are: (a) physical functioning and physiological stability; (b) psychasthenia and seclusiveness; (c) attitudes towards religion; (d) moral posture; (e) sense of reality; (f) personal adequacy, ability to cope; (g) phobias, infantile anxieties, and (h) miscellaneous.

High scorers among the 40 male graduate students tested by Barron were subjectively judged by staff members of the Institute of Personality Assessment and Research, University of California at Berkeley as conveying "... great resourcefulness, viability and self-direction", or generally an excellence of ego function while low scorers were more "effeminate" and introverted. He further relates ego behavior to intelligent behavior, which follows from the idea of the ego having mastery over the intellectual and cognitive functions of the personality. One inherent difficulty with this line of reasoning is the tendency to then assume that ego strength is somehow related to intelligence. Barron suggests that a scale purporting to measure ego strength should correlate with intelligence, (p. 330). Frank Barron (1953) describes the personality characteristics of ego strength as a sense of reality, physical health and stability, and personal adequacy, liberal morally, and ethnically, spontaneous, outgoing and intelligent.

Within the model we see that ego strength is the relationship of the mental format to the apperceptive mass. This, however, is not self-esteem. An individual may make a good adjustment between the mental format and the apperceptive mass and still have low self-esteem. He may have a degree of spontaneity, a sense of reality, etc. He may be aware of his relationship to his environment, but this does not of necessity imply that he is happy with or that he accepts this reality. A simple way of stating this is that an individual may be aware that others consider him a jerk and be unhappy with it, or he may be aware that others consider him a jerk and not care, or others may compliment him on his intelligence, on his physical attractiveness and yet he may interpret this to mean that they do not really mean this, they are just being nice. Self-esteem is not proportional to an understanding of an individual's relationship to reality. By utilizing Barron's ego strength scale as a measure of ego strength, and Brownfain's self-concept test as a measure of self-esteem, we are able to show empirically that self-esteem and ego strength have a different denotatum. By defining self-esteem as the distance between the self and the mental format, and ego strength the distance between the mental format and the apperceptive mass, we see that the two concepts are related but not coincidental. A person may have good ego strength and good self-esteem, or good ego strength and low self-esteem, but the converse is not true: he will not have poor ego strength because in order to maintain good self-esteem, an individual's concept of reality must be reasonably in line with the true reality of the social situaton vis-a-vis the apperceptive mass. It is clear from the author's counseling (see Figure 2) that many very bright students manifest ego weakness (No. 1, 2 & 5) and that there is generally a strong negative correlation between ego strength and schizophrenia.

Figure 2

	Ego Strength	Schizophrenia[1]	I.Q.[2]	Self-Esteem[3]
1	35	63	130	
2	30	55	128	
3	42	98	130	
4	47	69	128	28
5	38	80	135	
6	46	72	128	
7	56	55	140	55
8	50	52	120	71
9	48	52	140	73

1 and 2 — Schizophrenia and I.Q. source obtained from MMPI and Wais.

Numbers 4, 7, 8 & 9 are examples of good ego strength with self-esteem varying tremendously.

The difficulty with the concept of ego strength, and intellectual and cognitive function is not a theoretical problem but an operational one. We refer to intellectual function as behavior appropriate to the situation (common sense) but our notion of I.Q. measures the individual's abstract intelligence at the expense of an assessment of practicality. I.Q. in this sense is not a measure of concrete functioning, but rather an abstract dimension (see Hallowell, 1955).

III. *Status*:

Sociologists and anthropologists have long been aware of the importance of status to an understanding of human behavior. The full impact of the concept of status has long been overlooked by psychology even though it has been fundamental to Adler's theory of individual development. The simplistic S-R theory of behaviorism clearly overlooks the role of society in shaping the individual. Society's role in developing personality is fully explicated in the sociological literature under the heading of "socialization" and therefore we will not attempt to define the concept in this chapter except insofar as status relates to the socialization process.

Roszak (1975) argues that consciousness is rarely achieved by most people. This aphorism indicates just how much human behavior is a reflection of the culture in which the individual lives. This can be expressed further by stating that each of us lives in his own world, a world constructed by him as a result of his social perceptions and the function of the apperceptive mass. Before continuing, it is probably appropriate to define and discuss status briefly. Status has been defined by Linton (1963) as a position in a particular cultural *pattern*. Status is the position assigned to an individual by the society while his role (the dynamic aspect of status) is the part he plays in reference to the assigned position. This is further delineated by saying that man has both ascribed and achieved status. Ascribed status is a position based on inherent characteristics of "who" a person is and the part described by society whereas achieved status, in an open culture, is based on the accomplishments of the individual. For example, he is born into the status of "lower class" but due to his own accomplishments he achieves the much higher status of "upper class". Status also has a double meaning: in the singular context, we have a status basically due to sex, age, family relationships and class structures. The sum of these individual statuses, is also referred to as status in the sense of class or caste.

In complex modern societies, the list of ascribed and achieved statuses is much broader than that in a primitive culture. We have status in terms of not only sex, age, family and class, but many further subdivisions in these various areas. We are not only males but sons, brothers, students, church members, various secondary group members, etc., and each of these ascribed or achieved statuses requires a role performance in terms of the normative system of the culture, from which variations are frequently classified as deviance. Role performance is further a function of deliberate cognition, innovation, or inadequate performance as a result of sociocultural chem-physio- intellectual inability to perform to society's set standards.

A further complicating factor in modern society is that various statuses are never clearly delineated for the individual but rather are implied through the teachings of the "American Credo" by such institutions as the family, the schools, the churches, and so forth. In this respect, we also find that different institutions do not all provide the same definitions and frequently are even in conflict with each other.

Under the topic heading of institutional variation, Robin Williams (1970) comments that our analogy of the structural fabric of society being similar to the framing of a building are figurative and that norms are not a line but a zone with variations in perception and application. Robin Williams develops a set of criteria for what he calls "patterned evasion" of the normative patterns. In summary, he says the situation is handled by...(a) public affirmation; (b) covert acceptance; and, (c) token punishment (p. 421). One of his examples is prohibition vs. boot legging, while a contemporary case might be society's marijuana laws vs. widespread use by the youth culture.

Another important concept of Williams is what he calls "regularized" evasions of the typical normative patterns which are used as a means of filling the gap between society's norms and behavior.

The important theme of Robin Williams' chapter is that while normative patterns provide the blueprint for role behavior, not all deviance is damaging to the social order. Deviance in the sense of innovation is frequently seen as beneficial to the dynamic development of the culture. Further, under the concept of patterned evasions, we find that while society establishes a normative blueprint on one hand, on the other it provides the patterned evasions for a large segment of the society to follow. These patterned evasions frequently vary further in reference to the social class structure.

Norms are briefly defined as the rules that specify appropriate and inappropriate behavior within the social fabric. Norms can only be understood in terms of goals which are broken down into the cultural and individual level. Merton (1938) in his theory of social structure and anomie discusses the role of the American Credo in establishing goals which are then inculcated into the individual by the social institutions. These goals are then further broken down into a normative pattern for the individual.

Adler's basic proposition that striving for success can be consistent with or against social interest can only be understood in terms of the social concept of status. Status is that social prescription which is the cultural given which provides the cultural patterning from which the institutional goals may be inculcated in the individual. Fundamental then to the development of man as a social animal, society provides both achieved and ascribed statuses. While achieved statuses are of relatively little importance in regard to social adjustment in primitive culture, the more complex and mobile societies place greater emphasis upon achieved status allowing for greater deviance through pattern evasions of the normative system.

IV. *Social Flexibility:*

We find that as we move from a primitive folk culture to a modern urban culture, society becomes more complex and social flexibility becomes important. Modern man is placed in a position of rapid social change and can only maintain his psychic equilibirum by becoming flexible in his interpsychic relationships. (See Toffler, 1970.) Rigidity of thought and action are the earmarks of the neurotic individual.

Social flexibility becomes our third cornerstone in the mental format. Man is a forward moving individual and this movement towards socially useful, and/or attainable goals can only be accomplished in a complex society by remaining flexible. Each social situation is evaluated in terms of the apperceptive mass and is reminiscent of all past social situations but also contains an element of uniqueness. It is this uniqueness which requires flexibility in thought and action. As we have indicated, the need for flexibility has become and is becoming increasingly more important due to the complexity of modern society. In past primitive cultures, a rigidity of thought and action was not undesireable because the number of possible choices of behavior was limited in terms of the normative behaviors prescribed by the group. Such rigidity led to stability and would be tantamount to the personality adjustment in such societies.

Lack of flexibility was responsible for many American male youths being either rejected for military service or being discharged for neuro-psychiatric reasons (see Philip Wylie's concept of Momism," Wylie, 1942). This inability to adapt to an "alien environment" created such adjustment problems that the individual could not fit into the Army environment. We would further suggest that in the framework of our model, the individual would have low self-esteem as a result of this lack of flexibility, since he would see himself as incapable of adapting to new and different situations. The individual with low self-esteem can function in a safe, 'closed' milieu but comes apart when the choices become too great. Future shock (Toffler 1970) then, affects the individual in inverse proportion to the degree of social flexibility which he has integrated into his personality.

V. *Courage*

In developing our model of self-esteem, courage is the idea of facing reality instead of withdrawing from it. We have previously defined the trait of courage as the ability to cope with and perform cultural roles. Our traits of courage and status are intricately linked through roles. A role may be defined simply as the dynamic aspect of status or the part the individual plays in society. These individual roles are defined by society through the definitions of status, through the normative systems of the culture, and further, by the individual through his apperceptive mass.

To understand the apperceptive mass and its relationship to courage we turn to phenomenology. Marvin Farber (1943, p. 215); suggests that while psychology is concerned with the real conditions of the organism (perceptions, judgements, etc.), phenomenology is not interested in this but rather in their prior nature, their essences.

This begins to clarify the importance of the apperceptive mass in understanding human behavior. From the perspective of phenomenology, man responds to his perceptions of the stimulus and not in essence to the stimulus itself. A physical object exists in the real world, but it is our perception, our cognition, of that object which is then reassessed, and it is our judgment which then becomes the real stimulus for behavior. An example might be the fear of snakes which is so evident in western culture. We find that the snake becomes an object of fear, dread, aversion and revulsion, not necessarily by virtue of its physical form, but from the Judeo-Christian tradition in which the snake is identified as an object of evil rather than merely as another creature placed on the earth by God (it becomes identified with the Devil and all that which is considered evil in this religious framework). We clearly see that the snake as an object is not what is feared, but rather the snake as a symbol of evil, the judgment which becomes the basis for this cultural fear. We can give many other examples in which the actual stimulus is not the stimulus for the behavior, but rather in which the interpretation, the apprehension, the judgment, is the stimulus for the response. As W. I. Thomas said, "Situations which are perceived as real are real in their consequences".

In our previous section, we saw the importance of status in understanding behavior. An additional aspect of status crucial to our model can be defined in terms of Brentano's proposition that cognition apprehends the very existence of the general" (Farber, 1943, p. 11). In applying this proposition, we can see that the apprehended status of the individual becomes the basis for the existent (the behavior). In a chapter on "Opinions and Social Pressure" by Solomon E. Asch (1955, p. 324), we find the following: Society requires consensus, the tendency for conformity today is so strong that reasonably intelligent young people are willing to call white black as a matter of course, and the greater the status of the group or the individuals, the greater is the individual's propensity to alter his judgments in line with the perceived judgment of the leader. Status plays two vital roles in affecting behavior: (a) by prescribing the role behavior for the individual; and, (b) through cognition as an existing thing.

Courage, then, plays a very special role as a determiner of personality. The ability to hold to one's convictions in the face of adveristy becomes a very special trait that can be defined as "individuality"—a disposition of personality. This quality becomes an important component of self-esteem. An individual who constantly backs down in adversity, who always gives way to the importance of the status of others, who always conforms to group norms even though he may perceive them as wrong is prone to see himself as of little consequence. When behavior is always determined by judgments which are made in relationship to the perceived status position of other individuals and groups (as with Reisman's [1950] Other-Directed person) rather than in terms of an individual's own perceptions of the situation, he is prone to develop a poor self-concept or poor self-image. Although the group always exerts pressure towards conformity, adversity also allows for "patterned evasion" which take a courage of conviction.

Courage becomes a very special trait in our theory of self-esteem. We see ourselves as having the courage to stand by our convictions or as constantly succumbing to the consensus of the group. This perception itself becomes a function of ego strength. That is, we evaluate our position, an assessment which may be true or false. To the extent that our assessment is "real", we have good ego strength, whereas our self-esteem is contingent upon the balance and strength of the traits.

V. *Social Milieu*:

Merton's theory of anomie postulates disjunctive means-ends scheme (1938). The American Credo is taught by the educational institution and suggests that everyone has equal opportunity for material success. While the success goals are inculcated in the individual, the social structure fails to provide the legitimate means whereby these success goals may be obtained by everyone. This disjunction between means and ends is then postulated as the basis for the emergence of delinquent subcultures where opportunities for attaining the success goals of the American Credo are blocked by a failure of the social structure to provide the legitimate means for their attainment. Although anomie theory provides an explanation for many forms of deviance (e.g., alcoholism, drug addiction and mental disorders), it fails to provide for many other forms: statutory rape, common law marriage, marijuana use, violence of running amuck, gambling). Anomie theory, however, is of importance in our concept of self-esteem. From a sociological perspective we would postulate that expectation over aspirations equal self-esteem. To further delineate, if we call aspirations goals and expectations means, we can then fit this into the anomie typology. On an empirical level, we find that where the greatest discrepancies exist between aspirations and expectations, and we find the greatest amount of delinquency. James F. Short (1964) states that boys who perceive closed educational opportunities have the highest delinquency rates. Adler discusses the low self-esteem which results from the setting of goals above any possibility of attainment, or to use his phraseology, "god-like" goals. This directly fits the anomie typology (high goals but low perceived means) and is reflected in Short's statement, in that the highest rates of delinquency are found among those individuals who perceive the means "the educational opportunities" as being closed, which is seen as a discrepancy between the means and ends. These "god-like" goals are not only a result of the primary group socialization process, but a function of the social milieu (mass media).

Education becomes a means for the attainment of success goals, and consequently, those individuals who perceive educational opportunity as blocked further perceive the means as blocked as well. The disjunction between the aspirations and expectations (the means-ends) is clear: individuals aspire to success but expect failure, and this process effectively lowers self-esteem. Society, through the educational institution, the communication media, etc., has inculcated the success goals into many of its members. The chance of achieving these goals, however, are then not equally offered to all. Low self-esteem then, according to Adler, becomes a protective mechanism by which the individual resorts to such compensatory maneuvers as suicide, delinquency, sexual deviance, etc., all as a means of protecting his fragile self-esteem. This is particularly true of the lower class segment of the population in the American culture.

If we continue teaching the American Credo in a society which is moving towards a rigid caste system based upon intelligence, we will be fostering a society in which low self-esteem will become prevalent among a very large segment of a total population, specifically the lower class. Low self-esteem will then be a direct result of the discrepancy between aspirations and expectations in a theoretically mobile class society.

Another area in which low self-esteem becomes a direct function of a discrepancy between aspirations and expectations is a segment of the upper-middle class society. In this particular social class, it is not the social structure in the form of inequality which creates low self-esteem but rather the socialization process of the primary group. In middle class society, the family puts direct pressure upon their children to succeed and along with the internalization of success goals through the socialization process, they also provide the means of education by sending their kids to college. Thus, it would seem in a subculture where the goals are internalized and the means are provided, high self-esteem would normally be the end product. This is not necessarily the case however. The offspring are frequently placed in a position where they cannot hope to achieve the expected levels of success and consequently the goals become again "god-like" in perspective. This is particularly true among the upper-middle class Jewish youth where many of the fathers had moved from a relatively lower class status to a much higher class as a result of the mass mobility of post WW II. Many of the parents went to college for the first time through the GI Bill and as a result of a real striving had achieved a great deal of success in terms of the normative prescriptions. Their children, unable to duplicate this mobility, develop low self-esteem. As a result of this, we find drug abuse a common form of deviance within this segment of the college youth population.·

VII. *Self-Acceptance*:

The literature rarely discusses self-acceptance in relation to self-esteem, but it is our contention that self-acceptance is vitally important as a component part of true self-esteem. The dynamics of self-acceptance became evident through a clinical case history. John had a very low self-esteem which was manifested in his obsessive-compulsive behavior, his constant striving to be number one, and his free-floating anxiety. He is a tall, handsome young man with a very high intelligence. His performance in college was always within a 3.8/4.0 GPA although he never gained any real satisfaction from his success. As a result of a hypnotic procedure designed to develop self-esteem, we were able to raise this dimension greatly. Interestingly, his perceptions of his self-image did not change greatly; he did not suddenly change his self-image from feeling as though he were unattractive to now feeling that he was handsome. The change, which was readily observable to his firends and acquaintances, was an acceptance of himself. In his own words, he was able to describe it in this fashion:

> Q: How do you feel about yourself now?
> A: It doesn't really matter . . . laugh . . . it is just kind of stupid . . . when I used to think about self-esteem, I thought it was really feeling good about yourself . . . liking yourself. Now when I think about it...it's dumb to have to either like yourself or dislike yourself...because you just are anyway...whether you like it or not. I just feel much more sensible. I used to picture people who really liked themselves as getting the biggest kick out of feeling better than someone else.

That is what I associated self-esteem with. You cannot really feel better than someone else. Now I don't feel less or better than someone else. When I used to get good grades, I would feel good because I did better. Or looking at my physical appearance and always thought it was much worse than everyone around me. If I happened to come upon some poor leper, I would feel better, but that doesn't matter anymore. I never really thought of it in this way . . . you don't have to feel better in order to feel good.

This clearly demonstrates the concept of self-acceptance. Now John is able to accept himself in relationship to his social milieu. His acceptance is not, as was stated, based on his self-image (as being good or bad) or his self concept (how he feels about himself) but rather, is in relationship to his being able to accept himself among his peers without having to make any evaluative judgment.

This is further brought out by another individual in which the Brownfain was used in a pre-and-post test fashion. A pretest score of 42 was obtained at the beginning of the therapeutic process. Although the client and the therapist agreed subjectively that the individual had developed a much better self-esteem the post-test score on the Brownfain was 52, an increase of 10 points showing a rather significant decrease in self-esteem. This raises the question of why the objective measure shows one thing whereas the subjective evaluation by the individual and the therapist indicate an entirely different change. Some discrepancies in the scores between the items changed in both directions; on some items the individual saw himself as being higher; on other items he saw himself as lower than he did on the first test. On such items as social poise, sportsmanship, flexibility, etc., he was able to handle the discrepancy between how he sees himself and how he thinks others see him, whereas in the past, this was source of consternation, i.e., before he would be concerned about the fact that others might not see him as poised as he would like to be, whereas now, as we stated in terms of the first case history, it doesn't really matter. He is able to accept himself.

VIII. *Goals*:

All behavior becomes the function of a complex set of motives, a motive being a goal-directed drive. Hans Selye has been *reported as having said* the malaise of our culture is purposelessness or, more explicitly, that many people lack a goal orientation. Alfred Adler has proposed that the basic striving for success goes with social interest. Success striving which is in line with social interest leads to adjustment whereas success striving which is against social interests leads to maladjustment. Unfortunately, from the point of view of maladjusted individuals who lack social interest, the achievement or attainment of a goal for personal enhancement is by far more important than keeping in line with the social norms. Such individuals often do not consider the social repercussions which may develop as a consequence of their form of striving for success. In summary, all forms of deviance are nothing more than individual efforts for enhancement.

The individual cannot exist in isolation but always exists in the framework of a social milieu and his success striving takes place within the framework of a given social structure, affected by the *Volkgeist* and *Zeitgeist*. This success striving can also be conceptualized as goal orientation. Adler has indicated that a common form of neurosis exists by virtue of goal orientations which may become "god-like" as the result of a familial emphasis upon success. In such a situation, it is impossible for the individual to ever obtain these goals, since they are unattainable by definition. When goals become unattainable, we see a diminution in self-esteem because the individual can never feel truly good about himself. He is never capable of attaining anything worthwhile in terms of his own perceptions. As we have said the basic striving for success goes with or against social interest and it is in the framework of this social interest that the individual develops high or low self-esteem. Returning to our model, we then find that we have a mental format functioning in a *fluid* state within the framework of a given social structure. However, when the goal orientation of the individual is blocked or to the extent that he perceives this blocking, as a result of his particular apperceptive mass, the individual may develop maladjusted techniques for goal attainment, s/he may seek out deviant means to achieve his goals.

IX. *Self-esteem*:

   C. I. Lewis (1946) comments that knowledge ameliorates experience by guiding behavior, and it is precisely this action which the individual is pursuing. All action is goal oriented; he pursues goals which he perceives as bringing satisfaction (self-esteem) and these goals are culturally inculcated through the socialization process. In light of our model, there are various behavior orientations which may lead to deviance or normative behavior. Normative behavior successfully* pursued leads to high self-esteem whereas normative behavior unsuccessfully pursued leads to low self-esteem. Our theory posits the premise that low self-esteem leads to deviance and that the type of deviance is the result of the individuals orientation toward action which is determined by the social milieu.

Function

   Self-esteem involves a totality of the individual's perceptions of himself; consequently, it includes self image (physical), self concept (mental), and social concept (cultural). In the framework of our model it is composed of status, courage, flexibility, ego, ego-strength and self acceptance—the action taking place within the social milieu.

   In order to understand the model we need to see how it functions. We will begin with the Mental Format, and discuss the concepts in terms of their function. The ego (the self, the I, the consciousness) is the core of the triangle, not the zenith of the pyramid as in the Freudian model. In our model, it is concomitant with consciousness since self- esteem can only exist in a state of awareness. In essence, this is a *given* and the ego as normally perceived is a result of the function of the other factors. The points of the triangle (status, courage and flexibility) are situational; status is one of the prime motivators of the organism. Status initiates action and the product is then evaluated; perceived

---

   * Successfully here refers to the individuals evaluation of his own behavior, thus the individual with 'god-like' goals may be seen as successful by his contemporaries but unsuccessfully by himself.

low status will tend to reduce self-esteem.

Status may be perceived in terms of two social milieus — the milieu of the immediate social environment (the peer group) and the cultural milieu. The gang delinquent may well have status within his group and yet lack all the symbolic trapping of having status in a broader cultural sense. Here we have the individual operating under two umbrellas — the umbrella of the peer group where he achieves status in the group (W.F. Whyte's, Street Corner Gang) and status in terms of the broader society (J.P. Getty). Most of us strive for a balance between these two crucial areas of status achievement; however, it is possible to have high status in one area and not another. If the individual perceives status within one area as being sufficient, then his self-esteem may be high, as in the case of the delinquent with high self-esteem and no social interest; in this case he would have high status in only one area.

Courage, a psychological disposition, also results from social participation and develops through the socialization process; when we fail to have the courage of our conviction we lower our self-esteem.

Flexibility is that psychic dimension of being able to change. A healthy personality is one which is able to change. The opposite of flexibility is rigidity and a person who is rigid cannot feel good about himself because he is a threatened individual.

In our triangle the distance between points A-B-C are also vital and this is determined by the relative strength of the components, i.e., if status is low it reduces the distance and changes the shape of the triangle directly affecting the ego function.

Ego-strength is the reality orientation of the actor and is determined by the apperceptive mass and the mental format and is seen as the distance between these two points. If the individual's perceptions of himself are similar to those of his significant others then he has good ego-strength. This is similar to Cooley's "looking-glass self" and depends upon our ability to interpretate accurately the behavior of others. In our model good ego-strength is essential for good self-esteem, a necessary but not a sufficient cause.

The mental format is always moving forward; man can only go forward, he can never go back. He may mentally live in the past (regression), but he can never go back into the past. When the mental format moves to the left we reduce self-esteem; the more god-like or useless the goals, the less the self-esteem and this movement also distorts the shape of the triangle. The direction of movement is still forward but lagging behind the axis. When the axis is perpendicular, the goals are perceived as useful and attainable.

Now the distance between the mental format and the organism is seen as self-acceptance and this distance is affected by the structure of the mental format and is further affected by what we might call a transcendence of the ego, a spiritual reality. We have seen people coming from an adverse environment, with 'broken' bodies, who have an inner strength which allows them to transcend the material and to accept themselves while others with lower self-esteem cannot. Crucial to good self-esteem is self-acceptance. This distance is also a balancing agent and helps give stability to the format. For some individuals status may never be very high as a result of an adverse environment and flexibility may be low because of lack of an opportunity for education or training yet, these individuals are able to sustain their self-esteem — they maintain their self acceptance. This is a true transcendence, not the Freudian Pollyana but the ability to look at material life as only one dimension of a total reality, situational and spiritual.

Tension and stress as perceived by the individual also directly affect the shape and function of the mental format. Any feeling of inadequacy at any point in our model will be perceived as stressful and have an inordinate effect upon our self-esteem. Social stress may well result when our status, courage or flexibility are threatened and result in low self-esteem. An individual who, because of age, experience, etc., is boxed into an occupational slot will feel threatened and have a resultant decrease in self-esteem. A second occupational choice in modern society is an insurance policy for flexibility and good self-esteem. A similar case can be established for status and courage. Self-esteem now is a result of the mental format (shape and structure), ego strength, slope of the axis and self acceptance.

For illustrative purposes we shall translate the paradigm into a mathematical model as follows: $A + B + C + D = E$

A = 20% ego-strength
B = 30% mental format (status, courage, flexibility)
C = 20% slope of the axis
D = 30% self acceptance
E = self-esteem

It is clear that the assigned values are relative and that they will vary from individual to individual and be affected by the social milieu.

In Merton's Paradigm, success is translated into monetary gain within the American Credo where success = \$; the underlying assumption is that the individual has been successfully acculturated. If, for whatever reason, a different value system has been internalized the individual may be able to develop good self-esteem outside the system. This is a case in point in which the individual has good self-esteem but little or no social interest, *Gemeinshaftsgefuhl* (community feeling) or, in the broader sense, Adler's social interest. Here we have a situation in which we can have deviant behavior and good self-esteem — a delinquent.

Self-esteem provides the basic motivation for the organism. It is not the sex drive, the libido, as Freud throught, but rather, sex is used to sustain self-esteem. In this model the function of the format is a dialectical process whereby the individual needs to reconcile opposing forces. High or Low status, high or low courage and flexibility vs. rigidity are not dichotomies but opposing forces to be worked out and integrated into the individual's personality. The striving for self-esteem is a true dialectical process and therapy should focus upon helping the individual to come to grips with these oppositions. An understanding of the past is not essential to, and may actually be detrimental to, good therapy.

References

Asch, S. E., Opinions and Social Pressure. *Scientific American*, 1955, 193 (5) pp. 31-35.

Barron, F., An Ego-strength Scale Which Predicts Response To Psychotherapy. *Journal of Consulting Psychology* XVIII:5, October, 1955, pp. 327-333.

Benedict, Ruth, *Patterns of Culture* New York: The New American Library, 1948.

Farber, Marvin, *The Foundation of Phenomenology*; Edmund Husserl and *The Great Quest for a Rigorous Science of Philosophy*. Cambridge, Massachusetts: Harvard University Press, 1943.

Gittler, Joseph B., *Social Dynamics: Principles & Cases in Introductory Sociology*. New York: McGraw-Hill, 1952.

Hallowell, A. I., Some Psychological Characteristics of the Northeastern Indians in *Culture and Experience*, Philadelphia: University of Pennsylvania Press, 1955.

James, W., *Habit*. New York: Henry Holt and Company, 1890.

Kinsey, A. C., Pomeroy, W. B., and Martin, C. E., *Sexual Behavior in The Human Male*. Philadelphia: W. B. Saunders Company, 1948.

Lewis, Clarence Irving, *An Analysis of Knowledge and Valuation*; LaSalle, Illinois: Open Court Publishing Company, 1946.

Liebow, E., *Tally's Corner*. Boston, Toronto: Little Brown and Company, 1967.

Linton, Ralph, *Acculturation in Seven American Indian Tribes*. Glouchester, Massachusetts: P. Smith, 1963.

Maslow, A. H., *Self-actualizing People: A Study of Psychological Health*. Brooklyn, New York: Brooklyn College Book Store, 1951. Reprinted from Personality Symposium, No. 1, 1950, W. Wolff, ed., published by Grune and Stratton.

Merton, R. K., *Social Structure and Anomie*, reprinted from the American Sociological Review, Vol. III, No. 5, October, 1938."

Morgan, Clifford Thomas, *Introduction to Psychology, 3rd ed.* New York: McGraw-Hill, 1966.

Reisman, D., *The Lonely Crowd*. New Haven, Connecticut, Yale University Press, 1950.

Robinson, J. P. and Shaver, P. R., *Measures of Social Psychological Attitudes*. Ann Arbor, Michigan, Institute for Social Research, 1969.

Rogers, C., *On Becoming a Person: A Therapist's View of Psychotherapy*. Boston: Houghton Mifflin, 1961.

Roszak, T., *The Unfinished Animal*. New York: Harper Colophon Books, 1975.

Shaver, P. R., *Measures of Occupational Attitudes and Occupational Characteristics*. Ann Arbor, Michigan, Institute for Social Research, 1969.

Short, James, F., and Henry, A. F., *Suicide and Homocide*. New York: Free Press of Glencoe, 1964.

Thomas, W. I., *Social Behavior and Personality: Contributions of W. I. Thomas to Theory and Social Research*. Ed. by E. H. Volkart. New York: Social Research Council, 1951.

Toffler, A., *Future Shock*. New York: Random House and Company, 1970.
Wallace, Anthony, F. C., Cultural Determinants of Response to Hallucinatory Experience. *AMA Arch. Gen. Psychiatry*, 1959, July 1, pp. 58-69.
Williams, Robin M., *American Society: A Socialogical Interpretation*. 3rd ed., New York: Alfred A. Knopf, 1970.
Wylie, P., *Generation of Vipers*. New York: Farrar Publishing Company, 1942.
Wylie, R. C., *The Self-concept; A Critical Survey of Pertinent Research Literature*. Lincoln: University of Nebraska Press, 1961-1968.

R. A. Steffenhagen Ph.D
Department of Sociology
University of Vermont

6

SELF-ESTEEM AND STRUCTURE:
HOW DOES SELF-ESTEEM DEVELOP?

This chapter examines the importance of structure in the development of self-esteem. Self-esteem is defined as "the totality of the individual's perceptions of self, his self-concept (mental), self-image (physical), and social concept (cultural)." These perceptions develop only in a social milieu. We sometimes think of nature as a structure of evolving processes; so we may think of self-esteem as an ongoing process unique to each individual, which takes place in an *Uwelten*, (a milieu). Opler (1956) suggested that phenomenology has shown us that the differences in the meanings attributed to symbols within the symbolic processes among human groups suggests that the differences between personality and environment are artificial abstractions. For the individual, psychical phenomena exist intentionally and actually, whereas physical phenomena exist intentionally and merely phenomenally; our emotions are much more real and existent than a tree a mile away. Our self-esteem emerges out of our perceptions and it is this reality which becomes the basis for conscious behavior.

The thesis being presented here is that structure, personal and social, is important for building self-esteem and that self-esteem develops situationally (socially) and spiritually (transpersonally). This can be shown with the following diagram:

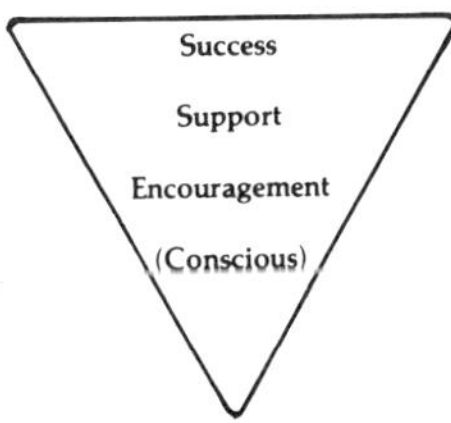

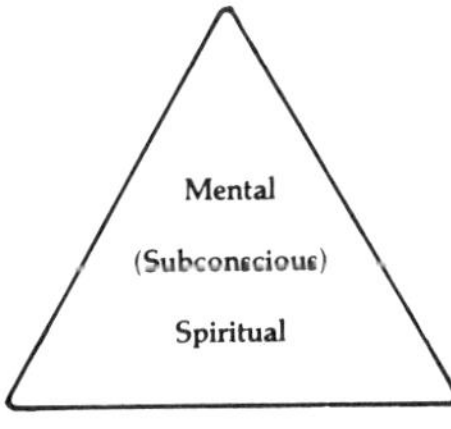

Structure means to organize, to provide a guiding principle for the individual to follow. The concept of structure in education has been a source of debate in recent years: when we provide structure do we curtail spontaneity? Dr. Spock suggested we provide as 'free' an environment as possible for the individual to grow up in so s/he is as free as possible to develop creativity.

We shall look at structure in the personality from the perspective of norms, values, freedom and responsibility, socialization, roles, symbolism and cultural heroes and further examine how the family, school and society are responsible for developing self-esteem.

Norms and Values

Norms are society's prescriptions for social action, they are the standards which describe the course an action should take. Weber (1947) defines action as all human behavior which the actor attaches a subjective meaning to, and which is social by virtue of this subjective meaning and that it takes into account the behavior of others.

How is behavior oriented toward social action? The norms provide the standard or the guide for the action to be social since the norms are derived from society's values, those objects, ideas, and actions which are defined as desirable or preferable. Robin Williams (1970) comments that social action is always oriented towards specific social situations (Time & Place), oriented by interests, values, etc. Norms then become the *Leitlinie* (guiding line) for group action and for individual action.

In order for these norms and values to become of value to the individual, for the development as a *Leitlinie*, for social actions of the individual, they must be meaningfully integrated and this integration we shall refer to as structure. Structure, or order, must first be superimposed from without by the parent or parent surrogate, societies, norms, and values. To provide a common reference point let's call this structure the Freudian 'superego' which represents the morals of society. The function of the superego is to inhibit the id impulse, and the substituting of moral goals for immediate goals and the striving for perfection. What this involves is the need for the personality to internalize the norms and values of the society (the morals) into a structure which gives satisfaction vis-a-vis the ego, the secondary process. Societal norms and values then become the raw material from which the individual develops his own system which is in keeping with the idea of individual psychology with the idea of unlimited *Unwelten*.

Society needs a *Leitlinie* but does not need common rules and regulations for everything. The more complex the society the more variations may be allowed without threatening the system. The primary group provides the more clearly defined standards while the secondary group provides more variation. Institutions, at times, may actually be in conflict with each other with respect to value systems, e.g., the role of the conscientious objector (wartime). Society may actually provide for patterned evasions. Opler (1959) quoted Frank as saying the real patient is society and Fromm as saying that patterned defects are as common in culture as in the individual. While the Freudian system allows for these patterned defects (the superego), it has tended to ignore the 'Unwelten' in favor of the individual deviations.

Freedom and Responsibility

It would appear that the more complex the society, the more room there is for varying behavior. At first blush this would seem desirable, as it would broaden the range of behavior which could be acceptable and reduce the range of deviance. Pushed too far, all behavior becomes permissible (deviance becomes the norm) and anomie ensues. While freedom is a much cherished value in modern American democratic society, the meaning is less clear. We are free as long as we don't impose on the rights of others. Also, with freedom comes responsibility for our actions. The social structure, through norms and values, gives us the internal structure to make these responsible decisions. Culture teaches us how to perceive reality, see LeShan (1976). Freedom means responsibility to vote and in order to vote we have the responsibility to know our candidates so our decisions will be rational and meaningful.

When we study the psycho-socio-political-historic-cultural context of the rise of Nazism, we see that in the perceptions of the symbol "卐" freedom was a basic issue in the development of Nazism. Culture depends on man's ability to symbolize, to give abstract meaning to signs, and to have signs function as symbols. After the crucifixion of Christ the ⋈ became the symbol used to identify an ideology for the initiates. This sign became an abstraction so powerful that men were willing to die for it, so that they might live. What does this mean in terms of freedom? It means that freedom to Christians meant a spiritual freedom. Social and physical freedom bought at the price of renouncing their beliefs was bondage. Not only does this cultural structure become a reality for the individual but, in the Hegelian context, culture is capable of developing its own anthesis (deviance) which restructures reality. In our example, the early Christians were deviants; Christianity was a cult, equally as defiant as the Moonies, Children of God, Divine Light Mission, Scientology, etc. A society which provides political and religious freedom must of necessity provide the foundation for its destruction, i.e., it must allow for deviant ideologies to emerge and offer them freedom of expression. Our culture provides freedom for its members to join these cults; however, many of these cults express true totalitarian views and do not allow their members freedom of belief, but express rigid dogmas. Now we can begin to see why the Nazi movement had such an appeal for the Germans. Most important, the German culture was a strong patriarchy, the father's word was law and similarly the Kaiser's word was law. Then the Weimar Republic came into being and people were supposed to accept responsibility for their government. They had freedom at the price of responsibility. They were not acculturated to accept this responsibility and easily gave up political freedom for the freedom from responsibility. It should be apparent by now that what we are postulating is that for any uniformity of behavior to occur, we need to have a structure which provides a framework, a pattern within which the individual can operate. This social structure then provides the basis for the development of a social science based upon the predictability of behavior. So far, we have looked upon this from a socio-dynamic perspective and now need to translate this into a psychodynamic perspective.

Socialization

We have pointed out that the child is acculturated into his society vis-a-vis the socialization process and that this process is accomplished within the primary group. The cultural norms and values are inculcated into the individual through this process and internalized by him into his own philosophy. These values make up Freud's superego, the super structure. What we are really concerned with is the ego function where the impulses of the id, the primary process, are satisfied within a world of objective reality. The ego is the reality principle, the secondary process, so that id impulses are satisfied with the framework of the superego — the culture. The individual has to create a structure to organize the norms and values of society into his own *Weltansicht* which provides the *Leitlinie* for his behavior. This is first superimposed from without and then later may be imposed from within. It is this latter process which gives us the *Unwelten*; the superstructure is provided by society, the substructure by the function of the apperceptive mass.

"Man is his Choices," is a proposition in keeping with modern existentialism; the greater the cultural alternatives, the greater the variability of behavior. Gustov Ichheiser (1970) has pointed out that the value of prejudice is manifested through ethnicity. The belief in the superiority of one's own group is a positive value and helps one to structure his reality in a meaningful fashion. One's reality is cultural bound, and ethnic beliefs (nationalism) help give order to our existence and provide a map of reality. Science provides us with another map of reality based upon other premises and in a sense transcends the ethnic map which is superceded by a still more abstract map based upon religious ideals. Cultural relativity has been helpful in reducing prejudices but at the same time, while it has reduced rigidity and increased flexibility, it has also increased the number of choices. An increase in choices results in an increase in the number of decisions one has to make; the inability to make decisions is, without equivocation, the mark of the neurotic in our culture. Decisions can only be made by having guide posts, maps, which generally are derived from the norms and values of society.

How values are transmitted may be as important as the values themselves and at times what is internalized may be the direct antithesis of the value held. Bateson & Mead (1942) argue that what we learn is conditioned by the method of learning as well as the content. In his article, "World View and Self-view of the Kaska Indians," Honigmann (1949) shows how the world view of experience as manageable and life as threatening, is offset by the personal ethos of self-reliance and helplessness and how these views are the result of the socialization process. He subdivides these into infant care, emotional rejection, parental attitudes and authority, identifications and activities of later childhood. Here we see how one set of values is communicated and how another set is developed through the socialization process.

These dichotomies are seen in our culture when the child is told that honesty is the best policy and also sees his father engaging in income tax evasions (legitimate or illegitimate). Similarly, injunctions against drinking may be followed by weekend cocktail parties, etc. We find that these conflicts in values are the most flagrant examples, but more subtle examples exist. Teachers may present one set of values explicitly, and another implicitly. In therapy, it is becoming increasingly evident that there is no such thing as value-free therapy and that the values of the therapist are picked up by the client, which further supports our contention that personal values are transmitted overtly or covertly.

Modern man in the Western World has developed a concept of reality based upon science which gives us a narrow sense of reality since it is confined to the physical world. A reality based on the physical world, (a sensory mode of being) is very limited, deriving from the senses, and postulates that only stimuli which can be sensed are real. The suggestion is that everything which is experienced is on a time-space continuum and can be measured. A value system based upon scientific principles is a pragmatic system and can only determine what works or doesn't work; it can never deal with good or evil, right or wrong, etc.; it can never truly deal with 'truths' but is grounded in probability. We have postulated that values are essential to the individual for creating his maps for social action. However, the maps may become loose and indefinite because there are no eternal truths to act as a *Leitlinie* for actions; rather, actions must be evaluated in terms of their own time-space continuum. Freedom and individuality can be as much a bane to existence for modern man as it has been deemed a virtue. LeShan (1976) refers to four modes of being: the sensory, the clairvoyant, the transpersonal, and the mystic. The sensory mode provides techniques; the clairvoyant mode gives meaning; the transpersonal provides guidelines; and the mystic provides a psychological adrenalin, a spiritual meaning. Ellsworth Faris, in *Nature of Human Nature*, comments on the fact that we become human in terms of self and it is the self which is responsible for building self-esteem. Crucial to our perceptions of our self is the apperceptive mass.

Roles

A further aspect of structure in the school and family is the crucial component of the role model. During the socialization process the neophyte needs a role model to provide guidance (structure) for the development of the personality. In the Freudian model the ego ideal, as a subdivision of the superego, is often underevaluated by psychologists while being emphasized by sociologists, who rarely use the term "ego-ideal" but rather refer to the role model. Certainly, 'the conscience,' the evaluation of behavior in terms of the norms and values, is probably most often examined because when deviance is viewed in terms of a departure from the norms, it is the most observable and definable. It becomes the basis for psychiatric and psychological decisions of normalcy or abnormalcy. More important than the conscience is the function of a role model (ego ideal), since the actor's decisions to conform to, or ignore, the norms are frequently made on the basis of evaluation and interpretation of a model's decision. Sutherland's (1947) differential association speaks directly to this issue. We are not building a case for the function of the role model but rather mean to set the stage for how the role model affects the self-esteem of the individual.

The role model provides a structure for the individual to emulate; when he behaves in the manner in which he believes his role model would, he pats himself on the back and when he doesn't, he feels guilt. The conscience — this ego ideal (role model) — also sets the stage for the conscience part of the superego.

Erik Erikson, among others, has emphasized the fact that the male child in modern Western culture lacks a role model within the family. The father is away from home such a large part of the time that social interaction is greatly reduced; television further reduces this time period. In America, the situation is worse in that the grammar school teacher is most often female. The attributes which define manliness must then be obtained from the peer group, where the same confusion prevails. Shevin (1978) cited the fact that on an average a middle class father has less than a 2 minute interaction with his infant children per day. He further suggests that probably more interaction takes place between the father and the T.V. set than between father and child. Does one then wonder why Philip Wylie discusses the role of "Momism" as a serious problem in American society?

We need to further consider the role of the conscience and ego ideal in the development of the superego and the interrelationship between these two components. It is clear that the conscience must develop or the child would remain a little "id" running around the house—a situation most intolerable to the most permissive of parents. He must be reasonably socialized if the family is to survive. According to Cooley (1956), it is within the contact of the primary group that the child becomes socialized and humanized. The primary group is characterized by intimate face-to-face association and cooperation. Further, the primary group is characterized by the highest degree of ego involvement, thus it is within this group that the individual receives his humanness.

Symbolism and Cultural Heroes

The conscience, the negative prescriptions, is largely on the verbal plane of interaction. Man's most notable feature which differentiates him from the animals is his ability to symbolize, to interact on the symbolic level of action. If mother says "No, that's naughty," the child then feels he is naughty because he has been told so; he feels guilty because he hasn't lived up to the expectation of his significant others as superimposed upon him vis-a-vis the values and norms. These values and norms are explicitly impressed upon him through the use of symbols. The use of symbols is what distinguishes man from animal, a distinction well made by Ernst Cassirer in his *Essay on Man* (1944). Cassirer felt that as symbolism increases, the distance of man from his physical reality decreases. Symbolism is the basis for the development of the superego— the ego ideal—and the conscience; and the conscience can only exist by the virtue of symbols.

An important component of this ego ideal is the cultural hero—or cultural figure—who, in myth or actuality, stands for those values most prescribed by the culture—in Judeo-Christian tradition, Jesus Christ; in early mid-20th century America, the American Cowboy; the white uniform and white horse standing for good (*The Lone Ranger Rides Again*). What we have here is a situation in which the cultural hero reinforces implicitly, through his action, the values explicitly conveyed through the verbal symbols of the values and norms of the culture. Ernest Becker (1962) suggests that the appeal of Nietzsche and Emerson is largely due to the fact that they saw heroism as essential to man. He felt that one of the reasons why modern youth opt out of the system is because we have failed to offer the possibility of real heroism. He further expressed the notion that culture breaks down when it fails to offer "meaningful hero-systems." These meaningful heroes present and reinforce, implicitly and explicitly, the values and norms which provide man with his *Leitlinie* for action. Becker feels that modern day theorists are increasingly aware of the role of self-esteem as an etiological factor in the development of disease.

We must understand that self-esteem is vital to the personality. We have indicated that guilt is the negative and that the ego-ideal (the cultural hero) is the positive component of the superego — "a true dialectical process." If, as Becker suggests, we are losing our cultural heroes; if, as Wylie and Erickson say, we are lacking in male role models during the socialization process, we are creating a situation in which building self-esteem into today's culture is becoming eminently more difficult. The dialectic process of the superego is crucial to building good self-esteem. What we are creating is a situation in which we are inculcating the norms and values into the youth only through explicit verbalizations. We are not balancing the conscience (the negative) with the cultural heroes (the positive). This produces a situation in which the building of good self-esteem becomes more and more difficult. Max Scheler (1928) says:

> "In no other period of human knowledge, has man ever become more problematic to himself than in our own days . . . We no longer possess any clear and consistent idea of man."

Cultural heroes play an important part in building this consistent idea of man; cultural heroes are role models on a higher level of abstraction. The cultural heroes are positive and help us balance the negative in a true dialectic fashion. No one would deny the negativism of our modern culture, the mass media seems to emanate from a negative bias, with individual negativism feeding into group negativism. This lack of balance in the superego is another manifestation of a lack of an integrating structure in the personality and constitutes a further manifestation of the lack of Alder's *Leitlinie*.

Ego

The ego (the administrator of the personality, secondary process, or rational component) is meant to maintain a balance between the id and superego. This balance is another example of the dialectic nature of the personality. The id is the basic energy, the pleasure principle which is balanced by the superego the cultural prescriptions. Ruth Cavan (1975) in discussing different delinquency types among social classes, distinguished between the id-operated delinquent, the lower class delinquent, and the middle class delinquent. The lower class delinquent is governed by the pleasure principle. He is concerned with immediate pleasures, resents cultural authority (police, teachers, etc.), but does not resent his parents who he feels are also at the mercy of structured society. The middle class delinquent, governed by an abundance of superego, lives in a straight jacket of negative prescriptions laid down for him by his parents, i.e., their interpretations of society's values. Because of all the "nos", the adolescent feels unable to express himself in a self-actualized manner and when he rebels, it is not against society, but rather against his parents, whom he sees as the jailors. Here we have examples of an incomplete dialectic. These are examples of how a system with too much or too little internal or external system can effect self-esteem. The M-C delinquent would be the case of too much internal structure, further complicated by the incomplete dialectic of the superego. Too much internal structure can, then, be as bad as too little in effecting the development of good self-esteem. In the former case of the L-C delinquent, we have a more complicated situation. The incomplete dialectic in this instance is a necessary condition but not a sufficient cause for delinquency. As a result of the lack of structure (external), the adolescent may develop low self-esteem resulting in delinquency. We can also have a case of delinquency in which the delinquency, as a behavioral mechanism, can itself bring about self-esteem, e.g., by creating a peer group support system. This would be a case in which the individual is able to develop a functional self-esteem, through the group structure but with a lack of social interest.

Phenomenology and Conclusion

We have discussed the role of the individual's philosophy as a unifying personal philosophy of life, a philosophical underpinning which provides meaning and structure for the individual. We have quoted Scheler as saying modern man lacks a clear and concise idea of himself, a well-structured Weltansicht. In the age of reason, science has replaced religion in providing a superstructure and we have replaced a transcendental reality with a physical reality. Karl Marx says religion is the opiate of the people; he has, in his own inimical way, replaced religion with science and then deified science. It is interesting that the very nature of symbolism is to transcend the physical. Animal is a sign being with a 1:1 relationship (concrete reality) whereas man is a symbolic being with a 1:infinity relationship and so losing contact with physical reality. Religion, art, myth, and language are as much parts of our reality as are physical artifacts; they are the threads which weave the web of human existence. The apperceptive mass even changes the nature of the physical universe. Cassirer (1944, p. 43) argues, that as symbolic content increases the effect of physical reality decreases.

The advances in science tend to move us away from the spiritual, yet these advances (these increases in symbolism) tend to take us beyond the physical into the abstract. The more we move into the abstract, the more we move beyond the immediacy of the physical reality, which becomes a negation of the very reality posited. In essence, Hegel freed history from mysticism and 'throw out the baby with the bath water' as Ichheiser would say. For Hegel, every phenomenon has an opposite, the opposing entities making up a dialectic. The dialectical method is itself a method which transcends the physical, goes beyond science. The phenomenological method, in like fashion, also goes beyond science. Farber presents the idea that the real content (subject matter) of phenomenology are those judgements perceptions, feelings, etc., which transcent the material world, their essences, their a priori nature. What we have attempted to do here is to show how both the dialectical movement and phenomenological movement are both involved in a broader judgment of reality, a transcendent reality, and how, in this reality, the nature of man, the inner essence, is being distorted. This is Scheler's notion of the plight of modern man: an emphasis upon the physical at the *exclusion* of the spiritual.

Theodore Roszak in *Unfinished Animal* (1975), speaks to this same issue. He illustrates it as follows:

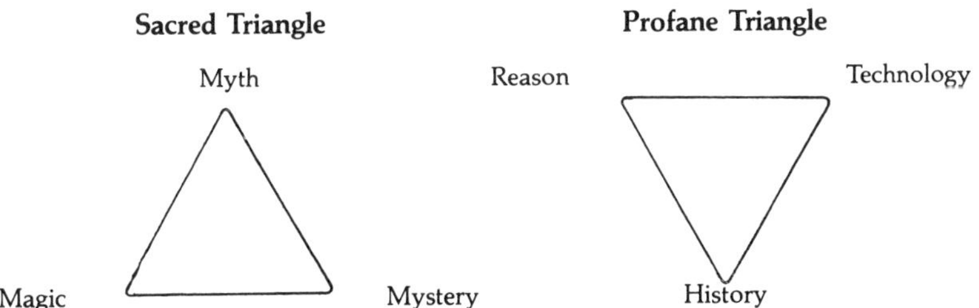

he suggests, a profane triangle oriented away from transcendent experience. To integrate the material in Chapter V & VI we need to create a type of developmental sequence or a hierarchical sequence of levels of abstraction.

Level				The Integrated
I	Situational and Spiritual			Personality
II	Self-Concept	—	Mental a	
	Self-Image	—	Physical b	
	Social-Concept	—	Cultural (Interpersonal) c	
III	Status	1	Ego Strength	
	Courage	2	Goals	
	Flexibility	3	Self-Acceptance	

It is important to develop a theoretical framework for the development of self-esteem because therapy can then be geared to the model.

REFERENCES

Bateson, Gregory an Margaret Mead. *Balinese Character: A Photographic Analysis.* New York: a Special Publication of the New York Academy of Sciences, 1942, p. 84.

Becker, Ernest. *The Birth and Death of Meaning.* New York: The Free Press, 1971, p. 76-77.

Cassirer, Ernest. *An Essay on Man:* New York: Doubleday and Company, Inc., 1944, p. 42-43.

Cavan, R. *Juvenile Delinquency.* 3rd Ed. New York: Harper Row, 1975.

Cooley, C. H. *Social Organization.* Ill.: The Free Press, 1956.

Farber, Marvin. *The Foundations of Phenomenology.* Mass: Harvard University Press, 1943, p. 215.

Faris, Ellsworth. *Nature of Human Nature: And Other Essays in Social Psychology*. New York: McGraw-Hill, 1937, Ch. 2.

Honigmann, John. "World View & Self-View" from *Culture and Ethos of Kaska Society*. Yale Universiy Publications in Anthropology #40, Yale University Press, 1949, p. 305-315.

LeShan, L. *Alternate Realities*. New York: Ballantine Books, 1976, p. 11, 84.

Opler, Marvin, K. *Culture and Mental Health*. New York: The Macmillan Company, 1959, p. 15, 16.

Roszak, Theodore. *Unfinished Animal*. New York: Harper Colophon Books, 1975, p. 178.

Ichheiser, Gustov, *Appearance & Realities: Misunderstanding in Human Relations*. San Francisco: Jossey-Bass, 1970.

Scheler, Max. *Die Stellung des Menchen im Kosmos*. Dormstadt, Reichl, 1928, p. 13.

Shevin, Robert. Breakdown of Family Life Behind Delinquency. *U.S. Journal of Drug and Alcohol Dependence*, April, 1978, p. 4.

Sutherland, E. H. *Principles of Criminology*. Philadelphia: J.B. Lippincott, 1947.

Weber, Max. *The Theory of Social & Economic Organization*. Trans. by A.M. Henderson & Talcott Parsons. New York: Oxford University Press, 1947. p. 88.

Williams, Robin. *American Society: A Sociological Interpretation*. 3rd Ed. New York: Alfred A. Knopf, 1970. p. 414.

Wylie, Phillip. *Generation of Vipers*. Georgia: Larlin Corp. 1979.

Julia Flynn B.A.

and

R. A. Steffenhagen Ph.D
Department of Sociology
University of Vermont

7

ANOREXIA NERVOSA AND SELF-ESTEEM

When society's values advocate the attainment of power, strength, health and perfection of physical form, the denouement for many individuals is dis-ease, powerlessness and personality disintergration, or anomia. One of the manifestations of this dis-ease is anorexia nervosa-a psycho-physical form of starvation. The impact of our society's values upon the individual, the values of power, self-esteem, and the emphasis upon physical form become of etiological significance in understanding anorexia.

Anorexia nervosa is a model of a disease of fragmentation within our society. It exemplifies the personal deviance that arises in attempting to fulfill Western cultural values and the customary perpetuation of those values through treatment. 'Anorexia nervosia', literally meaning 'loss of appetite', was identified by Sir William Gull over 100 years ago: Gull (see Drossman, 1979) attributed the emaciated condition to the presence of hyperactivity in patients whose "want of appetite is due to a morbid mental state." Though food intake is sharply curtailed, this is not because of poor appetite or lagging interest in food, but on the contrary, because of a preoccupation with concerns about food and eating. Anorexics consider self-denial a virtue (see Bruch, 1978). Why the preoccupation with food? In order to understand this we need to look at the culture.

Cultural Values
The disease of today is society. The source of our disconnection and imbalance is specialization. Viewed from the standpoint of the social system, without focusing upon the underlying assumptions, the benefits of specialization are noted with pride: with specialization the responsiblities of government, law, medicine, engineering, agriculture, education, etc., are given to the most skilled, the best trained people. However, when we look at specialization from the standpoint of the individual, we begin to see the fragmentation that arises when the idea of a skill is separated from the idea of the person as a whole. Wendell Berry (1977) suggests that today's average citizen is very unhappy, probably one of history's unhappiest. His only source of power is money which is rapidly inflating. He is at the mercy of other people. The theme

underlying modern despair is powerlessness - one of Seeman's (1958) five conditions for alienation. This feeling of powerlessness is crucial to our development of the theory that anorexics have low self-esteem resulting from feelings of powerlessness.

I. A Question of Boundaries: Enmeshment

A primary belief, one which influences all others, concerns sovereignty-the concept of mankind's place in relation to the universe and each individual's place in relation to his fellow man. Historically, man's view of his place within the universe was one of symmetrical sovereignty. He believed himself to be above the animals and below the divine creator. He accepted his responsibilities and limitations; there was a sense of mutuality among men in their connection to a higher power. Through the acceptance of boundaries, man received the protection and security which enabled him to accommodate to changes.

However, a redefinition of humanity has appeared which allows man to claim, a sovereignty absolute in the order of things. This belief undermines the whole chain of being. In a world of available resources, man's purpose, it is assumed, is to wrest from his context whatever is most beneficial for the development of his separated self. He assumes, as he has been taught to assume, that as a member of the human race, he is sovereign in the universe, and then, when he cannot control his environment he feels powerless.

II. The Future

Another concept which accompanies the idea of absolute sovereignty is a linear notion of time. Time is no longer cyclical, with past, present and future intertwined in a spiritual sense but distinct. The past is looked upon as casual, yet separate from the present. The present is rejected because the great aim of life is to improve the future; the biblical admonition, "Think not of the morrow for the evil of today is sufficient thereof," no longer applies to modern man. The future is the time when science will create a new garden of Eden. This belief creates the foundation for an overwhelmingly goal-oriented society, a society preoccupied by materialism with little or no thought of the spirit. Kierkegaard (1974) says:

> Furthermore, the vulgar (materialistic) view overlooks the fact that, as compared with sickness, despair is much more dialectical than what is commonly called sickness, because it is a sickness of the spirit. And this dialectical quality, rightly understood, again brings thousands under the category of despair. (p. 157)

In his effort to create a 'better world', endless problems and paradoxes arise. In his limitless quest to relieve himself of the drudgery of 'work' and 'inconveniences of daily life', man abdicates to specialists the various competences and responsibilities that were once personal. The bounaries between society and self become so blurred, that most of his 'power' is dependent upon external domains. His *one* chance to live is based on his expertise in his own small speciality. He cannot imagine himself without socially approved aspirations. His source of strength is obtained from 'without' not from 'within'; thus when approval is withdrawn, he is powerless.

Because man's self-esteem is so tied up with achievements and success, a sense of community is destroyed; the rule is never to cooperate, but rather to follow one's own interest as far as possible. An inevitable result is that rigid boundaries must be created to protect man's tenuous power. In order to maintain his niche in the universe, constant vigilance over regulations is needed to protect him from the threatening, unlimited interests of others. An example of this fear is the increasing number of regulatory agencies that have been created to protect the rights of the individual. As a result, the individual must keep tabs on the 'regulators' as well as the 'regulated', creating a further dependency.

III. Mind vs. body vs. spirit

At some point man began to assume that the life of the body would be the business of the scientists who take no heed of the spirit and that the spirit would be the business of church leaders who, at best, would have only a negative interest in the body. The struggle between body and spirit produced such paradoxes as despising the body yet longing for its resurrection. In modern society, 'spiritual' values, no longer able to explain the world in any meaningful or useful way, have been cast off as unnecessary. The source of 'salvation' today is the body in total exclusion from the soul. Material existence, in union with spiritual values, is impractical and uneconomical. The denial of the spirit removes another dimension of power.

Physical health, as a union of body, spirit, and mind, as a natural and appropriate condition for the human body, is no longer satisfactory. Satisfaction with the body as it exists naturally has been replaced by exclusive physical 'models'. As Berry (1977) suggests, boys should be broad-shouldered, narrow-hipped, tall, athletic and handsome. Girls should be slim, leggy, large breasted, curly-haired and beautiful. Both sexes should look sexy in a bathing suit and should, above all, look young.

Many healthy people are 'beautiful' but, few resemble these ideal models. The result is widespread dissatisfaction and the continuation of absurd paradoxes. One such paradox is the pseudo-ritual of 'accepting one's body' which may take years or be the source of anxiety for a lifetime. One means of dealing with the non-acceptance is to spend one's life dressing and 'making up' to compensate for one's supposed deficiencies; the modern guru is the "Cosmetician'.

Another paradox is the denial of the body for the sake of maintaining the fashionable model of luxurious slenderness. The desires to live in material luxury and idleness and yet to be slender and good looking are incompatible. The ideal presented in modern society is the sexy woman in the television commercial who drinks only diet soda; slenderness without effort. Then there are those who angrily denounce the sexism inherent in such models: they assertively comfort and over-indulge the body with equal disdain for its health.

IV. Role Division

Indeed, the fact that the dictates of fashion and beauty affect the lives of females more than males, is an important reflection of sex role differences. A preoccupation with weight is much more likely to occur in the female but with the new trend toward unisex and a breaking down of some of the older concepts of masculinity and femininity, more and more males are becoming diet conscious. With the tremendous emphasis upon 'body beauty,' we are also witnessing an increase in anorexia. Cultural values repeatedly promote a disconnection from the whole and entrap people in the freedom of their autonomy.

By rejecting the concept of 'self-within-the universe' and substituting 'self-in-control-of-the-universe' and through preoccupation with the future, and separation of body, mind, and spirit, man repeatedly shuts himself off from the earth, his fellow man, and himself. He suffers from the dis-ease of fragmentation. His symptoms are a sense of powerlessness and loss of community, freedom, autonomy, and self-esteem.

Anorexia Nervosa

Anorexia is a psychosomatic syndrome characterized by both physical and psychological symptoms. Physical symptoms include a loss of over 25% of the body weight as well as one or more of the following conditions: hyperactivity, amenorrhea or hypothermia. Psychological symptoms include a pursuit of thinness, a fear of gaining weight, a denial of hunger, a distorted body image, a sense of ineffectiveness, and a struggle for control (Minuchen, 1969). Anorexia is potentially fatal with reported mortality rates of 10 to 15%. The disease usually occurs in middle and upper-middle class families, with a ratio of 19 females to 1 male (Drossman, 1979). Social class and incidence figures are a physical reflection of the cultural values of beauty previously discussed. The middle class women would be the most receptive to an internalization of these values. It generally starts in adolescence, although other known precipitators include separation or loss of family member, family illness, and marriage. The prevalence of anorexia is rising, even adjusting for the increasing awareness of the illness by physicians (Drossman, 1979).

I. Enmeshment

Anorexia is a disease occuring primarily in 'ideal' American families-middle, upper-middle class families with stable marriages, manifesting successful occupational achievement. In cases of lower class families, one usually finds a high degree of achievement motivation. The parents tend to be protective and to provide excellent educational opportunities and cultural exposure. They speak with pride of haveing provided a happy, harmonious home environment. The mothers are characteristically self-assured, conscientious and devoted. They are guilty of invidious nurturing comparisons and anorexic children, up to the point of illness, exemplify their mothers' beliefs in their superior methods. Often, the mothers had been career women who felt they had sacrificed their career aspirations for the good of the family. They are submissive to their husbands in many ways, yet do not truly respect them. The fathers, despite social and financial success, tend to feel 'second best', thus exemplifying low self-esteem. They are enormously preoccupied with physical appearance, admiring fitness and beauty and expecting proper behavior from their children. The fathers value their daughters for their intellectual achievements. Rarely do they compliment them but they may criticize them for being plump. The child, in the Veblenian sense, becomes an object of invidious, pecuniary comparison and ostentatious display. Since the adolescent experiences family members as focusing on her actions and commenting on them, she develops a vigilance over her own actions; she becomes too' responsible. The parents frequently control with guilt: "We only want the best for you, it is only for your good." Therefore, non-compliance engenders guilt. In this manner the denial of 'self' for another's benefit and loyalty to family takes precedence over autonomy and self-realization.

The Future: Need for Rigid Boundaries

The result of this enormous concern for each other's well-being (child to family) is a fear of the outside world, as well as of disease, accident or change which threatens the shaky foundation of security and happiness. The parents' self-esteem stems largely from the fulfillment of their familial expectations and in turn the child's self-esteem derives largely from pleasing the parents. Within such a tenuous balance any outside threat is a source of anxiety.

The familial emphasis is upon present behavior as a means of becoming someone who is acceptable and as a means of establishing a life that will be conflict free. This concern is reflective of a society in which man is in control of creation-the rejection of anything that does not fit into the utopian model of a trouble free life and the preoccupation with the future.

When threats to harmony appear, the response is to establish rigid boundaries that swiftly and comprehensively restrict undesirable deviations. The purpose of this structure is to regulate any internal or external pressure for change, to protect the parents and child from confrontation which threatens the transactions within the social unit, thus protecting the family from loss of its tenuous self-esteem. Whether it be on the individual, family or societal level it is this continual reinforcement of dependency upon others for one's sense of self-worth which perpetrates powerlessness and despair.

It is not surpristing, therefore, when an adolescent from within this type of family structure finds her views differing from the picture of harmony and happiness painted by her parents, she suffers from an all-pervasive fear of being ineffective, of having no control over her own life or her relations with others. Bruch (1978 p. 45) points out that a basic rule of life for these adolescents is to please and not to give offense. Bruch further describes these individuals as giving the impression of great stamina and pride, while they really feel ineffective, have difficulty making decisions, constantly worry about what others think of them and thus try to outguess others and do what they think others expect of them. The anorexic is thus at the mercy of the social milieu.

These adolescents constantly try to please. They accept authority and rarely question; thus they fail to develop any autonomony. The importance of pleasing may even lead to deceitful behavior. In one case, an anorexic recalled that, at the time of starting school, she one day discovered a box containing a beautiful Indian headdress. She correctly concluded that this was meant to be her Christmas present. Although she was no longer interested in anything Indian and felt embarrassed at the idea of wearing such a headdress, she was more concerned about making her mother feel good about the gift. She got out her old books and started drawing pictures of Indians to reassure her mother about the appropriateness of the intended gift.

Later on, these children usually place a high value on academic performance as a result of an internalization of the achievement motivation of the parents, especially the father. However, an excellent academic record may be achieved only as the result of great effort. However, still feeling their work to be unpraiseworthy, these children are vulnerable to feelings of low self-esteem. Rigid boundaries conceal and protect while masking and perpetrating the underlying anxiety; with a lessening of these boundaries anxiety may break through.

Adolescence
With the onset of adolescence, the troubled child is confronted with new social pressures and physical changes which trigger a greater sense of powerlessness. Because of her over-involvement with her parents, the child frequently fears that association with peers might lead to parental disapproval. Wanting to deserve their parents' love and admiration by excelling academically and in sports, they frequently withdraw from social events and contact with their peers. Also, due to their deficient sense of self, these youngsters are often paralyzed with fear of not being able to meet others on equal terms. Extemely vulnerable to anything that sounds like criticism, they live by the rule of never drawing attention to themselves. To leave home is to risk destruction of what little bit of power they have maintained through transactions with their parents.

Another change during adolescence is that physical growth fosters body-image awareness. In the case of a girl, the additional weight, developing curves, and roundness, trigger a fear of not even being able to control one's body - the last arena of control in a world where everything else seems to be dependent upon external forces. Under healthier conditions, adolescence should be a time of individuation (developing self-esteem) and psychological growth. In the past, tradition, ceremonies, rituals (the rites-de-passage) helped adolescents through this stage of transition. Today, there is no longer an emphasis upon a return to the inner self and a reaffirmation with the tribe. In modern society, transitions to adulthood fail to consider the obvious and ancient realities of doubt and self-doubt inherent in adolescence, as well as the authentic conflict created by social values. Today one needs to acquire the skills and education necessary to control one's environment within a highly specialized social system.

Expectations of her parents and demands which the young girl makes on herself to become a super-achiever conflict with the submissiveness and fidelity associated with females. Her conception of herself as a female is influenced by the role model, her mother. In many cases of anorexia, the mother has resentfully sacrificed her career for the family, conforming to the cultural housewife role. To further compound the problem, if the parents really wanted a boy, this message may be conveyed explicitly or implicitly.

Sexually, the girl is confronted with an array of messages, all of which deny any respect for the self, either by advocating unlimited freedom or demanding total denial of the body, all of which she confronts with the fear that she may not choose correctly. The social ideal (today) is for the young girl to be slender, beautiful, independent, career-oriented, and a swinging single. These pressures to be 'liberated' conflict with the need for a sense of community, a sense of belonging and commitment. They also conflict with the desire to be accepted and noticed for just being, rather than to have to look and be perfect in the social context.

Suffering from the need for inner power and control, from the need of a sense of self, it is not surprising that the demands and confrontations of adolescence create a crisis in the life of the unprepared adolescent. The cure for crisis which has been modeled for the child by the parents is to eliminate, neglect, or deny the cause of concern, thereby removing it from the responsibility and control of the individual and the family. The source of self-worth and power for the parent lies in career-oriented achievement and social status. Any conflict within the family is quickly suppressed under the guise of concern and the protection of its members from threatening forces. The children become enmeshed with parents because all decisions are made for them and for their own good.

The false sense of autonomy created by the "problem-free" world of the parents becomes the child's source of despair and loss of independence. The subsequent "identity crisis" is a condition of society at large and if the protected child were to turn to "solutions" outside the family circle, the popular recommended means of resolving the crisis would be "finding yourself". As Berry suggests, the modern seeker becomes a tourist of cures looking from one guru to another for an external source of the well-being for which he is searching. Filled with fear and self-doubt, and confronted with the confusion of conflicting external demands, expectations and solutions to her problems, the pre-anorexic adolescent turns to control of food - the most direct means of contact with the world as an illusionary path to power - "If I can't control anything else, at least I can control what I put in my mouth".

Anorexic's uniformly say that they began to restrict their food because they were too fat. Only a few, at the beginning of their diet were actually overweight, with a weight excess in the five to ten pound range, rarely more.

The idea of a diet initially emerges as a means of striving for the model of ultra-femininity. Society's emphasis upon fashion and slimness, messages from family magazines, movies, and television suggest that one of the conditions for obtaining love and respect is slenderness. The additional weight occasioned by puberty may be a source of despair. In most cases, anorexics are concerned with food, frequently regarding it as a means of meeting nutritional needs, rather than a means of satisfying appetite.

Many anorexics say they remember a definite remark or event that made them feel too fat. Frequently the preoccupation with weight and diet begins when confronted with a new experience such as going to camp, changing to a new school or going away to college. In these new situations they feel at a disadvantage, afraid of not making new friends or not being athletic enough, and worry about being overweight. The seemingly sudden dieting always occurs after a long period of self concern which actually represents an impasse in the lives of these adolescents.

One of the first things that serves to reinforce the dieting is that they usually receive praise and admiration for their initial weight loss. Taking pride in looking slimmer and enjoying it, they then decide to lose more weight to earn more respect. Self-imposed rules, which in the past had focused on academic performance, and unquestioning compliance as a means of obtaining respect, now take on the additional dimension of strict adherence to diet. Any violation of their self-imposed harsh rules causes them to feel guilty for having given in to gross, vulgar demands of the body.

With continued dieting, the biological effects of hunger begin to take place and body sensations get transformed, similar to intoxication. Most anorexics experience a new keenness of senses and some aspects of a disturbed sense of time - both related to the physiological effects of starvation. Later, other more unpleasant changes occur which also are common to involuntary starvation. These include constant preoccupation with food, wide mood swings, decreased sexual activity and disturbance in body image. Mood swings involve a drastic switch from the sweet, obedient, considerate child to the demanding, irritable and arrogant daughter. Due to biochemical changes, patients also experience disturbed perceptions and characteristically overestimate their body width, particularly the face, chest, waist, and hips.

Anorexics maintain a rigid determination not to eat; by controlling their eating, many feel a sense of self for the first time. The longer the illness lasts and the more weight they lose, the more anorexics become convinced that they are special. They feel that being so thin makes them "worth-while," "significant," "extraordinary," or "outstanding" - each one has a private word to describe her state. Feeling that they are no longer able to communicate with ordinary people, who won't understand, anorexics become increasingly isolated, especially from their peers. They ruminate only about weight and food which prevents them from focusing or concentrating on anything else except food.

One sub-group of anorexics, estimated by Bruch (1978 p. 11) to be about 25%, goes through a binge-eating syndrome. Binge eating, referred to as bulimia, adds a more deliberate component of deceit and those who have given in to it tend to be more resistant. They periodically ingest massive amounts of food in short periods followed by self-induced vomiting, laxative or diuretic abuse. Initially it is a means of giving in to an urgent desire for food and still lose weight. However, as time passes, pride in "outwitting Nature" gives way to the feeling of being helplessly under the domination of a compulsion. Gorging on food is no longer a way of satisfying hunger but a terrifying, dominating compulsion.

Associated with binge eating are various notions about food, all of which have in common the idea that the food they feel compelled to gulp down cannot be integrated or would be damaging, and therefore has to be removed from the body. Although these notions are often bizzare, they may also stem from dissatisfaction with foods that are genuinely unhealthy. Many behavioral modification treatments have focused on weight gain by whatever means is quickest without consideration for nutrition.

Anxiety about weight also commonly results in excessive exercising. Most anorexics had been interested in sports before the illness and had participated in athletic activities of their group, but with the onset of anorexia, exercising becomes a solitary way of burning off calories and showing endurance. They typically drive themselves to unbelievable feats to demonstrate that they live by the ideal of "mind over body." They develop a whole range of justifications for their ultimate thinness.

It is apparent from the studies on anorexia that physical and mental self-destruction are both the cause and effect of these desperate youngster's efforts to acquire and maintain an internal feeling of power. Moreover, the destructive symptoms of anorexia support and are supported by the social unit in which the initial loss of autonomy occurs. Feeling both protected and helpless, the child continues to approach all interpersonal situations as a weak, crippled person. As her dependent demands increase, family members respond by increasing their protective control. Many anorexics explain why they cling to the illness with the simple statement, "If I were well I would lose support."

For the family, the illness provides a focus of concern that diverts attention from the unresolved and unnegotiated conflicts that might shatter the 'harmony' if the child were to mature and leave the family transactions. Challenged by the chronicity, the unpredictability, and the life-threatening danger of anorexia, the family eventually attempts to have the 'adolescent's problem' cured by a physician or therapist. No other problem can gain salience. They feel everything would be all right if their daughter would just be well.

The child's and the family's longing for a cozy, anxiety-free environment parallels the desire for a return to the garden of Eden. The individual in this attempt to maintain a model of absolute control and harmony may choose inappropriate techniques. The unity of mind, body, and spirit are natural sources of power, independence and healing not seen by many people. Instead they blindly maintain the fragmentation by assuming that the only way to obtain security, happiness and success is by control of the physical.

A. Linear Model

The assumptions underlying the *Weltanschauung* of Western culture are:

1. Man's position is that of "self-in-control-of-universe"; he has the potential to transcend all undesirable human conditions by means of his domination and control.

2. Time is linear.

3. Mind, body, spirit and community are separate entities and though interrelated their union is not important. Within this framework, focus upon the various divisions of spirit, mind, and body has shifted through the ages.

In early Christianity the struggle focused upon domination by the spirit with rejection and denial of the body and mind. But, with 'victory' of the spirit in isolation from the world, spiritual values began to lose their meaning. In modern times the battle has raged on between body-mind, and spirit, this time with body and mind the 'victors' and spiritual values suppressed. Through human intellect, science and technology has granted man unlimited access to resources and material wealth. Yet despair, strife and discontent abound amid abundance.

The most recent struggle focuses upon the mind, first in competition with body and spirit, and ultimately divided against itself. Paradoxically, the division between mind and body was strengthened by the recognition, in the early 20th century, that the two were interrelated. When it was discovered that the state of mind of an individual could produce physical illness it was never considered that the reason for this might be an underlying disconnection between mind and body rather than the interconnection.

Illness created by the mind could only mean that the mind was not functioning properly; there was something 'wrong' with the mind as it presently existed and the 'disorder' would have to be eradicated if the individual were to be able to control his physical health and his behavior in the future. The assumptions of this 'linear approach' (that, with the application of scientific knowledge, the individual will be able to overcome his 'imperfect' human condition) have formed the basis of Western treatment of illness.

Treatment

Minuchen et al. (1978) has described three types of treatment within the model of a 'linear approach': (a) medical, (b) behavioral, and (c) psychodynamic. These three types recognize various factors as being significant in the exploration and treatment of psychosomatic disease, but ultimately they all converge on the model of a self as transcending the relationship of which it is a part.

1. Medical

The fact that anorexia comes to professional attention only when it has become so severe as to be life-threatening at least partially accounts for the fact that most of the literature on the subject and the treatment of anorexia has been in a medical setting. A medical focus is based on the idea of health as an absence of illness - a physiological condition. Illness is believed to result from germs or some other external cause which must be kept under control or eradicated if the patient is to regain health. In the medical model, the individual is first of all a patient rather than a whole person. She is diagnosed and her illness defined. The doctor, as an authority figure, will protect her from illness and 'cure' her only if she obeys and follows his directions. Through the control and elimination of the physical disorders which appeared at some time in the past, the doctor will be able to restore the body to health. The patient's spirit, mind, and sense of connection to the community are not within the bounds of his speciality, nor should they be for they are believed to be unrelated to the problem.

However, studies of anorexia were not long restricted to the purely physiological aspects of the disease. It was early recognized as a psychosomatic syndrome. According to Weiss and English it was one of the diseases most responsible for understanding the role of psychological factors in the development of disease (see Minuchen 1978, p. 13).

2. Behavior Modification

Behavioral Modification is the psychological approach most closely relted to the medical model. The goal is for the patient to gain control over her body by means of the therapist's manipulation of her environment. The behavioral therapist focuses on the 'what, not the why', seeking to remove the psychological symptoms rather than the underlying causes. Symptom removal occurs by reducing anxiety in the presence of the stimulus.

The function of the therapist is to explore and map the client's behavior and then develop a therapeutic procedure in which reward and punishment for desired and undesirable behavior can be provided. If the client fails to improve, the behavioral therapist attributes this not to the client's resistance, but to improperly developed procedures. The behavioral therapist's role is that of an objective scientist; his goal is to structure the milieu exterior so behavior will change.

The relationship between therapist and client is the same as between doctor and patient. The therapist, by controlling the client's environment on behalf of her own best interest, is totally responsible for the 'cure'. The process of setting up rewards and punishments reaffirms the importance of the mind's control over the body. It also reaffirms the isolation of self from the rest of the community, for there is no consideration of the social milieu outside the hospital. The success of behavior therapy in the hospital environment is good but a sustained change back in the family is not accomplished.

The importance of weight gain should not be ignored. However, when a patient's weight is below a critical level of 90-95 pounds, there are psychological changes which precipitate rigid preoccupation with food and which make therapeutic exploration of underlying problems virtually impossible. Also, there are serious distrubances in electrolyte balance as well as acute danger from severe emaciation. However, after the critical level of weight is reached, therapeutic treatment should begin.

3. Psychodynamic approach

In the psychodynamic approach, the focus is on the psychological causes of behavior and how these causes are related to the mind's failure to properly control its own functioning. According to the Freudian view, the mind in its totality, is dangerous and undesirable; parts of it must be suppressed and controlled. If totally released, nothing but destruction can be expected.

The causes of the patient's illness are seen to be historical -experiences that occurred in early childhood are considered to have significant impact upon the patient's mind. The therapist takes on a paternalistic role; the goal is to bring the patient's mind into the right state. The therapist works to tease the childhood experiences out during the therapeutic process, interpret them for the patient, and in so doing, enable her mind to understand and thus control the unwanted behavior.

On the basis of this model, early studies of anorexia centered upon a search for the etiology of the illness. For a time, the specific psychodynamics took precedence over empirical findings. Cases exhibiting the usual symptoms of anorexia - loss of weight, lack of appetite, amenorrhea, and hyperactivity - were not considered anorexia if the psychodynamics of the case did not fit the schema. Eventually the causes were understood to be multiple. For Falstein et al. (1956), the possible causes were almost unlimited. Food and the ingestion of food may be seen as symbolizing impregnation, performance, gratification, killing, destroying, castrating, engulfing etc.

In recent years, psychotherapy has begun to acknowledge the interpersonal nature of the therapeutic process, in which the client sees herself as part of the process. This approach gives the client greater responsiblity for her own growth. Yet, the importance of interpersonal relations in anorexia has not generally extended beyond the dyad of therapist and client. Although, the input of parents and the social context is recognized, few efforts have been made to include them in the therapeutic focus. The goal is to help the client overcome the problems of the system to which she belongs rather than trying to change the social context. If therapists involve the client's parents, it is ususally as 'management' rather than 'therapy'.

Another related development in more recent psychotherapeutic techniques has been a greater respect for the client's present reality and subjective experience. Nevertheless, current conflicts in the client's life, though well observed and clearly described, are still interpreted as recurrences of conflicts in the early childhood.

The psychodnamic model has provided valuable insights into the inner world of the client, but it is still bound by the framework it shares with the medical and behavioral models. In all models, the underlying assumption is that the patient is sick, the family is helpless, and the expert will to bring about change. In all three models, the expert, by means of his specialized knowledge, strives to help the client successfully confront his environment. Within the framework of a linear concept of time, past experiences or present behavior are processes* important only as a means to a future end - the anorexic's ability to transcend her condition by winning control in the struggle against undesirable aspects, whether they be of the mind, body or social milieu.

The psychodynamic model involves certain dangers. First, the focus on exploration of the past may bar fast recovery. Psychotherapy frequently takes months or years, at considerable financial cost. Second, by focusing solely on the individual and problems of food and eating, the method is likely to reinforce rather than cure the symptom.

Outcome

The value of any treatment can only be established on the grounds of its efficacy. Unfortunately, methods of evaluating treatment within the linear model have reflected the same values under which the treatment were established. Therapeutic procedures have been unquestionably adhered to as the only means of obtaining vague benefits. There has been little in-depth focus upon the effectiveness of results or upon the negative side effects of the means used.

Evaluative studies indicate that even with the best practitioners, cure rates have been no better than 70% and seems to average closer to 40 - 60%. However, even these results are tenuous. Getting well' is often poorly defined.

---

* If past, present and future behavior are seen as processes, then a dialectic approach would be crucial.

Sheer weight gain is often the sole criterion for evaluating treatment outcome. Other important questions are frequently ignored. For example, see Blitzer et al. (1961), Gladston (1974), Lesser (1960), Lucas et al. (1976), Reinhart et al. (1972), Silverman (1977), and Warren (1968).

B. Systems Model

Only since the 1950's have investigators viewed anorexia in terms of a systems orientation. This approach represents an entirely different framework based on the following assumptions:

1. Man is in the position of 'self-within-universe'; he must learn to cooperate rather than dominate.
2. Time is cyclical; the present is a creation of the past and the past is a creation of the present.
3. Union of mind, body, spirit, and community are essential for the maintenance of health.

Treatment

The systems model does not discard the linear model's focus upon the individual but includes and goes beyond it to consider the client in her social context. The systems therapist focuses upon the individual as a member of a social group, usually the family. The function of the social group is seen as twofold: (a) to provide individual members with a supportive network, and (b) to provide individual members with a margin of choice within the range of that system's rules. The source of pathology of anorexia is believed to be the overdependence and total enmeshment among family members. When this occurs, the freedom of choice of individual members is diminished to the point of powerlessness. Amid the 'freedom' created by a lack of boundaries or restraints among members of the social group, anorexia becomes a desperate attempt to maintain a sense of autonomy. The goal of therapy is to facilitate the growth of a social group so as to allow independence of its members.

For the systems therapist, change comes about by the formation of a new social structure; all family members need to be freed. The therapist's aim is to uncover and foster the use of more effective transactional patterns among family members and in their interactions with society (see Carl Rogers 1977, p. 80).

In working to facilitate growth, it is the process rather than the end which is important for the systems therapist. His focus is upon the present. He recognizes the influence of the past but he also views it as a creation of the present; within this system it is unnecessary to seek causes. Thus, the past is incorporated into the present. The self is expanded to include its place in the universe and in accepting that position, freedom and health are attained.

Outcome

In his work with psychosomatic illnesses, Minuchen (1978) and his colleagues saw, over a seven-year period, an increasing number of anorexic patients. All were treated on the basis of a systems model. He drew up a detailed study o the first 53 cases treated and analyzed them according to: (a) The presenting characteristics of the patients, (b) course of treatment, and (c) follow-up data. The patient population was essentially adolescent (60%), with 25% of the group pre-adolescent and 15% of the group falling in the range of 17-21 year olds. The median age for the entire group was 14½ years. Eleven percent of the group was male. The median interval between the onset of illness and the start of family treatment was six months, the range being from 1 month to 3 years.

All patients were involved in family therapy, conducted at weekly intervals. Three families dropped out of treatment after 1 to 2 sessions. For the 50 families who remained involved, the median course of treatment was 6 months, the range being 2 to 6 months. The therapy was conducted by 16 different therapists including staff psychiatrists, psychologists, social workers, and psychiatric residents. All treatment was conducted within a systems framework, but specific goals of treatment varied with the developmental status of the child in the family context. A survey conducted among the therapists revealed the emergence of a different treatment plan for each group: (a) Pre-adolescent patients and their parents, (b) Adolescent age group, and (c) Young adults. The outcome was evaluated in two areas: (a) a medical assessment of the degree of remission of anorexic symptoms and (b) a clinical assessment of psychosocial functioning in relation to home, school, and peers. The evaluations were based on the client's conditions at termination of therapy and also on information obtained through follow-up studies ranging from 1½ to 7 years. Eighty percent of the sample was followed for two years or more.

The two assessments revealed that 86% of the cases were recovered from both the anorexia and its psychosocial components. In comparison to other studies, Minuchen's use of therapy within a system approach has been dramatically successful.

Use of Hypnosis in Systems Model

It is interesting to note that, in developments of both the linear and systems model, the lack of self-esteem has only been referred to, never being the central area of focus. Within behaviorial models the central focus was merely upon correction of specific manifest behaviors. Within the psychodynamic model, therapists searched for the underlying cause of anorexia by focusing upon the client's personal, past experiences. Few attempts have been made to explore the underlying cause of anorexia by focusing upon the client's personal and present experiences - the lack of self-confidence and self-esteem. While Minuchen acknowledges individual therapy, he moves on to advocate the exploration of the client's present experiences through the social context. No mention has been made of the value of focusing upon present experiences through an individual approach. Would the exploration of individual therapy within the systems model increase its effectiveness?

One means of working with present experiences in individual therapy is with the use of hypnosis. Hypnotherapy has traditionally been used in the context of a linear approach, its sole function being to facilitate the memory of past experiences for use by the psychoanalyst, or to control specific actions as a means of implementing the program of behavioralists. Within a systems approach, hypnotherapy could be used to improve current feelings of self-esteem. With this technique, autonomy could be achieved more rapidly than with reliance upon traditional methods of psychotherapy. Although shorter than a strictly linear approach, Minuchen's therapeutic sessions still lasted approximately six months. The use of hypnosis would be advantageous in regards to both time and effectiveness, particularily with young adults, where individual therapy was Minuchen's primary method of treatment.

REFERENCES

Berry, W. *The unsettling of america: culture and agriculture.* New York Avon Books, 1977.

Blitzer, J.R., Rollins, N. and Blackwell A. Children who starve themselves: anorexia nervosa. *Psychosomatic Medicine* 1961, *23*, 369-383.

Bruch, H. *The golden cage: the enigma of anorexia nervosa.* MA.: Harvard University Press, 1978.

Drossman, D.A. Clinical conference: anorexia nervosa. *Gastro Enterology,* 1979; *77*, 1115-31.

Falstein, E.I., Feinstein, S.C. and Judas, I. Anorexia nervosa in the male child. *American Journal of Orthopsychiatry,* 1956, *26*, 751-772.

Gladston, R. Mind over matter: observations on fifty patients hospitalized with anorexia nervosa. *Journal of American Academy, Child Psychiatry,* 1974, *13*, 246-263.

Kierkegaard, S. *Fear and trembling and sickness unto death.* New Jersey: Princeton University Press, 1974.

Lesser, L.I., Ashender, B.J., Debuskey, M. and Eisenberg, L. Anorexia nervosa in children. *American Journal of Orthopsychiatry,* 1960, *30*, 572-580.

Lucas, A.R., Duncan, J.W. and Piens, V. The treatment of anorexia nervosa. *American Journal of Psychiatry,* 1976, *133*, 1034-1037.

Minuchen S. Roseman, B. and Baker, L. *Psychosomatic families: anorexia nervosa in context.* Ma.: Harvard University Press, 1978.

Reinhart, J.B., Kenna, G.D. and Succop, R.A. Anorexia nervosa in children: outpatient management. *Journal of Academy of Child Psychiatry,* 1972, *11*, 114-131.

Rogers, C. *On personal power: inner strength and its revolutionary impact.* New York: Dell Publishing Co., Inc. 1977.

Seeman, M. On the meaning of alienation. *American Sociological Review,* 1958, *24*, 783-791.

Silverman, J. A. Anorexia nervosia: clinical and metabolic observations in successful treatment plan. in Vigersky, ed. *Anorexia Nervosia* New York: Raven Press, 1977.

Warren, W. A study of anorexia nervosa in young girls. *Journal of Child Psychology and Psychiatry, and Allied Disciplines,* 1968, *9*, 27-40.

CASE HISTORY: ANOREXIA NERVOSA
R. A. Steffenhagen

Instead of presenting one rather detailed history I am going to present two shorter case histories of clients I have dealt with who presented the anorexic sydrome.

Case A had been medically diagnosed as anorexia nervosa and had received medical and psychiatric care. I saw her for the first time two years ago when her complaint was no longer that of dealing with anorexia but a complaint of stamina.

As was presented in the chapter, it is evident that many anorexics are very athletic young women and that athletic prowess is important in their role identification. This particular case involved a long-distance runner who had been running in high school and college competition.

Susan first came to me asking if I would be willing to hypnotize her to deal with the symptom of her inability to run. She had made excellent progress medically and emotionally and theoretically her condition was adequately under control. Psychiatric counseling had been terminated.

She had been practicing and after a ten-minute run, for no apparent reason, she collapsed. It became evident, as our discussion proceeded, that she manifested all the syptoms of low self-esteem. There was a tremendous need to excel academically and physically, and her family background had all the criteria that one would anticipate in the case of anorexia. The family was upper middle class, both parents professionals, and Susan was an only child. She had never had any difficulty with her family, spoke extremely highly of her parents and gave no indication whatever of any conflict within the family structure. Although her symptoms had abated (she regained her body weight), the feeling of powerlessness remained. We discussed the relative merits of using hypnosis and I explained my self-esteem theory in detail and suggested that this would be the modus operandi I would use, that we would not deal with running explicitly, as I felt her problem was one of a feeling of powerlessness and of low self-esteem. We proceeded with hypnosis, using a relaxation technique with the program centering around self-acceptance on a spiritual level. At the second session we went immediately into the deeper hypnotic state and worked intensively on the self-esteem. The problem of her inability to run was totally corrected after two sessions; she had no more difficulty during practice and was able to make competitive meets. It should be noted that several months later she ran the Boston marathon with no difficulty whatsoever. This case does not suggest that two sessions are sufficient to cure anorexia but rather to point out that a problem which had not adequately been dealt with therapeutically in the past was the source of difficulty in running. Moreover, Susan was happier and was performing better socially and academically than previously.

Case B deals with Carol. This particular case had not been diagnosed anorexia. From the symptomology manifested the anorexic label would not have been applied.

Due to an unusual set of circumstances, Carol had lost a great deal of weight over a period of time when she was visiting a relative on the west coast and had not been provided with an adequate diet. The year's experience of going to another school, etc., was very enjoyable, but occasioned this dramatic weight loss. From counseling it seemed evident that a girl of her stature and body weight should not have lost that much weight. Upon returning home she had been put under medical management to regain her health and in no time she was back to 'normal'.

Carol came to me stating that she was aware of my theory of deviance and that she felt she had a problem with self-esteem, that school was not progressing properly, that she was concerned about gaining weight (certainly symptomatic of the anorexic) and generally felt depressed and unhappy. Carol was a good hypnotic subject. In the first session we proceeded by working on self-esteem and during the second and third sessions we utilized the spiritual approach to which she responded beautifully. I did not see Carol again until the end of the semester when she came in and spent a couple of minutes telling me how great she felt; in fact, she informed me that after the first session her parents came to visit her and her mother had commented on the fact that she was like her old self; she was astounded and pleased by the results. She went on to indicate that she could not believe how good she felt or how much in control she was over her social and physical well being and how pleasant the semester had become. I did not see Carol again until late in winter when she came in again with a concern about body weight; it seemed she was again beginning to eat compulsively and was concered about weight gain, especially since her particular athletic interest required low body weight. She had taken a job of some responsibility and was situationally under a great deal of pressure. We discussed the nature of the situational pressure and I suggested that a reinforcement session or two would certainly be appropriate. We had one deep session and apparently this was quite adequate to bring her back into a homeostatic balance emotionally and physically. Carol is another example of a girl with tremendous interest both academically and physically; she is a very fine athlete, is more apt to compete in rough contact sports with males than with females. She is an excellent equestrian and is generally an all around good athlete.

These two case histories illustrate the role of self-esteem in anorexia and how self-esteem therapy can be utilized effectively in dealing with this particular malady. It is the author's opinion that feelings of powerlessness are by far the most important element underlying anorexia. In both cases we have seen the sociodynamics underlying anorexia. In the first case, self-esteem therapy was used to deal with a residual problem after the anorexia was seemingly under control. The second case was more indicative of anorexia in its initial stages. This is not to suggest that two to four sessions will 'cure' anorexia but to show the use of self-esteem therapy in treating anorexia and that anorexia is a special case of deviance resulting from low self-esteem.

Nicholas Danigelis Ph.D

Department of Sociology
University of Vermont

8

SOCIAL INTEGRATION:
SELF-ESTEEM AND YOUTHFUL SUICIDES*

In the latter part of the nineteenth century, Emile Durkheim (1951) proposed a sociological theory of suicide as a dramatic vehicle to highlight his break with the moral statisticians of his day and to establish the unique value of sociology for the study of suicide. Focusing on the social bonds which tie individuals to one another and to their society, Durkheim applied his arguments to a wide variety of social contexts, including religion, marriage and the family, the military and political change, and the economy. Today, some eighty years later, Durkheim's name and ideas continue to be invoked in research aimed at explaining both variation in suicide rates (toward which phenomenon his own work was aimed) and individual suicide (about which he tried not to concern himself) (see his 1951:51 discussion about the differences between the two phenomena). Ironically, what Durkheim admitted to be an important social correlate of suicide rate variation — age — is a concept he treated with brevity, and he did not attempt to explain the relationship between age and suicide (Maris 1969:162; Pope 1976:147-8). Furthermore, aside from referring to the positive correlation between age and the tendency toward suicide, he ignored the general question of why people at certain chronological stages in their lives are apparently more vulnerable to suicide than at others, and he never dealt with the specific question of why youths commit suicide.

The thesis of this paper is twofold. First, Durkheim's theory, though ignoring the general relationship between age and suicide and the specific phenomenon of youthful suicides, nevertheless is an extremely useful tool for understanding both the overall problem of why youths suicide and the recent trends toward increased youthful suicides. Second, in order to make Durkheim's theory "work" in this area, it is necessary to reverse the process Durkheim followed by proceeding from the sociological to the social psychological and to use a recent theory with demonstrated application in the area of deviance — Steffenhagen's (1978; 1980) theory of self-esteem. What follows is, first, an examination of the present state of research on youthful suicides, followed by quick sketches of Durkheim's theory of integration as applied to suicide and of Steffenhagen's theory of self-esteem, and last, a tying-together of these two theories in an effort to understand better the phenomenon of youthful suicides.

Research on Youthful Suicides

The Published Data

The underpinning of most research on suicide, including the study of youthful suicides, has been official government data on suicides cross-classified by different social categories (e.g., sex, age, race) and converted into rates (suicides per one hundred thousand population). Recent works on childhood and adolescent suicides, in fact, generally have started with references to the rapidly increasing suicide rate among young people (see e.g., Toolan, 1968; Lester, 1972; Hendin, 1975; Diggory, 1976; Duncan, 1977; Holinger, 1977, 1979; McAnarney, 1979). Indeed, official U.S. government data on suicide rates cross-classified by age, sex and race show that between 1960 and 1977 the suicide rate among 5-14 and 15-24 year olds has at least doubled for white males and females and for black males and females while the overall rate increase for each sex-and-race-specific category has been marginal during this time period (see Tables 1 and 2). Interestingly, if one goes further back in time, the period between 1940 and 1960 tends to show a curvilinear trend (decrease in rate followed by increase) for each sex and subgroup both among the 5-24 year olds and the population in general. (The only two exceptions are the general population of white males for which there is a decrease in rate between 1940 and 1960 and the 15-24 year old group among non-white males for which there is a slight increase in rate between 1940 and 1960). Official suicide data, therefore, show a recent dramatic increase in youthful suicides which appears not to be a part of a long-term increase in either the overall suicide rate or the suicide rate among young people.

In the last few years official suicide data have come under heavy fire (Douglas, 1967; Baechler, 1975) and their validity and reliability questioned. While there has been no lack of defenders of the use of official government figures on suicide (e.g., Sainsbury and Barraclough, 1968; Gibbs, 1971; Besnard, 1976), two points need to be made regarding the validity and reliability of official figures on youthful suicides. First, while official suicide figures generally underestimate the number of actual suicides, this is an especially serious problem in the case of children's and adolescents' deaths for two reasons: first, many youthful deaths (e.g., poisoning, are likely to be termed accidents rather than suicides because of children's greater vulnerability to errors of judgment concerning what constitutes dangerous behavior. Second, there is likely to be much guilt and fear of stigma among parents whose child has died; they in turn are likely to press for a diagnosis of "accident" (Holinger, 1979; see also Duncan, 1977; Toolan, 1968, 1975). Thus overreporting probably occurs for accidents because of both unintentional and intentional misreporting of cause of death.

The second important point has to do with the implications of the apparent underreporting of youthful suicides. Obviously there is no problem if underreporting youthful suicides more than underreporting adult suicides remains constant over time, because the youthful suicide rate obviously has increased dramatically relative to the overall suicide rate in recent years. If, however, the recent rise in reported youthful suicides represents merely an increased accuracy in reporting the actual cause of youthful deaths, then the 'rise' in children's and adolescents' suicide rates really is not an increase in suicides but an increased tendency toward better reporting. While argument and evidence can be marshalled to support either side of the argument, the main point to remember is that attempting to understand why youths commit suicide is the fundamental issue; whether there have been dramatic increases or not in the number of actual youthful suicides (a point to which this paper will return later) may help direct us to the explanations beyond youthful suicides but should be considered carefully. As Haim (1974) points out, we don't know how many adolescents commit suicide, and having a better idea than we have now would be of some utility. On the other hand, he questions whether such an endeavor should be of central concern. He fears that in the search for better data the critical issues of how and why children kill themselves would be lost.

The Arguments

The Correlation Between Age and Suicide

For many scholars, the question of why children and adolescents kill themselves is tied up with the question of why the tendency toward suicide increases with advancing age.[1] For this reason, a quick look at the arguments generated to explain the age-suicide relationship is in order.

From analysis of clinical and anecdotal data, Menninger argues that suicide is a death involving three internal elements: dying, killing, and being killed (1938:26). Suicide notes analyzed by Farberow and Shneidman (1957) indicate that, while the wish to kill and be killed decreased with age, the wish to die increased. The factors apparently making the wish to die an especially important correlate of age range from biological to social. For example, O'Neal et al's (1956) comparison of attempted suicides among over 60 year olds and those 59 and younger led them to argue that chronic brain syndrome and manic-depressive illness more than loneliness and ill health increase the likelihood of suicide attempts. More recent evidence (Buchsbaum et al, 1977) points to a relationship between platelet MAO levels and average evoked response (AER) augmenting and suicide attempts and suicides, suggesting possible genetic connections to psychiatric disorders. Other works have looked for links between cancer, depression and suicide (see, e.g., Plumb et al, 1977; Whitlock, 1978). On the other hand, different researchers have found neuroticism (Pallis and Jenkins, 1977) and family role relationships (Cazzullo et al, 1974; Howe and Robinson, 1975) to be correlated with suicide attempts.

The bulk of the evidence suggest, however, that older people kill themselves more often than younger people for a variety of reasons, including especially those of poor health and social isolation (see, e.g., Batchelor, 1957; Bohannan, 1960; Stengel, 1964; Maris, 1969; Robins et al, 1977; a good overview is Weiss, 1968). Related to factors of health and social relationships are the arguments which focus on life cycle changes. For example, Sainsbury (1968) argues that suicide tends to be most common for women during menopause and for men at retirement, times of important biological and social changes (see also Porterfield's 1965:ch 13, measurement of stress in the life cycle in the context of the age-suicide relationship).

The arguments for why youths suicide less than adults represent the complements to the above points: Objectively children are less likely to suffer serious physical and mental illness; they, in turn, are integrated into society and dependent on their elders in such a way that aggression tends to be vented against others rather than oneself; consequently, the younger the age category, the lower will be the suicide rate (Maris, 1969; see also Lester, 1972). Therefore, whether we look at the tendency toward suicide from Menninger's paradigm based on the three components of suicide or from explanations based in the physical or social sciences or from a view based on life cycle changes, all available clinical and official governmental suicide data and the arguments concerning the data make the positive correlation between age and suicide a hypothesis writ in stone — in fact, law-like. But official data suggest that youthful suicides are dramatically rising; and, even if only reporting of them is becoming more accurate, the fact still exists that youths are killing themselves and the question that remains is why.

Theories on Youthful Suicides

One important link to the above discussion on the general relationship between age and suicide is the degree to which stresses become severe at certain points in one's life. As Cavan (1965:310) points out, it is not only in one's later years that stress occurs, but also during the period of adolescence, a time during which rapid physiological change is accompanied by serious psychological and social change (e.g., increasing independence and conflict with parents) (see also McAnarney, 1979). The evidence on suicide rates for Europe during the end of the nineteenth and early part of the twentieth centuries, she continues, tends to support this pattern (1965:310-11).

The data in Table 1 support the idea that life stresses and the suicide rate are correlated for both young and old. In 1977, for example, among white males there is a dramatic increase from the 5-14 year old rate of 1.0 to the 15-24 year old rate of 22.9 and a similar, though not as dramatic rise in the rate after retirement age: 30.9 for 55-64 year olds vs. 41.3 for those over 65. For white females during this year the increase in the early years is also large (0.2 to 5.5) and the rate among the 45-54 year olds, when adult life changes — e.g., menopause — are apt to occur, is the highest. The data on non-whites in Table 2 shows different trends but could be interpreted to reflect life stresses when one realizes that employment problems are particularly severe for young blacks and may have implications for both young black males and young black females (see Davis, 1979, for an overview and bibliography regarding recent trends of black suicides and the reasons for them).

As with other similar concepts, however, the term stress touches upon a multitude of sociological, psychological and physiological correlates. In order to be more precise, we should look at the most important. Fortunately, good overviews of research on adolescent suicide exist. Seiden, for example, lists fifteen "psychodynamic characteristics (which) have been causally linked to adolescent suicides," including "chronic depression," "guilt," "desire to control environment," "feelings of helplessness," "feelings of hopelessness" (1972). He then proceeds to classify them with respect to whether they are individual, social or cultural determinants. A slightly different classification scheme is Haim's (1974) distinction among psychiatric, circumstantial, and sociological factors (see also Klagsbrun, 1977). Variables which have been studied in relation to adolescent suicide are:

Genetic and familial tendencies
Puberty
Mental disorder
Identification, imitation, suggestion
Death concept
Aggression
Spite, revenge, or manipulation
Impulsivity
Drugs (Seiden, 1972:158-66)

While much documentation exists to connect these factors to excessive risk-taking and attempted (but not completed) suicides, the tie between them and actual suicides is quite tenuous for many. One exception is "mental disorders." While depression, as a mental disorder, may be less important in younger age groups than in adults (Seiden, 1972), schizophrenia has been demonstrated to be present in a substantial proportion of youthful suicides (see Seiden, 1972:160 references for relevant studies). Another possibly important individual factor in completed youth suicides is drugs (Seiden, 1972).

Social determinants studied in the context of adolescent suicide include:

Family relationships
Social isolation
Communication
Socio-economic status
Religion
Education - especially student suicide
Mass media (Seiden, 1972:166-78; a more recent discussion
    of social determinants is McAnarney, 1979).

For the last four determinants in the above list the relationship between the determinant and adolescent suicide has been found to be non-existent or the determinant and adolescent suicide has been found to be non-existent or complex enough to warrant substantial reservation concerning the question of causality. On the other hand, of all the non-biological predictors of life-threatening behavior, human isolation seems best to separate out those who will commit suicide from those who will not commit suicide (Seiden, 1972). Closely connected to isolation are family relationships (e.g., family break-up, loss of family member) and communication. For all of these determinants a central idea is that the ties which bind individuals to one another (especially to significant others) provide a kind of protective barrier if these relationships are healthy ones. This idea is closely related to Durkheim's theory of integration and will be discussed later (for clinical examples of the importance of family and other significant ties for the suicidal youth see, e.g., Toolan, 1968; Jacobs, 1971; Hendin, 1975; Holinger, 1977).

Finally, there are cultural determinants connected to adolescent suicide reflected by the following questions: How much pressure is brought to bear on the members of a society? How acceptable is suicide? Does the culture provide alternatives to suicide? (Seiden, 1972). The evidence on cross-cultural comparisons of suicide rates suggests that, in fact, different cultures answer these three questions differently and that the differences in suicide rates between cultures may be attributable to differences in stress, acceptability of suicide, and alternatives to suicide. Again Durkheim's theory of integration is relevant here.

In sum, the literature on youthful suicides, containing as it does a potpourri of social- and individual-level explanations, as well as official government and private clinical data, presently provides the researcher and clinician with a good cataloging of factors related to youthful suicides. But while theories of varying degrees of specificity have been offered (see, e.g., Haim, 1974; Jacobs, 1971), the link between sociological and psychological perspectives on youthful suicides is still lacking (see, e.g., Krauss, 1976). The next two sections will examine two concepts the relationship between which provides an important key for understanding the social and individual links in youthful suicides.

Durkheim's Theory of Integration[2]

As indicated at the outset of this paper, Durkheim's theory of integration applied to suicide focuses on the social bonds among individuals. While complex and often self-contradictory, Durkheim's theory contains a consistent message: Different levels of integration into and regulation by society produce bonds of differing strength between the individual and the social milieu and thus suicide rates of differing magnitude between different social categories. These differences in social pathology occur generally for two reasons. One, too little integration or regulation produces individuals whose ties to society are weak and consequently whose vulnerability to suicide high. Suicides resulting from low integration or regulation are labeled egoistic and anomic by Durkheim (1951). A social category likely to produce egoistic suicides is the religious category "Protestant," because Protestants, more than Catholics, place a greater emphasis on the individual conscience over the collective conscience, which in turn permits greater free inquiry and a lessening of (traditional) social bonds (Durkheim, 1951). Another social category which will tend to produce egoistic suicides is the family category of "married without children" because larger families (i.e., those with children) are very dense (the rate of interaction among the members is high), which in turn increases the collective conscience and the protection of family members (Durkheim, 1951). Finally, an example of a social category encouraging anomic suicides is the situation of economic crisis in a society; whether it's a time of boom or bust, economic dislocation represents a de- regulation of human passions, because the preserving force of society's rules is at a low point and the vulnerability to suicide is thus heightened (Durkheim, 1951).

A second problem leading to high suicide rates involves too much integration or regulation which produces too strong a tie to society and the subsequent denigration of the value of human life and, again, increased vulnerability to suicide. Too much integration produces the altruistic suicide, while too much regulation produces the fatalistic suicide. Some examples of the former, cited by Durkheim (1951), are the self-inflicted deaths of very old or very sick men, women whose husbands have died, servants whose masters have died, religious martyrs, and soldiers. While Durkheim distinguishes several varieties of altruistic suicide, the essential common demoninator is the concept of duty: Social norms in the form of law or religious doctrine or public pressure encourage and, in some cases, demand suicide from certain individuals at certain times. The Kamikazee pilots of Japan during World War II are a more contemporary example. So also could one label the suicides in Guyana among the Reverent Jim Jones' religious followers as altruistic suicides, because of the sect's requirement that members kill themselves when the group's existence was threatened and the willingness of at least some members to follow organization doctrine. Too much regulation produces a type of suicide Durkheim called fatalistic but which he dealt with only in a footnote at the end of a chapter (1951:276, fn. 25). The self-inflicted deaths of slaves whose lives were far too regulated, and, in a sense, strangulated, represent fatalistic suicide in the sense that their only perceived escape lies in death.

Given Durkheim's substantially more detailed discussion and analysis of egoistic and anomic suicides, the almost identical nature of egoism and anomie, and his marginal treatment of both altruistic and fatalistic suicides, Johnson (1965) has argued that Durkheim's theory of integration- regulation really is a theory of integration based on the notion that too little integration results in too high a suicide rate. More recently, Pope (1976) has refuted both Durkheim's and Johnson's positions by arguing that, while egoism and anomie are indistinguishable in empirical, if not theoretical, terms, there is an important conceptual difference between egoism-anomie and altruism-fatalism. Thus Pope postulates a U-shaped relationship between integration and suicide, too little or too much integration resulting in high suicide rates.

While Durkheim's name is mentioned briefly in a few works on youthful suicide (e.g., Haim, 1974; Klagsbrun, 1977) and his ideas concerning social integration utilized (e.g., McAnarney, 1979), the modal response among suicide researchers has been to acknowledge the importance of social facts in creating stresses among youths but to deny that these facts are sufficient to explain or predict individual suicides in cause and effect terms (Haim, 1974; Klagsbrun, 1977). One approach is to argue that social and psychological factors together are important and leave it at that; another is to acknowledge that point but then to go further in an effort to look for the connecting links (Haim, 1974). This paper will follow the latter path.

Steffenhagen's Theory of Self-Esteem

Proposed as a means of predicting and explaining drug abuse, Steffenhagen's self-esteem theory of deviance (1978, 1980) is based on the writing of Alfred Adler and utilizes both sociological and psychological perspectives in the spirit of Adler. The relevance of self-esteem, or self-worth, for deviant behavior is explained thus:

> Associated with self-esteem are the important Adlerian
> concepts of inferiority and superiority. The individual
> who feels inferior has a poor regard for himself and
> generally withdraws from meaningful social participation.
> He tends to see the group as valuing him even less than
> it in fact does (Steffenhagen 1978:2).

Steffenhagen goes on to point out that an individual who thus perceives the social environment as being antagonistic might well lash out in an equally hostile manner and elicit further enmity from the group. In any event, an individual with low self-esteem is not *ipso facto* a deviant but rather more vulnerable psychologically than an individual with high self-esteem to the stresses which emanate from particular social contexts. In terms of drug abuse this means that both low and high self-esteem individuals will not use drugs if there is no "reason" to use them (social situation not pressuring) but, while the high self-esteem individual might use drugs when there is pressure to do so, it is the low self-esteem individual in that high pressure situation who will most likely become the drug abuser (Steffenhagen, 1978: 2-3).

Three variable concepts which Steffenhagen borrows from Adler are important for clarifying the relationship of self-esteem to social context; they are goal orientation, lifestyle, and social milieu (Steffenhagen, 1978: 3-7; 1980: 159-61).[3] Goals attainable by the individual are not so much a problem, but unrealistically high goals coupled with low self- esteem are likely to lead to coping behaviors like drug abuse. With respect to lifestyle, a child who is treated even-handedly by parents is again not a focus of concern; but the overly indulged, pampered child and the forgotten, neglected child are both problems, because they are likely to have developed low self-esteem and to look to coping mechanisms like drugs to deal with problems stemming from their deviant lifestyles. Finally, assuming that deviant behavior is learned and that differential association is an important mechanism for understanding the learning of deviant behavior, Steffenhagen argues that, in addition to the low self- esteem individuals pressured to use drugs, individuals with a fair amount of high self-esteem might become drug abusers within a social milieu which encourages heavy drug use and provides no other reasonable alternatives and which therefore becomes an important mechanism of group cohesiveness (e.g., young soldiers using drugs in Vietnam).

While Steffenhagen (1980) mentions self-esteem and suicide in the same breath only in passing, the basic components of his theory would appear to have relevance for the study of youthful suicide. For one thing, both drug abuse and suicide are (in recent years especially, it would seem) deviant behaviors participated in by youth to an alarming extent. Second, some evidence exists to connect general youthful deviance with suicide (Moschel and Haberle, 1977). Finally, an effort already has been made to analyze the suicidal individual within an Adlerian framework emphasizing suicide as communication with one's social environment (Adler, 1970; Ansbacher, 1969). Throughout these Adlerian analyses of suicide there is a thread connecting self-esteem to suicide such that the latter is seen to be a solution to low amounts of the former in the suicidal individual (Adler, 1970:252; Ansbacher, 1969). In the next section, a search is begun for the connections between self-esteem, social integration and suicide. While substantially less than a complete theory results, the tying together of the two perspectives facilitates our understanding of both the existence of youthful suicides and the recent dramatic increase in the reported youthful suicide rate.

Toward A Theory of Youthful Suicide

Basic Assumptions

Any theory aimed at analyzing youthful suicides should take into account both the preponderance of evidence which suggests that social isolation is a key variable in predicting vulnerability to suicide and the lack of any clear correlations between vulnerabilities or tendencies attributable to social forces and the psychological process resulting in the actual suicide. This can be accomplished by looking at the relationship between social isolation and Durkheim's theory of integration and between Durkheim's argument and Steffenhagen's theory of self-esteem. These ties are represented by two sets of assumptions. In terms of the first, social isolation really represents one part (albeit an important one) of the general problem of social integration. While the literature on family breakups, teenage runaways, and broken romances among the young suggests that alienation from significant others (Toolan, 1968:225, calls it "loss of the love object") is quite central as a precondition for suicide, the other end of the integration spectrum is also represented. For example, Hendin's (1975) study of student suicides shows the extraordinarily *high* degree to which one suicide attempter ("Larry") was integrated into his family. The relationship with his parents was unhealthy but nevertheless highly bonded—what Hendin (1975: q.328) calls a "death knot." In such cases, loss of a love object (e.g., death of a parent) does not produce a release of ties to one's environs as much as it encourages the search for a "quick fix" substitute to the intense relationship one had with one's parents (e.g., burying oneself in one's academic work). Another example of overintegration within a family context is the "family tombstone" studied by Howe and Robinson (1975). Here the death of a parent precipitates the acquisition of different roles by family members as a way of coping with the family's grief. The person who becomes the living reminder of the deceased may, in conflict with other members of the family, be pushed toward suicide. Finally, as mentioned in the section on Durkheim, membership in cults appears to represent overintegration into a subculture, in some cases producing suicide (see Stoner and Parke, 1977, for a general description of cults and the problems ensuing from membership within them). Therefore, social conditions making youths more vulnerable to suicide are of two types: social isolation—indicative of too low social integration—and, for lack of a better term, social suffocation—indicative of too high social integration. For each condition, stress may provoke one of two types of reactions: either a tendency to swing back and forth between social isolation and suffociation (e.g., turning from drugs or alcohol to a cult) or fluctuating between different forms of suffocation (e.g., turning from the smothering ties within one's family to a romance).

The second set of assumptions concerns the connection between Durkheim and Steffenhagen in an effort to go beyond vulnerabilities and tendencies. If Steffenhagen's use of social milieu is left aside, several important connections between self-esteem and integration can be made. For one thing, neglected and pampered lifestyles really represent socialization examples of social isolation and social suffocation respectively. Hendin's (1975:331-3) clinical case, "Larry," is a perfect example of the former; the cases Seiden (1972) reviews in his section on social isolation contain many examples of the latter.

Another connection is the way in which Steffenhagen's discussion of goal orientation helps us to understand how Durkheim's generalizations can be made more concrete. What is it which makes those socially isolated or suffocated take the step toward suicide? While it's only a partial answer, the idea that setting unrealistically high goals for oneself (or having them set by someone else) is likely to promote deviant behavior like drug abuse to compensate for failing to meet one's goals suggests that failing to meet unrealistic goals may also be a form of stress triggering suicide attempt or actual suicide. But, Steffenhagen argues, the problem of unrealistic goal setting is not to be considered in a vacuum; it occurs as a producer of and co-worker with low self- esteem. Stress by itself, we are told, does not cause drug abuse (or any other form of deviant behavior, for that matter), nor does unrealistic goal-setting. But if one has low self-esteem and one is confronted with stress or failure in reaching one's goals, then, in terms of Steffenhagen's paradigm, drug abuse is a likely result. Based on similar reasoning, the argument here is that low self-esteem coupled with high stress in the social context of isolation or suffocation, in fact, likely will produce suicide if one's means of coping (e.g., drugs, alcohol, delinquency) fail and no alternative means are seen to be available. This suggests that, among youth, suicide may be an outgrowth of deviant attempts to cope with the joint problems of isolation/suffocation, high stress, and low self-esteem; also, however, suicide may be a first choice when conventional, acceptable means like thinking, talking, working hard, etc., fail to produce appreciable change.

A final connection between Durkheim and Steffenhagen relates to the dramatic oscillation between isolation and suffocation or between different forms of suffocation many suicidal youths experience. Why are these changes possible? One very plausible answer is: They occur only among low self-esteem youths, and it is precisely because such youths have low self-esteem that they are without the personal resources to find real solutions to life stresses and thus end up alternating between isolation (e.g., resignation, alienation) and suffocation (e.g., excessive dependence on family, peers or some reference group) or between different forms of suffocation. But these solutions merely substitute group esteem and denial of self or barriers to real communication for the low esteem youths and, as such, exacerbate their problems.

A Working Model

The basic assumptions described above can be graphically presented in the context of a working model of youthful suicide (Table 3). Measurement problems of the main variables are by no means trivial, and dichotomizing or trichotomizing these variables does not solve the measurement problem and, in fact, might obscure subtle but important distinctions in variable relationships. Nevertheless, the main independent variables are posited to be self-esteem (low versus high), social stress (low versus high) and social integration (too low, moderate,[4] too high); and the main dependent variable is behavior (ranging from stable to unstable to quite deviant to suicidal) (See Table 3). None of the independent variables, by itself, predicts suicidal behavior, but in concert they appear to. For instance, analogous to what happens in Steffenhagen's theory of drug abuse, high self-esteem protects one from suicidal behavior, as represented by the relatively stable behaviors anticipated in all six categories in Table 3a. On the other hand, low self-esteem promotes suicidal behavior *only* if stress is high *and* integration is too low or too high, as the first and last categories of the bottom row of Table 3b show — low self-esteem and high stress with moderate integration promoting unstable but not necessarily suicidal behavior (Table 3b, last row, middle category).

From the point of view of integration, a moderate amount has a prophylactic effect generally; note the unstable situation when self-esteem is low and stress is high, however. Too little and too much integration, of course, produce suicidal behavior by itself, only when self-esteem is low and social integration too little or too much. Therefore, each independent variable is necessary but not sufficient to promote suicidal behavior.

An observation about the relative probability that an individual would be in any particular category should be made at this point. Specifically, the likelihood that an individual with high self-esteem is socially isolated or suffocated is probably low, because a positive self- image will encourage contact and interaction of a relatively egalitarian nature in a variety of normal social relationships. Such an individual will probably not "hide out" from the rest of the world or attempt to lose his/her identity through domination by others in a group context. Thus, the four outside category outcomes in Table 3a are probably rare.

Table 3b contains two other examples in which rare outcomes can be expected: Low self-esteem probably will not allow many individuals to develop healthy relationships with important significant others, so that the middle column in this table also will not be heavily populated. This table is important for another reason, however, because all of the likely remaining outcomes (as well as the rarely occuring low self-esteem, moderately integrated individual under great stress) are clearly probemmatic for the individual. The poorly integrated loner and runaway and their overly integrated counterparts (the cult members, living tombstone, and mama's boy) would appear to be only some serious stressful events away from suicide. Similarly, were the integration patterns to change for the rare low self-esteem individual under great stress who is moderately integrated, the individual's behavior likely would become suicidal.

Several questions of theoretical and clinical importance arise from this model. For one thing, while it earlier was suggested that low self-esteem probably facilitates movement between isolation and suffocation, how easily does an individual's self-esteem change between low and high, integration between moderate and too little or too much, and stress between low and high? With respect to integration how does one measure the relative importance of various integration contexts like family, peers, school, work, etc.? Given data which consistently show males to have a higher rate of completed suicides than females but the reverse to be true for uncompleted suicide attempts, what are the implications for this model's applicability to young males versus young females? Are any changes necessary for either group in the theory? Finally, while it has been intimated, no explicit relationship between suicide and other forms of deviant behavior has been drawn; how precisely does one come to predict suicide after a long history of drug abuse or, in some cases, instead of drug abuse? Does the difference lie in the nature of the group into which one is integrated (the differential association argument comes into play here) or the kind, duration or frequency of the stress one is under (perhaps Erikson's, 1968, analysis of identity crisis should be invoked here)? Or does it have to do with goal orientation, lifestyle or social milieu?

Obviously these and many other questions remain about youthful suicides, but space does not permit an adequate exploration for their answers in this paper. What should be evident in this paper is at least as important as these unanswered questions, however; and a summary statement about the questions it has attempted to answer and the directions in which future research might follow from the model developed here will be addressed briefly.

Conclusion

One major thesis of this paper has been that Emile Durkheim's eighty-year-old theory of suicide is relevant for understanding youthful suicides. Through discussion of the clinical and theoretical literature on youthful suicide, it has been possible to show how too little or too much social integration, in fact, creates strain for the individual and makes a youth more vulnerable to what Durkheim called egoistic/anomic suicide or altruistic/fatalistic suicide. Because his argument was developed to explain variation in suicide rates rather than to predict individual suicides, little has been done to incorporate Durkheim's or any other sociologist's arguments on suicide into a theory of youthful suicide. The second thesis of this paper has been that Steffenhagen's theory of self-esteem as applied to drug abuse could be combined with Durkheim's theory of integration to help us understand individual youthful suicides. The distinction between low and high self-esteem was then used to develop a model relating self-esteem, social integration, social stress, and suicidal behavior among young people.

If the model is a fair representation of reality, then it has relevance for the data on the youthful suicide rates discussed at the beginning of this paper. Concomitant with the recent dramatic increases in the suicide rates of children and adolescents has been a similarly large increase in the divorce rate, proportion of women heading households and working in the labor force, geographic mobility, and pressure to achieve in school (McAnarney, 1979). All of these measures in one way or another speak to social disintegration and stress. While McAnarney emphasizes that her work is hypothesis-generating and meant to be understood in the context of analyzing youthful suicide rates rather than predicting individual suicides, her findings are very suggestive in light of the model presented here. The model posits an increased likelihood of youthful suicide if social integration is diminished or strengthened in a pathological manner and if stress is increased; furthermore such changes in integration patterns and stress levels might very well negatively affect self-esteem among young people (e.g., "Mommy and Daddy are divorcing—it's my fault." "I can't get into college—I'm stupid"). If all of these propositions are true, then the recent dramatic rise in reported youthful suicides does not represent more accurate reporting; it represents a real increase in youthful suicides.

These propositions, of course, should be addressed by future research. One strategy would be to proceed at the clinical level by content analyzing past case histories of suicidal and non-suicidal individuals in an effort to compare self-esteem, integration, and stress profiles. An advantage of this procedure is that there are many such case histories in the public record. The disadvntages, however, are serious. First there is the measurement problem discussed earlier in this paper; how does one accurately indicate an individual's self-esteem, integration, and stress? Second, even if good measures existed, those writing up the case histories may not, in all cases, have deemed it necessary to include data which would allow future researchers to determine self- esteem, integration and stress levels very accurately. Third, there is the problem of being able, in most cases, to analyze the case histories only of suicide attempters, not of completed suicides. While Hendin (1975: 329) strongly argues that this creates no problem, Seiden (1972: 170) sees important differences between the two in terms of social isolation.

Another clinical strategy, obviously aimed at the problems inherent in secondary analysis, is for psychiatrists and psychologists to begin efforts to collect as much information as possible relating to self-esteem, integration and stress in their sessions with clients. While problems remain, it's possible that such a data collecting strategy will encourage clinicians and researchers alike to attempt to generate better measures of self-esteem, integration and stress and to continue efforts to compare attempted with completed suicides.

Social scientists, too, can orient research efforts toward testing the societal analog of this model by examining systematically relationships between macro-level measures of the independent variables and the youthful sucide rate through multivariate data analysis techniques. Altogether, there is much that scientists can do to pinpoint better the causes of the self-inflicted death of young people. It is hoped that the model presented here will encourage that effort.

FOOTNOTES

* Work on this paper was supported in part by a University of Vermont summer research grant. For research assistance I am deeply indebted to Jill White and Dick Garnett.

1. Recent work by Danigelis and Pope (1979), however, found that age contributed negligibly to suicide rate variation when sex and marital status were controlled. See also Lester's (1972: 117) summary of findings showing different age-suicide relationships for males than for females and Sainsbury's (1962) research which shows social class differences in the relationship between age and suicide for males over 65.

2. An excellent critical analysis of Durkheim's theory, his data, and the theory-data fit is Pope (1976).

3. Steffenhagen's argument includes more variables than are discussed here but

is not distorted through their omission, I believe; see his discussions of these other variables (1978: 10-1; 1980: 162-3).

4. By moderate is meant a number of moderate or healthy ties to different social environs rather than a single tie of moderate intensity.

Table 1

Suicide Rate by Age and Year for Whites in the U.S.

Age

Males	Year				
	1940	1950	1960	1970	1977
5-14	0.4	0.3	0.5	0.5	1.0
15-24	8.8	6.6	8.6	13.9	22.9
25-34	19.9	13.8	14.9	19.9	26.7
35-44	30.1	22.4	21.9	23.3	24.7
45-54	44.1	34.1	33.7	29.5	27.3
55-64	58.8	45.9	40.2	35.0	30.9
65 +	60.2	55.8	46.7	41.1	41.3
Total	23.5	19.0	17.6	18.0	21.4
Females					
5-14	0.1	0.1	0.1	0.1	0.2
15-24	3.9	2.7	2.3	4.2	5.5
25-34	8.6	5.2	5.8	9.0	9.3
35-44	11.5	8.2	8.1	13.0	11.2
45-54	14.0	10.5	10.9	13.5	13.6
55-64	13.1	10.7	10.9	12.3	11.2
65 +	11.6	9.9	8.8	8.5	8.3
Total	7.3	5.5	5.3	7.1	7.3

Sources: U.S. Bureau of the Census (1973, 1975, 1976, 1979)

Table 2
Suicide Rate by Age and Year for Blacks and others in the U.S.

Males	Year	Age			
	1940	1950	1960	1970	1977
5-14	0.4	0.1	0.1	0.2	0.4
15-24	5.1	5.3	5.3	11.3	15.5
25-34	11.5	10.1	12.9	19.8	25.7
35-44	10.6	11.3	13.5	12.6	16.0
45-54	14.8	11.7	12.8	14.1	11.7
55-64	12.6	16.8	16.9	10.5	13.3
65 +	12.0	13.3	12.4	10.8	12.2
Total	7.2	7.0	7.2	8.5	11.4
Females					
5-14	0.0	0.1	0.0	0.2	0.2
15-24	3.3	1.7	1.5	4.1	4.0
25-34	3.5	2.8	3.5	5.8	6.8
35-44	3.0	2.2	3.7	4.3	5.1
45-54	3.2	4.0	3.2	4.5	5.2
55-64	1.4	1.2	3.4	2.2	4.4
65 +	2.4	2.4	3.9	3.6	2.3
Total	2.1	1.7	2.0	2.9	3.5

Sources: See Table I.

Table 3
Posited Relationships among Self-esteem,
Integration, Stress, and Tendency
Toward Suicidal Behavior

a. High Self-esteem

Stress		Integration		
		Too low (Isolation)	Moderate	Too High (Suffocation)
Low		Stable (rare)	Stable	Stable (rare)
High		Probably Stable (rare)	Stable	Probably Stable (rare)

b. Low Self-esteem

Stress		Integration		
		Too Low (Isolation)	Moderate	Too High (Suffocation)
Low		Somewhat Unstable (warning signs evident)	Probably Stable (rare)	Somewhat Unstable (warning signs evident)
High		Egoistic/ Anomic Suicide	Unstable (rare)	Altruistic/ Fatalistic Suicide

Note: Arrows (→) (↔) show predicted tendencies to change social environment and level of integration among low self- esteem youth.

REFERENCES

1. Adler, A. *Superiority and Social Interest.* Ed. by H.L. Ansbacher and R.R. Ansbacher. Evanston: Northwestern University, 1970.
2. Ansbacher, H.L., "Suicide as communication: Adler's concept and current applications." *Journal of Individual Psychology,* 1969, 25: 174-80.
3. Baechler, J., *Les Suicides.* Paris: Calmann-Levy, 1975.
4. Batchelor, I.R.C., "Suicide in old age." Pp. 143-51 in E.S. Shneidman and N.L. Farberow (eds.) *Clues to Suicide.* New York: McGraw-Hill, 1957.
5. Besnard, P. "Anti- ou ante-durkheimisme? Contribution au debat sur les statistiques officialles du suicide." *Revue francaise de Sociologie,* 1976, 17:313-41.
6. Bohannan, P., *African Homicide and Suicide.* Princeton: Princeton University, 1960.
7. Buchsbaum, M.S., Haier, R.J. and D.L. Murphy, "Suicide attempts, platelet monoamine oxidase and the average evoked response." *Acta Psychiatrica Scandinavia,* 1977, 56:69-79.
8. Cavan, R., *Suicide.* New York: Sentry, 1965.
9. Cazzullo, C.L., Invernizzi, G. and A. Vitali, "Suicide, attempted suicide and the community." *Socijalna Psihijatraja,* 1974, 2:267-91.
10. Danigelis, N.L. and W. Pope, "Durkheim's theory of suicide as applied to the family: a contemporary test." *Social Forces,* 1979, 57:1081- 106.
11. Davis, R., "Black suicide in the seventies: current trends." *Suicide and Life-Threatening Behavior,* 1979, 9:131-40.
12. Diggory, J.C., "United States suicide rates, 1933-1968: an analysis of some trends." Pp. 25-69 in E.S. Shneidman (ed.) *Suicidology: Contemporary Developments.* New York: Grune and Stratton, 1976.
13. Douglas, J.D., *The Social Meanings of Suicide.* Princeton: Princeton University, 1967.
14. Duncan, J.W., "The immediate management of suicide attempts in children and adolescents: psychologic aspects." *Journal of Family Practice,* 4: 77-80.
15. Durkheim, E., *Suicide: A Study in Sociology,* Trans. by J.A. Spaulding and G. Simpson. New York: Free Press, 1951.
16. Erikson, E., *Identity: Youth and Crisis.* New York: Norton, 1968.
17. Farberow, N.L. and E.S. Shneidman, "Suicide and age." Pp. 41-9 in E.S. Shneidman and N.L. Farberow (eds.) *Clues to Suicide.* New York: McGraw-Hill, 1957.
18. Gibbs, J. P., Suicide. Pp. 271-312 in R.K. Merton and R. Nisbet (eds.), *Contemporary Social Problems.* 3rd ed. New York: Harcourt Brace Jovanovich, 1971.
19. Haim, A., *Adolescent Suicide.* Trans. by A.M.S. Smith. New York: International Universities, 1976.
20. Hendin, H., "Growing up dead: student suicide." *American Journal of Psychotherapy,* 1975, 29:327-38.

21. Holinger, P.C., "Suicide in adolescence." *American Journal of Psychiatry* 134: 1433-4, 1977.
"Violent deaths among the young: recent trends in suicide, homicide and accidents." *American Journal of Psychiatry*, 1979, 136: 1144-7.

22. Howe, B.J. and S. Robinson, "The 'family tombstone' syndrome: an interpersonal suicide process." *Family Therapy*, 1975, 2:17-21.

23. Jacobs, J., *Adolescent Suicide*. New York: Wiley, 1971.

24. Johnson, B., "Durkheim's one cause of suicide." *American Sociological Review*, 1965, 30: 875-86.

25. Klagsbrun, F., *Too Young to Die: Youth and Suicide*. Boston: Houghton Mifflin, 1976.

26. Krauss, H.H., "Suicide — a psychosocial phenomenon." Pp. 25-54 in B. Wolman and H.H. Krauss (eds.) *Between Survival and Suicide*. New York: Gardner, 1976.

127. Lester, D., *Why People Kill Themselves: A Summary of Research Findings on Suicidal Behavior*. Springfield, Ill.: Charles C. Thomas, 1972.

28. Maris, R., *Social Forces in Urban Suicide*. Homewood, Ill.: Dorsey, 1969.

29. McAnarney, E.R., "Adolescent and young adult suicide in the United States — a reflection of social unrest?" *Adolescence*, 1979, 14:765-74.

30. Menninger, K.A., *Man Against Himself*. New York: Harcourt, Brace and World, 1938.

31. Moschel, G. and H. Haberle, "The unequal distribution of juvenile delinquency and psychiatric disorders in Mannheim: a significant contribution of area to the unequal epidemiological backgrounds." *Social Psychiatry*, 1977, 12:157-69.

32. O'Neal, P., Robins, E., and E.H. Schmidt, "A psychiatric study of attempted suicide in persons over sixty years of age." *Archives of Neurological Psychiatry*, 1956, 75:275-84.

33. Pallis, D.J. and J.S. Jenkins, " Extraversion, neuroticism, and intent in attempted suicides." *Psychological Reports*, 1977, 41: 19-22.

34. Plumb, M.M. and J. Holland, "Comparative studies of psychological function in patients with advanced cancer: I. Self-reported depressive symptoms." *Psychosomatic Medicine*, 1977. 39:264-76.

35. Pope, W., *Durkheim's Suicide: A Classic analyzed*. Chicago: University of Chicago, 1976.

36. Porterfield, A.L., *Cultures of Violence*. Fort Worth: Manney, 1965.

37. Robins, L.N., West, P.A., and G.E. Murphy, "The high rate of suicide in older white men: a study testing ten hypotheses." *Social Psychiatry*, 1977, 12:1-20.

39. Sainsbury, P., "Suicide in later life." *Gerontol. Clinic*, 1962, 4: 161-70. "Suicide in depression." In A. Coppen and A. Walk (eds.) Recent developments in affective disorders. *British Journal of Psychiatry* (special pub.) 1968, 2:1-13.

40. Sainsbury, P., and B. Barraclough, "Differences between suicide rates." *Nature*, 1968, 220-1252.

41. Seiden, R. H., "Studies of adolescent suicide behavior." Pp. 153-91 in B.Q. Hafen (ed.) *Self Destructive Behavior: A National Crisis*. Minneapolis: Burgess, 1976.

42. Steffenhagen, R.A., "An Adlerian approach toward a self-esteem theory of deviance: a drub abuse model." *Journal of Alcohol and Drug Education*, 1978, 24: 1-13.
"Self-esteem theory of drug abuse." Pp. 157-63 in D.J. Lettieri, M. Sayers and H.W. Pearson (eds.) *Theories on Drug Abuse: Selected Contemporary Perspectives*. Abuse Research Monograph 30. DHHS Pub. No. (ADM) 80-967. Washington, D.C.: Supt. of Docs., U.S. Goverment Printing Office, 1980.

43. Stengel, E., *Suicide and Attempted Suicide*. Baltimore: Penguin, 1964.

44. Stoner, C. and J.A. Parke, *All God's Children*. Middlesex, England: Penguin, 1977.

45. Toolan, J.M., "Suicide in childhood and adolescence." Pp. 220-7 in H.L.P. Resnick (ed.) *Suicidal Behaviors: Diagnosis and Management*. Boston: Little Brown, 1968.
Suicide in children and adolescents. *American Journal of Psychotherapy* 29:339-44, 1975. U.S. Bureau of the Census, *Statistical Abstract of the United States*. Washington, D.C.: Supt. of Docs., U.S. Government Printing Office, 1973.
1975________________________
1976________________________
1979________________________

46. Weiss, J.M.A., Suicide in the aged. Pp. 255-67 in H.L.P. Resnick (ed.) *Suicidal Behaviors: Diagnosis and Management*. Boston: Little Borwn, 1968.

47. Whitlock, F.A., Suicide, cancer and depression. *British Journal of Psychiatry*, 1978, 132:269-74.

A CASE HISTORY: SELF-ESTEEM AND SUICIDE
R. A. Steffenhagen

This case history deals with youthful suicide and self-esteem. Jeff first came to my office in November, 1979. He is a middle-class, white, 20-year-old college male from Connecticut. Jeff had been at the University of Vermont since 1977 and had a good academic record. He has two siblings, an older brother and a younger sister, and lived at home until he came to college.

Jeff was one of my students. He came to my office one day and asked if he might talk to me. We discussed the course subject matter for about a half hour when it became evident that this was not why he came to see me.

He finally commented on the fact that he was depressed, unhappy and needed to see someone in counseling. We discussed the student services and then he asked if I would be willing to work with him. Jeff is a very quiet, unobtrusive young man, polite and considerate. He was depressed, and manifested a great deal of free floating anxiety. We discussed self-esteem and he commented on the fact that he felt inferior to his peers, that he wasn't good looking, when in reality he was very handsome. He admitted to the fact that he had been beginning to think about suicide as a way out of his unhappiness. There was no traumatic event precipitating the thought process.

In high school Jeff had been a very good student. He excelled academically and was well liked by his male peers, because he was a good athlete and participated in all the major sports. Jeff had minimal contact with girls and was very shy around them, to the point of being uncomfortable.

Jeff's father is a typical German patriarch who went to college following World War II, taking advantage of Veterans benefits. He is a mechanical engineer and put pressure on the boys to follow in his footsteps. He constantly stressed the need to excel, both academically and athletically. As a result of this, Jeff was continually under the pressure to succeed. The family unit was tightly integrated, typical of the German family unit, but this integration, because of the stress, tended to border on Durkheim's suffocation. He felt suffocated as a result of the tight control and the admonition to always do better. The tight control also produced an isolation from the peer group, since he had to spend so much time and energy on academics and athletics. This isolation was differential; he was continually in contact with family and male peers because of high school sports, but isolated from the social activities of the larger adolescent community. This isolation lay at the heart of Jeff's shyness and inability to communicate and associate with members of the opposite sex.

Jeff's father, while stressing college also put pressure on the boys to develop independence, which took the form of working part time to help support themselves. Thus, early in his college career he was also isolated from the college social environment because his time was largely accounted for through work, classes, and study, which continued to foster his shyness. As a result of these demands, Jeff was under constant stress.

Jeff's father would not allow the boys to attend high school social functions because of a highly moral religious orientation. He didn't trust his boys to socialize with girls because this could easily lead to sexual behavior and they might get a girl pregnant. He felt that modern morality was too loose and that high school functions were not adequately supervised. This further led to Jeff's shyness and feelings of inadequacy and isolation.

In high school Jeff had been a very good student. He excelled academically and was well liked by his male peers, because he was a good athlete and participated in all the major sports. Jeff had minimal contact with girls and was very shy around them, to the point of being uncomfortable.

Jeff's father is a typical German patriarch who went to college following

World War II, taking advantage of Veterans benefits. He is a mechanical engineer and put pressure on the boys to follow in his footsteps. He constantly stressed the need to excel, both academically and athletically. As a result of this, Jeff was continually under the pressure to succeed. The family unit was tightly integrated, typical of the German family unit, but this integration, because of the stress, tended to border on Durkheim's suffocation. He felt suffocated as a result of the tight control and the admonition to always do better. The tight control also produced an isolation from the peer group, since he had to spend so much time and energy on academics and athletics. This isolation was differential; he was continually in contact with family and male peers because of high school sports, but isolated from the social activities of the larger adolescent community. This isolation lay at the heart of Jeff's shyness and inability to communicate and associate with members of the opposite sex.

Jeff's father, while stressing college also put pressure on the boys to develop independence, which took the form of working part time to help support themselves. Thus, early in his college career he was also isolated from the college social environment because his time was largely accounted for through work, classes, and study, which continued to foster his shyness. As a result of these demands, Jeff was under constant stress.

Jeff's father would not allow the boys to attend high school social functions because of a highly moral religious orientation. He didn't trust his boys to socialize with girls because this could easily lead to sexual behavior and they might get a girl pregnant. He felt that modern morality was too loose and that high school functions were not adequately supervised. This further led to Jeff's shyness and feelings of inadequacy and isolation.

Within my theoretical framework, success, encouragement and support were all part of Jeff's social milieu. He achieved success athletically and was a high school star. He achieved success academically and had an SAT score of 1200. The father and mother, especially the father, constantly encouraged and supported him in his academic and athletic endeavors; however, while he achieved the encouragement and support, an important element of trust was lacking: "I cannot let you go to a high school dance because you might sexually get into trouble." Words of praise were never there: He was never told that he was doing a good job; he was never told that he had good athletic ability; he was never told that he was a handsome young man and many of the little things that are so important to the adolescent in his normal growth. The family is very religious and Jeff was required to go to church regularly although in college he began to break away somewhat from regular attendance.

Jeff is a tall athletically built young man, very handsome, and, if he had a modicum of self-confidence, would be a social success with the opposite sex. Because he was so shy, his social contacts were largely limited to males who were also athletes. This fact is important in that while he was totally at ease with members of his own sex, he had a rather narrow community perspective, a fact which has been referenced in the suicide literature.

The first session was spent allowing Jeff to talk about his problems, to bring them out into the open, and to clarify ambiguous thoughts and ideas. The second session was a mixture of my discussing my self-esteem theory and his relating to this, plus a hypnotherapy session. The beginning of the spritual foundation was established in the second session. The third session entailed the deep technique, the suspension of the ego. Jeff was very responsive to this technique and it proved very successful in building self-esteem. A couple of weeks later he came in for a fourth session and commented on the fact that he was feeling great. Before the fifth session, he called and cancelled and did not come to see me for a year. A year later Jeff came in commenting on the fact that he thought a booster session would be helpful. It became apparent that as he had begun to feel good about himself, he had begun to take on positions of responsibility in the college milieu, and his academic performance began to improve although even his first two years were good. With the increase in self-esteem Jeff was beginning to relate to members of the opposite sex. Because of his very high moral standard he was not sexually promiscuous but was able to have sex with a girl to whom he was able to establish a strong emotional attachment. He is still doing well, has been accepted into graduate school, and will be pursuing a graduate career.

This is another case of deviance-suicidal thoughts that were precipitated by low self-esteem. With the increase in self-esteem the suicidal thoughts totally dissipated and it should be noted that after the second session there were no longer any thoughts of suicide or any other forms of bizarre ruminations. Jeff is now enjoying life to its fullest and is well on his way to a very successful career. This is a case in which a minimum of five sessions over a period of two years was all that was needed to bring about a dramatic change in his personality, both overt and covert.

H. Gilman McCann Ph.D
Department of Sociology
University of Vermont

9

SELF-ESTEEM AND SOCIAL DEVIANCE THEORY:

A PRELIMINARY SYNTHESIS

The self-esteem theory of deviance developed by Steffenhagan and his associates (Steffenhagen, this book, chapter 4; Steffenhagen, 1974; 1978) makes use of and has implications for current sociological theories of deviance. The relationship is especially close with regards to the treatment of goals, status, social milieu, and self-esteem. In this chapter self-esteem theory is related first to theories of Merton and Sutherland and is then shown to complement later views (c.f., Wells, 1978; Hewitt, 1970). The basic argument is that deviance is highly dependent on social milieu, as noted by differential association, subcultural and other theories, but that certain forms of deviance, especially those that appear self-destructive (such as substance abuse), are due to and exacerbated by low self-esteem. Forms of deviance are learned from social interaction, but the meaning and extent of specific patterns are mediated by conceptions of self. For example, among some groups, use of alcohol or marijuana is normatively expected, but alcoholism or excessive, multiple drug use in which a person becomes dependent on the drug is not normal and may represent low self-esteem. The important point is that the *legitimacy* of the behavior is not the key but rather whether the behavior is extreme or abnormal *given the social milieu*. It may not always be clear to an observer whether some particular behavior is determined by milieu or by low self-esteem; the subjective meaning, which may only come out in discussion or therapy, is what is relevant.

Anomie

The most widespread and best known approach to deviance by sociologists is anomie theory. Developed by Durkheim to explain some of the deleterious consequences of industrialization, it was extensively revised and elaborated by Merton (1938). While Merton's version (as well as Durkheim's) has been amply criticized (especially Taylor et al., 1973: 105-109; Cohen, 1965), with modifications (Merton, 1957; Clinard, 1954) it persists as a major perspective (McCaghy, 1976; Cole and Zuckerman, 1964).

Merton's central proposition is that rates of deviance are the result of disjunctions between culturally determined goals and socially structured means; that is, when large segments of the population are excluded from access to the legitimate means of achieving the goals, we find high rates of deviance.

121

Although the theory is therefore a structural one, the focus is on individuals and their adoption of deviant behavior as a result of their being blocked from reaching desired goals through acceptable means. Individual adaptations may take one of four forms: (a) innovation, acceptance of the goals and rejection of legitimate means; (b) ritualism, rejection of the goals but continued use of legitimate means; (c) retreatism, rejection of both goals and means; and (d) rebellion, substitution of new goals and new means and rejection of the socially prescribed goals and means (Merton, 1957: 151-155). While the model should be applicable to any society, Merton's discussion is restricted almost entirely to the goal of the American Dream, material success, and assumes a general consensus on the goal (Merton, 1957: 146; McCaghy, 1976: 55).

Before turning to the principal problems with Merton's model, we note the important, although unelaborated, role of self-esteem and asso ciated concepts. Obviously, both Merton and Steffenhagen see human action as goal-directed behavior, following Weber's classic definition. Further, for Merton it is the social (or cultural) structure which sets goals and means and it is a person's position in the structure which determines the possible adaptation. Loosely, then, Merton's presentation of what happens on the social level parallels Steffenhagen's discussion of the intrapersonal process: goals are set in accordance with one's status and social milieu and failure to achieve those goals leads to "deviant" responses, illegitimate in the one case and pathological in the other.

Merton's typology, however, gives only vague clues as to the deviant adaptation to be chosen: illustrations, rather than detailed arguments, are presented. Innovation appears to be primarily a lower-class pattern[1] as this is the archetypal response of those denied access to legitimate means, while ritualism is characteristic of the middle-class bureaucrat who cannot make it to the top.[2] The social status of those who choose retreatism, however, is not at all clear, although the examples given are of types likely to suffer from low self-esteem: "psychotics, autists, pariahs, outcasts, vagrants, vagabonds, tramps, chronic drunkards and drug addicts" (Merton, 1957). Ritualism and retreatism obviously involve low self-esteem as the dynamic: persons of both types have given up hope of "making it" in society. The ritualist persists in going through the motions, compensating for low self-esteem by sticking to the "book" (lacking "flexibility"—Steffenhagen, "A Model" Ch. 5) and perhaps acting as a little god, much as the addict of alcohol or heroin turns to drugs to compensate for feeling bad about the self (Steffenhagen, 1974). From the point of view of self-esteem theory, the addict is someone who has turned to drugs due to social milieu but who abuses their use because of low self-esteem (Steffenhagen, 1974, 1978).

With respect to innovation, a social group which is systematically deprived of legitimate means to achieve its goals may well develop high rates of low self-esteem. Goals which are realistic for more advantaged members of society, and which may be presented as goals suitable for all by the media and other ideological organs of dominant members, will be unrealistic (godlike) for members of the deprived group. It is not assumed that all members of the group will develop low self-esteem, but only that self-esteem is more prevalent and is caused by the "neglected" life-style (Steffenhagen, 1974). Furthermore, not all of the deviance observed in the lower classes of society is due to low self-esteem; much of it is a realistic response to life conditions, a point to which we shall return.

In the case of rebellion more serious problems appear. It has been noted (McCaghy, 1976) that this category does not really fit the typology for it represents a substitution of *new* goals and means which, while not legitimate according to the dominant value system, are legitimate for the group(s) adopting the new values. Furthermore, it is very difficult in practice to tell whether given behavior is rebellion or innovation, even when the actors involved are questioned. Even some groups which might be classified retreatists may be rebels, such as the "hippies" of the late sixties.

Self-esteem theory alone cannot make the choice, for the source of *either* innovation or rebellion, as determined by the social analyst, might be low self-esteem. Merton suggests that rebellion introduces a new social structure, the cultural standards in which success would modify and provide for a closer relationship between merit, effort and reward, (1957; 55), making it sound as though the rebel is really a super-conformist introducing a meritocracy that would be the achievement of the ideals of the American Dream rather than its reality. From a larger perspective, however, Merton seems to be hinting at the possibility of more than one viable value system while maintaining the untenable view that there is a value consensus in American (or every) society.

This contradiction brings us to what are probably the two most serious criticisms of Merton's theory: its assumption of a single value system and its tacit assumption that official rates of deviance reflect true rates of adherence and nonadherence to legitimate values. Not only does Merton's presentation fail to indicate clearly the causal factors leading to one or another of the deviant choices, but it also makes the highly debatable assumption that a complex, industrial society has generally agreed upon goals. While Merton does note a basic cleavage in our society between the haves and the have-nots, he conceals this within the notion of a cultural-social "disjunction," a defect which can be remedied without basic change in the system. Since the assumption of value consensus underlies the dominant theoretical approach of American sociology, it probably contributed to the theory's attraction and persistence. Further, the theory tends to accept uncritically official rates of deviance and thus over-predicts lower-class deviance and under- predicts middle and upper-class deviance (Taylor et al, 1973) as do most American deviance theories.[3]

A final flaw in anomie theory is its mechanical nature, the failure to consider process and the interaction of the actor with his or his milieu (Taylor et al, 1973). The tendency to regard the actor as passive and the deviant response as automatic, given blocked avenues to success, also leads to lack of consideration for negotiated and collective responses to the problems faced by many people in similar social situations. Self-esteem theory, on the other hand, is a theory based on process and milieu-actor interaction. It assumes flexibility in the actions of people in the same social statuses such that those with low self-esteem will react differently from those with high self-esteem. More important in this regard, self-esteem is a variable: variations in self-esteem are expected from person to person and within persons over time. While low self-esteem may be in part self-reinforcing, especially given continual or frequent social stress, a person's experiences can raise as well as lower views of self.

Differential Associations

While Merton takes account of social milieu on a very general level, he ignores it on a more micro level. The theory which most directly treats social milieu is Sutherland's theory of differential association (1939), which draws on the observations of the Chicago School that different areas of the city and different social groups, not necessarily hierarchically ordered, are characterized by different rates of deviance (Shaw et al., 1929; Shaw and McKay, 1942).4

The core of differential association theory is that deviance is learned in the same way that conventional behavior is learned, in a process of interaction with others. Sutherland rejects the assumption of value consensus and notes that different groups in society have differing values. In contrast to anomie theory, the actor does not turn to deviance through frustration but because it is a part of the social environment. It is quite possible, according to Sutherland's discussion, to be a "normal deviant," someone without pathology who just happens to have learned different values from those of the dominant culture. In order to address the argument that the actor appears to be a passive calculator, merely counting the volume of deviant and non-deviant interactions (Box, 1971), Sutherland postulated that associations vary in intensity, frequency, duration, and priority (Sutherland and Cressey, 1974). That is, deviant interactions which occur early in one's life, often, for long periods of time and in primary-group situations, are the most influential. Thus therapists or policemen, who interact frequently with deviants, do not themselves become deviant.

These arguments are consistent with the emphasis on social milieu and goals in self-esteem theory. However, there are at least two interrelated problems with this formulation. One is that it does not appear to give the actor much choice or volition: he or she is purely the product of outside inputs (Box, 1971). We will return to this issue in detail in the discussion of labelling theory. A related issue is whether this theory can explain the existence of a deviant in the midst of non-deviants or the "straight kid" in a high delinquency neighborhood. Self-esteem theory suggests that the deviant in a non-deviant group is a person with low self-esteem, for whom the deviance serves as a coping mechanism, while the non-deviant in the midst of deviants may have particularly high self-esteem. In either case, it is clear that more than simple accounting of deviant and non-deviant interpersonal interactions is involved. Glaser (1956) introduces the concept of symbolic interaction, a view he calls "differential identification." People are not restricted to the values and attitudes of those with whom they directly interact but are exposed to roles outside their own experience with which they may identify. In a heterogeneous society such as ours there is a wide variety of role models or culture heroes from which to choose, both deviant and not, and self-esteem influences which are chosen.

Since life's pressures are more difficult for a person with low self-esteem, he or she is more likely to feel inadequate and to look for alternatives which provide gratification and help maintain fragile self-esteem. For example, the use of illegal drugs forces both normal and neurotic users into contact with more deviant persons who supply both the drugs and positive evaluations of their use (McCann et al., 1977). The abuser is particularly likely to become deeply involved with such a deviant group, increasing his or her level of deviance.

Subcultural Theory

Subcultural theories are an attempt to avoid some of the weakness of anomie and differential association by combining the strengths of both traditions. The two best known examples are Cohen's subcultural theory of juvenile delinquency (1955) and Cloward and Ohlin's theory of "differential opportunity" (1960). Both focus on collective responses to problems caused by the system. Cohen comes very close to explicit use of self-esteem in characterizing the problems of working class boys trying to succeed in a typical classroom setting. Unable to compete on equal terms with middle class youth, the lower class boy needs alternative ways to achieve goals and satisfy his need for self worth. Such an outlet is provided by the existence of a lower class youth gang culture which emphasizes goals that the boy can achieve and which can, therefore, lead to improvements in self-esteem, at least while he is in the group. Much as in Merton's theory, lower class youth are frustrated in their attempts to achieve the legitimate goals of society (school) and so turn to deviance. In addition, Cohen's theory provides an explanation for the particular type of deviance which results. He argues that the delinquent sub-culture has developed norms as a group solution to a common problem. The particular norms which he sees as guiding gang behavior are a rejection of the dominant norms of middle class society: they are nonutilitarian, a classic example of Merton's rebellion pattern. Low self-esteem clearly plays a part: in a society such as ours, which emphasizes performance and production, the "easy way out" will minimize production, leading to either the toughness, vandalism and drugs of youth gangs or the tranquilizers and alcohol of others.

Cloward and Ohlin (1960) develop their theory of differential opportunity along similar lines. Explicitly relying on Merton and Sutherland, they posit not only differential access to legitimate means but also differential access to illegitimate ones. Thus one can fail in either legitimate society, deviant society or both. The retreatist is a failure in both.

Structural factors and self-esteem are important and differentiated in both worlds, leading to an explanation for the well-known pattern (difficult to explain for Merton or Cohen) of many fewer adult criminals than juvenile delinquents. Whether we view delinquency as innovation or rebellion, some of those involved have or may develop high self-esteem. Those with high self-esteem may become successful criminals or non-criminals, depending on their contacts, while those with less self-esteem may turn to retreatism or become the less successful criminals who populate our prisons. In our experience, low self-esteem of prison inmates is commonplace, as are their problems with alcohol, other drugs and lack of education. Middle and upper class delinquents, who are much more prevalent than most of the literature indicates (Gold, 1970), may either become "useful citizens" (high self-esteem) or turn to alcohol, excessive use of legitimate drugs (particularly prevalent among doctors), child abuse, or corporate crime. The relative roles of milieu and esteem can only be unravelled through discovery of the subjective meanings of action.

Labelling, Social Reaction

In spite of advances over earlier theories, subcultural theories still tend to assume a single dominant value system and, as in Cloward and Ohlin's theory, a single deviant culture (Taylor et al., 1973: 134- 136). Further, they continue to treat the actors as passive, desiring to succeed in the legitimate world and turning to deviance mechanically when blocked. Labelling theory begins with a radical attack on the very conception of rules and deviance of the other theories. Labelling theorists argue that no given act is inherently deviant, it becomes deviant only by virtue of social constrictions placed upon it (Becker,1963; Erikson,1962; Schur,1971). Therefore, in a sense, societies and groups create deviance by creating rules.[5] Further, the mere breaking of rules (all rules, not just criminal laws) does not constitute "true" deviance, deviance only occurs when there is a societal reaction, the application of the label, deviant, to an "offender" (Becker, 1963). We all break rules but only some rule breaking and some rule breakers get labelled. Consequently, an important area for study according to the labelling approach is the processes of rule creation and rule application. Unfortunately, labellists have contributed few such studies (Erikson, 1966; Becker, 1963).

The actual focus of labelling theorists is the effect of labelling on people and the interaction between the labelled person and those around him. For this purpose Becker introduced the notion of "career deviance" (1963) and Lemert the distinction between "primary" deviance, which is frequent, normal, and unproblematic, and "secondary" deviance, which is an adjustment to problems caused by social reaction (1951). Taking their cue from Mead's conception of the development of the self, they look upon the development of a deviant self-identity as the result of the application of a deviant label by society and the reaction to that labelling by the rule breaker[6] (Lemert, 1951). One or even several acts of rule breaking do not make a deviant. Even being labelled a deviant does not automatically produce secondary deviance; acquiring a deviant self-identity is a process which may be successfully resisted at many points. Deviant labels, nevertheless, have several qualities which make such a consequence difficult to avoid, and labellists are fond of noting that applying deviant labels often has the paradoxical (since sanctioning deviance is intended to deter it) result of increasing deviance by making deviants out of rule breakers.

Primary among these qualities are stereotyping, generalizing, and stigmatizing (Goffman, 1963). Deviant labels are stereotypes, as are other social labels. They are categories which tell us how to react and interact with their bearers. Further, they tend to be generalized: we think of someone as a "criminal" or as "crazy," rather than as someone who has stolen a pocketbook or who sometimes hears voices. This generalizing characteristic is even embedded in the law. For example, a typical restriction on a parolee is that s/he cannot possess a gun, although the crime committed may have been check forgery or possession of cocaine; that is, the person is relegated to the category of "criminals." Even more serious is the stigmatizing quality, which is a major difference between deviant labels and others, for it is the stigma that is difficult to escape and which leads to defensive reactions.

As the person gets labelled, then, others react to the label, rather than the person. Since self-concept is created from interaction with significant others, the actor comes to see him or herself as a deviant. Others expect deviant behavior from a deviant and, consequently, the deviant does also. Since the label generalizes, the deviant generalizes his or her deviant behavior, associates with other deviants and engages in a wider variety of rule breaking. Once the person has been labelled, rule breaking is much more likely to be observed and to be labelled deviance.

In this process self-esteem has a major role, as do social milieu, goals, and status. Clearly, one's social milieu affects the probability of rule breaking and of consequent labelling. Social status also plays a major role in the type of rule breaking in which a person engages and in the likelihood of receiving a deviant label: in general, the higher the status, the less likelihood of being labelled deviant and the less deleterious the consequences. Self-esteem has the most important role in the production of secondary deviance, being closely related to self-concept. A person with high self-esteem who finds deviant behavior enjoyable and non-troubling is likely to continue his or her behavior in the face of efforts to bring it into line with dominant values. On the other hand, someone with low self-esteem is less able to resist the process of public labelling than someone with high self-esteem. Furthermore, since many deviant patterns are less demanding and are developed to solve social problems, it is rewarding for the person with low self-esteem to adjust his or her goals and turn to such avenues to self-enhancement (Steffenhagen, 1974).

Given a desire to "escape" the deviant identity, particularly criminal identities, a task which is often very difficult, the person with high self-esteem will find it easier to get rid of the stigmatizing label (Schur, 1971) and adopt a more conventional life-style. For example, there is evidence (cited in chapter above) that persons with high self-esteem who have used heroin due to its availability and to social pressure (e.g., soldiers in Vietnam) find it relatively easy to break the habit when it is no longer appropriate. A newly released prisoner with low self-esteem will find it very difficult to choose conventional, reasonable goals and to avoid "falling-in" with his old group and behavior patterns which led him/her to prison in the first place, while one with high self-esteem can more easily overcome the label and hold a "respectable job."

Clearly, then, from the perspective of labelling theory, self-esteem is of paramount importance. It can affect the tendency and the ability to avoid deviant labels and it can affect the ease with which one can escape such labels once they have been successfully applied.

Labelling theory adds new dimensions to our understanding of deviance, especially non-criminal deviance, where rules are not as clear-cut as in legal violations. It sensitizes us to the negotiability of rules, the ubiquity of rule breaking and the perniciousness of labelling; and it treats the actor as an actor rather than just a mechanical responder to outside forces. On the other hand, there are several ways in which it does not live up to its promise. (a) As noted above, although labelling theorists see rule creation as problematic, they provide almost no treatment of the process and social factors involved. (b) With their focus on secondary and career deviance, labellists tend to ignore primary rule breaking, that is, they do not treat the sources and patterns of rule breaking, whch is the primary concern of most investigations into deviance.[7] (c) There is serious question as to whether social reaction is either a necessary or a sufficient condition for the development of secodary or career deviance (Mankoff, 1971: 205; Box, 1971: 230-251; Irwin and Cressey, 1962). (d) Although particular acts are not inherently deviant, people generally do know when they are breaking rules.

In fact, deviants often develop "vocabularies of motives" (Mills, 1940) to justify their actions (Steffenhagen, 1974: 244). One response is to blame others. In a well known article Sykes and Matza (1957) elaborate five "techniques of neutralization" used by juvenile delinquents to justify their behavior, which they know is illegal. It is important to note that these are not mere rationalizations or *ex post facto* excuses; they are incorporated into the subculture of the delinquent and serve to neutralize social control mechanisms, including attempts to label them. Some prisoners claim to break the law to symbolize their rejection of the oppressive "privilege system" (Krisberg, 1975). At the other end of the stratification system, a defendant in the TVA electrical conspiracy case stated that they all knew that their meetings were illegal but felt that this was the only way to run a business in a system of "free enterprise" (Fuller, 1962).

Conflict theory

In recognition of the questionable status of the assumption that American (and other industrial) society is of a piece, with one value system to which we all subscribe, and of the obvious cleavages and differences among us, sociologists have recently begun to turn to theories of deviance in which deviance is seen to result, at least in part, from varying and conflicting groups and norms. It is convenient to divide conflict theorists into two types, one of which I call "general" or "random," and the other Marxian. The former sees that deviance may result from conflict between groups (Sellin, 1938; Turk, 1969; Vold, 1958) but does not see conflict as inherent in society. It is obvious that there are areas of conflict in society and deviance is often a result, but as with Merton's theory, deviance is viewed as the result of small remediable imperfections in the body social and in terms of a single dominate value system. Vold (1958), for example, sees only a few situations in which deviance arises from intergroup conflict: labor strife, war, and social protest. He notes that labor strife results in illegal activity, such as violence by both sides, but does not raise issues of the legitimacy of power or values. Sellin goes further and recognizes that some rule breaking stems from disagreements on values as groups compete, but does not see this as a systemic problem. Except for the explicit consideration of conflict, these observations add little to the discoveries of cultural differences within the city (Shaw and McKay, 1942).

The Marxian analysts, on the other hand, following Marx, regard conflict as essential in capitalist (and most preceding) societies. The basic underpinnings of the Marxian approach are the method of historical materialism,[8] and the focus on class struggle. Historical materialism means that concrete historical events must be taken into account and that the primary causal force in history is the material (economic) conditions of life in each historical epoch. The emphasis on class struggle implies that a conflict between a dominant or ruling group and a dominated group underlies all major social processes. For the purpose of explaining deviance in capitalist society, these assumptions imply that the causes lie in the historical development of capitalism and the forces involved in the struggle between the dominant capitalist class and the dominated working class. The material basis of capitalist society is the existence of private property, the driving force is profit, and the struggle centers around ownership (control) of the means of production of commodities (food, clothing, shelter, and all other goods produced for *exchange*). Capitalists are seen as owning the means of production and workers as owning only their labor power, which they are forced to sell to the capitalists in order to survive. Profit, it is argued, comes from the labor of the workers used to produce goods. Thus, in its most simplified form, the class struggle centers on profit: the capitalists must increase their profit, and this can only come at the expense of the workers since it varies inversely with their wages.

Marxian theorists take seriously the observations of the labelling theorists that rules create deviance, that rule breaking is ubiquitous, and that it is important to look at the societal reaction to rule breaking. Thus, an examination of laws, their history, their creation, and their function is a major concern (Balbus, 1973; Chambliss, 1964; Chambliss and Seidman, 1971; Kennedy, 1970; Piven and Cloward, 1971). Law is created by the powerful and its function is to protect the powerful. In capitalist society that means it functions to protect private property and the position of the capitalist class (Quinney, 1974). One way is to create the myth that we are all equal before the law. Historically, it was important to establish the principle of equality in order to bring the aristocracy under the same law as the rising bourgeoisie and to provide for free competition (Balbus, 1973). However, given the principle of legal equality and the reality of extreme inequality of resources, the result is oppressive as the law in its indifference maintains the inequality (Balbus, 1973).

Second, the law serves the interests of the capitalist class through unequal treatment of typical forms of rule breaking by the bourgeoisie (capitalists) and proletariat (workers). Examples abound of discrepancies in treatment: long prison sentences for minor crimes, such as smoking marijauna (there are people serving 15 years or more in Texas) or stealing small amounts of money (people have been imprisoned for stealing as little as one steak and the Supreme Court has ruled that it is constitutional to imprison someone for life as an "habitual offender" after being convicted three times for stealing less than $100), compared to relatively small fines (a few $1000's) for corporate crimes (such as pollution or price-fixing) involving millions of dollars. Probably the best known example of the latter is the electrical conspiracy case, referred to above, in which the largest 29 electrical equipment companies (including General Electric and Westinghouse) were convicted of price-fixing and conspiracy which resulted in a loss of more than $1 billion to the government — the people — over a ten year period. The corporations were fined a total of $1.8 million — one-tenth of a cent on the dollar — and the IRS allowed them to deduct it from their income as part of the ordinary expenses of doing business. In an unprecedented move, seven executives were sentenced to prison — for 30 days (Smith, 1961; Geis, 1968).

While the examples are striking, the more trenchant observation is that the law itself is unequally structured. The crimes which working- class people are driven to, those which anomie and subcultural theory are aimed at, are heavily penalized and stigmatized. They are the seven crimes which make up the FBI's Index of *Serious* Crime (emphasis added): murder, rape, robbery, assault, burglary, larceny, and auto theft. While some of these are violent (the first four), Marxists argue that there are crimes committed by large corporations equally as violent but which are typically not even treated as crimes: cars (Pinto) and tires (Firestone) which kill, industrial "accidents" which are preventable and which result from safety violations which continue even after they have been cited by Federal inspectors. As for the economic crimes, it is extremely difficult to get data on upper class crime; but Senator Hart estimated in 1970 that the public wasted approximately $200 billion on worthless goods or services, including $45 billion due to monopolistic price-fixing, many times more than all the Index crimes combined, and another $14 billion due to deceptive grocery labelling (Hart, 1970). The point is that rule breaking by those at the top is commonly treated as a civil violation for which consent agreements (an agreement to stop doing what you do not even have to admit that you were doing) or small fines are the rule, — a "tax" for stealing (Kennedy, 1970).

A third way that the law and the criminal justice system as a whole promotes bourgeois interests is by differentially applying deviant labels. The poor end up stigmatized as "criminal" while the rich get away with murder. And the ideological structure is such that the public is agitated about "crime in the streets" and apathetic about crime in the suites. Like the myth of equality, this is an example of what Marxists call "false consciousness." Furthermore, we are taught through the media and other propaganda organs of the state that criminals are violent (stigma) and dangerous, although most crimes do not involve violence and the most violent crime, murder, is most often committed by friends and relatives of the victims. The power to make laws is a key factor in the ability to escape deviant labels (Krisberg, 1975).

Marxist theorists obviously agree with anomie and subcultural theories that deviance occurs as a result of disjunctions within our society, but again they take the analysis much further and much deeper. They make it clear that the "disjunctions" are not small, remediable imperfections in an otherwise perfectly functioning whole, but that they reflect the basic schism in capitalist society between the owners of the means of production and those who own only their power to labor (which they must "rent" to capitalists). It is not an accident that some groups are "systematically" excluded from access to the means to achieve "agreed upon goals." First of all, the goals are those set by the ruling class, and can only be *dreamed of* by the mass of citizens (i.e. they are "godlike"). Second, by erecting artificial barriers to access, the ruling class is able to keep sectors of the population in a position where they find great difficulty finding work, which helps to depress the wages of all workers.

As a result, certain sectors of the population are forced by the system to engage in deviant economic behavior in order to survive, and these types of behavior are heavily sanctioned (Krisberg, 1975; Gordon, 1971). It is obvious that a businessman or a professional does not need to resort to burglary or robbery to obtain enough money to live a comfortable life. Nor does he need to resort to "street violence" in order to attain mastery over others or to boost his self-esteem since he can do so quite legally in his job. It is perfectly legal in our society to close a factory and lay off several thousand workers if profits are not high enough, but the laid off worker cannot legally turn out the owner(s) or take their property. Marxists are almost alone in trying to go beyond official statistics, although most criminologists are aware of the many defects of official crime statistics.

While other theorists note the existence of criminal behavior by upper class and middle class persons — white collar crime in Sutherland's description — they seldom pay much attention to it and their explanations of deviant behavior do not account for it (Liazos, 1972; Mills, 1943; Thio, 1973). Marxian analysts on the other hand are more likely to expose and discuss the crimes and non-criminal deviance of the upper classes (Gold, 1970) and to make an explanation of such deviance an integral part of their theory (Krisberg, 1975; Quinney, 1974). It is necessary to go beyond legalism and consider *harm to people* and who benefits in order to come to a full understanding of the process of deviance.

Self-esteem theory meshes well with the Marxist approach. Since self-esteem theory was not developed on the basis of official statistics on working-class criminality but from the analysis of middle-class pathology—drug abuse, alcoholism, problems with grades, the pampered lifestyle—its explanations complement Marxist ones and can be applied to upper- as well as lower-class deviance. Status, social milieu, goals, and self-esteem are all important for Marxist as well as self- esteem theory. One of the consequences of the structure of stigmatizing by criminal law is to contribute to the low self-esteem of the lower class, both as individuals and as a group. On the individual level we have seen how difficult it is for a lower class person to set attainable goals that meet bourgeois standards. Furthermore, social milieu is important, for the working class is bound to develop less respect, even active disrespect, for the law as a result of its position in society and, thus, produce a larger proportion of deviants, deviant values and deviant goals (as officially defined) than those groups which are the beneficiaries of society's wealth. Self-esteem also plays a part at the group level for, under capitalism, an entire class is stigmatized. The criminal "justice" process serves to discredit entire groups of people for both harmful and non-harmful acts. But the stigmatization is even more general. We learn that Blacks and members of other minority groups, if not all lower class people in general, are violent and dangerous, that welfare recipients are promiscuous, lazy cheats, that antiwar activists are dangerous revolutionaries agitating for mass riots, that marijuana users are crazed incipient heroin addicts. These stereotypes, together with the legal soft-pedaling of harmful upper class behavior, serve to keep the lower classes in a subordinate position (Piven and Cloward, 1971). Lower self-esteem also helps maintain divisions and "false consciousness" within the working-class: one group can maintain a fragile self-concept by denigrating another. Such action helps depress wages, increase profits, and maintain the dominant legal and moral positon of the ruling class.

Not all deviance within the lower class perpetuates low self-esteem, however. In contrast to the views of labelling theorists, Taylor et al. (1973) point out that, in the face of a demeaning and oppressive social structure, deviance (in the eyes of the dominant class) may result in a gain in self-esteem because it may lead to a measure of control: the opportunity to set meaningful, realistic goals, such as a strike or a demonstration.

There is evidence that among the middle and upper classes deviant behavior is not uncommon (Gold, 1970; McCaghy, 1976), which supports the observation of labellers that we are all "rule breakers," although we are not all labelled as deviant. Part of the reason for the deviance of the corporate class is, of course, the social milieu and status: being rulers they do not see their behavior as deviant. The primary justification is that it is in the interests of profit and that a business cannot compete successfully if it does not engage in price-fixing, shoddy design, misleading advertising, and other "sharp" business practices

(McCaghy, 1976).

While much of this behavior is "normal" for corporate executives, attributable to the status, social milieu and typical lifestyle of the corporate ruling class, extreme examples may well be due in part to low self-esteem. For this group low self-esteem probably results primarily from the "pampered" lifestyle and the development of godlike goals which can never be satisfied. (Steffenhagen, this book, Chapter 4). As Merton (1957) observed regarding aspirations in our materialistic society, the American Dream encourages godlike, unattainable goals within its ruling class, which helps explain behaviors which lie outside the normal bounds of corporate perfidy, such as wife-beating, child abuse, alcoholism, drug abuse by doctors, abuse of subordinates and extreme forms of sexism, ageism, and racism. Analogous to the distinction between drug use and *abuse*, we can distinguish between the normal discrimination and prejudice of the capitalist class, which contribute to the dominance of that class by perpetuating the "reserve army of labor,"[10] and extreme examples due to personal inadequacy. Of course the capitalist class, as a group, increases its esteem at the expense of the working-class as a group.

A Model

Now that we have briefly reviewed the major contributions of the sociological theories of deviance and the place of self-esteem within each of these theories, we shall sketch a model combining self-esteem theory, which provides a psychological dynamic, with the social explanations of the deviance theories we have considered.

Steffenhagen's self-esteem theory argues that a person's social milieu determines the kinds of behaviors to which a person is exposed and, therefore, the types of deviant patterns in which s/he is likely to engage. From an early age, a person develops a lifestyle which is in part a product of the goals set and success or failure in reaching those goals. This is a very complex process due to the variety of social milieux available. The most influential are the family and, later, the peer group. But there is the additional possibility of identification with many groups: through the media there is an extensive presentation of stereotypes, both deviant and not, in accordance with the dominant ideology. Due to the complexity of society, a person interacts, however fleetingly, with a range of groups, values, and subcultures, some of which are in conflict with the values of the dominant class.

What self-esteem theory gains from the sociological theories is more structure. Instead of a vague notion of social milieu, it is now clear that the social environment, although flexible, is highly structured. There are characteristic patterns of conformity and deviance for each class. Although the values of the dominant class are primary and are supported by the structure of the law, the power of the state, and the manipulation of the media, conflicting goals and values abound.

Those at the bottom of the structure are more likely to develop low self-esteem due to oppression and "neglect," while those higher in the social scale develop low self-esteem primarily due to a "pampered" lifestyle. The direction in which low self-esteem will lead, as well as the basic causes and directions of deviance, is strongly related to social structure. Low self-esteem, which can be the product of either neglected or pampered lifestyle is crucial in determining how likely certain patterns are to be engaged in, what alternative group associations a person will look for when trying to establish and meet goals, and whether or not the person will engage in *abusive* patterns, that is, patterns which deprive him or her of a desired lifestyle.

A good example of such abusive behavior, and the historical starting point for the development of the theory as applied to deviance, is the use of drugs. In their studies of drug behavior, Steffenhagen and associates realized that they had to distinguish between drug *users* and drug *abusers* within certain cultural groups (Steffenhagen, 1974). In particular, among college students, the use of marijuana was relatively common and users showed no pathology relative to non-users, whereas polydrug users and heavy users of strong drugs were found to be distinguishable from both users and non-users (Steffenhagen et al., 1969, 1971; McAree et al. 1972). The difference was found to relate to—and was possibly caused by—low self-esteem (Steffenhagen, 1974). Thus, given the presence of deviant patterns in the milieu, particularly patterns which represent an "easy way out," the person with low self-esteem is most likely to adopt those patterns, to persist in them even in the face of pressure both from within (desires to stop) and without.

This argument is reinforced by observation of prisoners in community correctional centers, who typically exhibit both objective and subjective signs of low self-esteem (Bennet, 1974). They tend to be from the lower rungs of society and to have had relatively deprived childhoods. They are typically poorly educated, so that one of the major "rehabilitation" programs of the institutions is tutoring for a high school equivalency degree. Many of the inmates also have alcohol and other drug *problems* (abuse) which are clearly related to their deviance, their tendency to "get in trouble."

On the other hand, high self-esteem may also lead to deviance if the society is oppressive or stressful enough. A possible example might be anti-war and counterculture people of the 1960's.[11] As respectable middle class youth (and a few elders) saw the hypocrisy and oppressiveness of the law and the rulers of society, they came to have less respect for the law. When they engaged in presumably constitutionally protected behavior such as mass demonstration, they learned that such behavior would not be tolerated by the ruling class (Lefcourt 1971; Kirsberg 1976: 46). When they came into close contact with illicit drugs and found that the prevailing official "line" on those drugs was misleading and unrealistic, their contempt for law increased. Many chose deviant labels willingly. When the drugs of the rulers—alcohol, valium, cigarettes—are highly promoted in spite of well documented harmful effects, while those of the outsiders—marijuana and LSD—are severely repressed with less documentation of harmful effects, it becomes evident that the law is a tool of the oppressors to subjugate the powerless—youth or the poor.

Finally, we must keep in mind that, while low self-esteem is seen as the psychological dynamic in certain types of deviance, it does not account for many other types of deviance. For example, the successful professional thief or organized crime figure, the drug user who is satisfied, performs his/her job satisfactorily, and uses drugs merely for creative mood altering. Even the heroin user who uses due to peer pressure or curiosity and who stops before it becomes a personal problem must be distinguished from the addict who cannot break the habit even though s/he wishes to do so.

Thus there is agreement with the labelling and conflict theorists that any given behavior pattern is not *per se* deviant or a sign of a low self-esteem person, but that meanings of acts are dependent on social definitions and conflicts among groups.

In sum, self-esteem theory adds a psychological dynamic to social structural theories of deviance that helps account both for deviance on a large scale or by groups and for deviant individuals who seem to violate the norms of their associates as well as those of the dominant class. It makes clear that many violations of legal norms are *not* due to pathology but are normatively guided responses to life situations. Self-esteem theory is particularly strong in explaining forms of middle and upper class deviance, which have been neglected by sociologists until very recently. Combined with structural theory self-esteem theory, can be *predictive*: given a social milieu and the knowledge that someone has low self-esteem, the pattern of deviance may well be clear. Finally, if self-esteem theory is correct, then therapy can change that predicted behavior and many undesirable (to the victim) patterns of deviance can be reduced.

Footnotes

1. Innovation can also be seen in the practices of those at top, such as the corporations involved in the "Great Electrical Conspiracy" (Smith, 1961; Geis, 1968), but upper class deviance is generally ignored by Merton and most other deviance theorists as we shall see further below.
2. It is logically clear, on the other hand, that the ritualist cannot come from a segment of the population that is systematically excluded from access to legitimate means and so would seem to contradict the theory. At this point, however, Merton relies on a more general version, harking back directly to Durkheim's concept of anomie, in which the American Dream tends to produce unlimited aspirations (Merton, 1957: 157; Taylor et al., 1973: 93), analogous to Adler's "godlike" goals (Steffenhagen, 1974: 248; Adler, 1956: 245).
3. While most deviance theorists and texts are aware of the many problems and defects of official statistics (McCaghy, 1976: 56- 57; Cohen, 1966),

they continue to focus on lower-class crime and ignore the prevalence of crime in other classes (Erikson, 1973; Gold, 1970; Lerman, 1967). This issue is raised most cogently by labelling and Marxist theorists.

4. The Chicago School also took official rates as given and therefore concentrated on explaining working-class deviance. Sutherland, on the other hand, was the first to seriously consider the criminality of the middle and upper classes (1949).

5. This basic assumption of labelling theory has been severely criticized (Taylor et al., 1973: 145-149; Gibbs, 1966; Akers, 1968). It is based on the observation that particular acts may be legal or illegal (or weird or normal) in different contexts, at different points in time, and from place to place. Typical examples are the killing of another human (a) in an argument, (b) by a policeman, (c) or in war; or prohibition and blue laws. The problem is that people are usually aware of the context of their acts: they know whether or not they are breaking rules, the knowledge does not occur as a result of a subsequent reaction, except perhaps in cases of more subtle forms of rule breaking such as mental illness or "weird" behavior. Furthermore the creation of a deviant category by "society" does not necessarily mean that any person will engage in behavior fitting that category.

6. It should be clear, of course, that mistakes can be made and a person may become labelled without breaking any rules. Becker also discusses the "secret" deviant (1963: 20), but this category creates severe logical problems and the combination of the two possibilities casts serious doubt on the entire scheme (Gibbs, 1966).

7. Cohen (1965) has attempted to remedy this serious problem by combining an interactionist approach with anomie theory, about which Taylor et al. (1973) comment that it moves anomie away from the consensus model to one in which reaction becomes dependent on the particular views of agencies of social control. Mankoff (1971) makes similar arguments.

8. Another important aspect of Marxian method is dialectical analysis, the emphasis on contradictions in all existing social processes and structures. However, the deep and difficult issues raised by this aspect of Marxism are beyond the scope of this paper and not essential to its analysis.

9. The reader should understand that this is a very simplified argument, which I present only because Marxist analysis is only a small, though growing, part of sociology with which most sociologists are relatively unfamiliar. For a more thorough presentation, see Marx and Engels, *The Communist Manifesto* (— simplified and highly polemical); or, for the ambitious, Marx, *Capital* (1976, or any other edition). An excellent presentation of the theory applied to crime is Krisberg (1975).

10. Reserve army of labor is a Marxian concept which refers to the sectors of the labor force which are sporadically employed or who are being squeezed out of a stagnant sector of the economy, such as welfare recipients in the former case and agricultural workers in the latter. They are

held "in reserve" as a threat to employed workers to help keep wages down. Discrimination against women, Blacks and other minorities contributes to this threat (Krisberg, 1975).

11. Of course, as Steffenhagen argues (1974), some of those involved may have "dropped out" due to low self-esteem. The actual situation can only be determined by ascertaining the subjective meaning of the action.

References

1. Adler, Alfred, *The Individual Psychology of Alfred Adler*, (ed. by H.L. and R.R. Ansbacher). New York: Basic Books, 1956.

2. Akers, Ronald, Problems in the sociology of deviance: social definitions and behavior, *Social Forces* 46: 455-465 (June), 1968.

3. Balbus, Isaac, *The Dialectics of Legal Repression*. New York: Russell Sage, 1973.

4. Becker, Howard, *Outsiders: Studies in the Sociology of Deviance,*; New York: Free Press, 1963.

5. Bennett, L., The application of self-esteem during incarceration, *Journal of Research in Crime and Delinquency* 11: 9-15, 1974.

6. Box, Steven, *Deviance, Reality and Society*. London: Holt, Rinehart & Winston, 1971.

7. Chambliss, William and Robert Seidman, *Law, Order and Power*. Massachusetts: Addison-Wesley, 1971.

8. Clinard, Marshall (ed.), *Anomie and Deviant Behavior: A Discussion and Critique*. New York: Free Press, 1964.

9. Cloward, Richard and Lloyd Ohlin, *Delinquency and Opportunity: A Theory of Delinquent Gangs*. Chicago: Free Press, 1960. Cohen, Albert, *Delinquent Boys: The Culture of the Gang*. Chicago: Free Press, 1955.
   — The sociology of the deviant act: anomie theory and beyond, *American Sociological Review* 30 (1): 5-14, 1965.

10. Cole, Stephen and Harriet Zuckerman, An inventory of empirical and theoretical studies of anomie, in Clinard, 1964: 243-283.

11. Erikson, Kai, Notes on the sociology of deviance, *Social Problems* 9 (4): 307-314, 1962.
    — *Wayward Puritans: A Study of Deviance*. New York: Wiley, 1966.

12. Fuller, John, *The Gentlemen Conspirators*. New York: Grove Press, 1962.

13. Geis, Gilbert (ed.), *White-Collar Criminal: The Offender in Business and the Professions*. New York: Atherton, 1968.

14. Gibbs, Jack, Conceptions of deviant behavior: the old and the new, *Pacific Sociological Review* 9: 9-14 (Spring), 1966.

15. Glaser, Daniel, Criminality theories and behavioral images, *American Journal of Sociology* 61: 433-444, 1956.

16. Goffman, Erving, *Stigma: Notes on the Management of Spoiled Identity*.

Englewood Cliffs: Prentice-Hall, 1963. Gold, Martin, Undetected delinquent behavior, *Journal of Research on Crime and Delinquency* 13: 27-49, 1966.

— *Delinquent Behavior in an American City*. Belmont, Cal.: Wadsworth, 1970.

17. Gordon, David, Class and the economics of crime, *Review of Radical Political Economics* 3 (3): 51-75, 1971.

18. Hart, Philip, Congressional Consumer Investigations: What Do They Tell Us? Remarks to New York Consumer Assembly, March 7, 1970 (reported in McCaghy 1976), 1970.

19. Hewitt, John, *Social Stratification and Deviant Behavior*. New York: Random House, 1970.

20. Irwin, John and Donald Cressey, Thieves, convicts and the inmate culture, *Social Problems* 10 (2): 142-155 (Fall), 1962.

21. Kennedy, Mark, Beyond incrimination: some neglected facets in the theory of punishment, *Catalyst* 5: 1-37 (Summer), 1970.

22. Krisberg, Barry, *Crime and Privilege*. Englewood Cliffs: Prentice-Hall, 1975.

23. Lefcourt, Robert, *Law Against the People*. New York: Random House (Vintage), 1971. Lemert, Edwin, *Social Pathology*. New York: McGraw-Hill, 1951.

24. Lerman, Paul, Individual values, peer values, and subcultural delinquency, *American Sociological Review* 33: 219-235 (April), 1968.

25. Liazos, Alexander, The poverty of the sociology of deviance: nuts, sluts, and perverts, *Social Problems* 20: 103-120 (Summer), 1972.

26. McAree, C.P., R.A. Steffenhagen, and L.S. Zheutlin, Personality factors and patterns of drug use in college students, *American Journal of Psychiatry* 128: 890-893, 1972.

27. McCaghy, Charles, *Deviant Behavior: Crime, Conflict and Interest Groups*. New York: MacMillan, 1976.

28. McCann, H.G., R.A. Steffenhagen, and G. Merriam, Drug use: a model for a deviant sub-culture, *Journal of Alcohol and Drug Education* 23: 29-45, 1977.

29. Mankoff, Milton, Societal reaction and career deviance: a critical analysis, *Sociological Quarterly* 12: 200-210, 1971.

30. Marx, Karl, *Capital*. Vol I, New York: Random House (Vintage), 1976.

31. Merton, Robert, Social structure and anomie, *American Sociological Review* 3: 672-682, 1938. — *Social Theory and Social Structure* (Rev. Ed.). New York: Free Press, 1957.

32. Mills, C. Wright, Situated actions and vocabularies of motive, *American Sociological Review* 5: 904-913 (December), 1940.

— The professional ideology of soial pathologists, *American Journal of Sociology* 49 (2): 165-180 (September), 1943.

33. Piven, Francis and Richard Cloward, *Regulating the Poor*. New York:

Random House (Vintage), 1971.
34.Quinney, Richard, *Critique of Legal Order*. Boston: Little, Brown, 1974.
35.Schur, Edwin, *Labelling Deviant Behavior: its Sociological Implications*. New York: Random House, 1971.
36.Sellin, Thorstein, *Culture Conflict and Crime*. (Report of the Subcommittee on Delinquency of the Committee on Personality and Culture, Bulletin 41). New York: Social Science Research Council, 1938.
37.Shaw, Clifford and Henry McKay, *Juvenile Delinquency and Urban Areas*. Chicago: University of Chicago Press, 1942.
38.Shaw, Clifford et al., *Delinquency Areas*. Chicago: University of Chicago Press, 1929.
39.Smith, Richard, The incredible electrical conspiracy, *Fortune* 63 (April): 132-180; (May): 161-224, 1961.
40.Steffenhagen, Ronald, Drug abuse and related phenomena: an Adlerian approach, *Journal of Individual Psychology* 30: 238-250 (November), 1974.
   —An Adlerian approach toward a self-esteem theory of deviance: a drug abuse model, *Journal of Alcohol & Drug Education* 24: 1-13, 1978.
41.Steffenhagen, R.A., C.P. McAree and L.S. Zheutlin, Some social factors in college drug usage, *International Journal of Social Psychiatry* 15: 97-101, 1969.
42.Steffenhagen, R., F. Schmidt, and C. McAree, Emotional stability and student drug use, *Journal of Drug Education* 1: 347-357, 1971.
43.Sutherland, Edwin, *Principles of Criminology* (3rd Ed.). Philadelphia: J.B. Lippincott, 1939.
   —*White Collar Crime*. New York: Holt, Rinehart & Winston, 1949.
44.Sutherland, Edwin and Donald Cressey, *Criminology* (9th Ed.). Philadelphia: J. B. Lippincott, 1974.
45.Sykes, Gresham, and David Matza, Techniques of neutralization: a theory of delinquency, *American Sociological Review* 22: 664-670 (December), 1957.
46.Taylor, Ian, Paul Walton, and Jock Young, *The New Criminology: For a Social Theory of Deviance*. London: Routledge & Kegan Paul, 1973.
47.Thio, Alex, Class bias in the sociology of deviance, *American Sociologist* 8: 1-12 (February), 1973.
48.Turk, Austin, *Criminality and the Legal Order*. Chicago: Rand McNally, 1969.
49.Vold, George, *Theoretical Criminology*. New York: Oxford University Press, 1958.
50.Wells, L. Edward, Theories of deviance and the self-concept, *Social Psychology* 41 (3): 189-204, 1978.

CASE HISTORY: INTERMITTENT EXPLOSIVE DISORDER
AND SELF-ESTEEM
R. A. Steffenhagen

The following case history is a classic example of Intermittent Explosive Disorder as a result of low self-esteem and is offered in support of the theory presented in Chapter III. (312.34* Intermittent Explosive Disorder (American Psychiatric Assoc.)

This is a new diagnostic category for individuals who have recurrent and paroxysmal episodes of significant loss of control of aggressive impulses, that result in serious assault or destruction of property. The magnitude of the behavior during an episode is grossly out of proportion to any psychosocial stressors which may have played a role in eliciting the episodes of lack of control. The individual may describe the episodes as "spells" or "attacks." The symptoms appear within minutes or hours, and regardless of duration, remit almost as quickly. Following each episode, there is genuine regret or self-reproach at the consequences of the action and the inability to control the aggressive impulse. Between the episodes there are no signs of generalized impulsivity or aggressiveness . . .

Case 1 — I first came in contact with Tom in his third year in college. He is an upper middle-class white college male, 20 years of age. Tom had a long history of intermittent explosive behavior dating back to the period he spent in boarding school before college. This was further complicated by periods of depression and borderline suicidal behavior. An aborted attempted suicide was made while he was in boarding school. During his high school period he saw a psychiatrist once but no follow-up of any sort was made. When Tom came to me I saw him in an entirely different light than the way he felt about himself. I saw him as a very intelligent young man who, because of inner conflict, was unable to perform to either his expectations or his true capabilities. I saw him as a handsome young man manifesting all the social amenities, a fine considerate human being. On the social level, Tom was capable of handling himself adequately and admirably but because of his low self-esteem he tended to be shy and retiring.

Tom came to college and was perceptive enough to realize his need for counseling. He began a counseling situation in his freshman year which continued through his sophomore year. It is important to understand that this counseling situation was essential for Tom as he would not have been able to stay in college without its supportive nature. While the support system was essential in order for Tom to maintain a borderline equilibrium, it did nothing to alter the dynamics underlying the symptoms.

Tom is an only child who exemplified Adler's upper middle-class pampered lifestyle. Both parents were extremely bright professional people, successful in

---

*The International Classification of Diseases. 9th Revision Clinical Modification, ICD.9.CM.

the arts. His mother did everything to instill in Tom her interest and ability in the theater. She encouraged him to read Shakespeare at a very young age and to perform Shakespearean roles before friends in the home environment. Tom hated both the time spent studying and the social performances. It is reasonably safe to say that at this time Tom developed an intense dislike for reading which has continued to the present. He has always been shy, unobtrusive, well-mannered, and considerate.

Tom's father has always played a very important part in Tom's life as an ego-ideal role model. He is a very busy and successful artisan who works long hours and extended periods of time which has prevented him from spending much time with Tom. Tom looked forward with great anticipation to the periods he would spend with his father. Frequently, however, he was hurt when his father, due to his professional commitments, would renege on promises made. Tom developed compensatory mechanism whereby he learned never to look forward to anything; then, if it didn't happen, he couldn't be hurt. However, this contributed to an inner feeling of worthlessness: "If I were worth something then things would go well, but since nothing happens the way I want, the way I anticipate, the way I desire, then I must be worthless." His feelings of lack of trust in others also intensified: "I am not worth anything; why would anyone want to do anything for me?"

Tom is a very intelligent young man but, due to his intense feelings of worthlessness and low self-esteem, he has never performed adequately in the academic milieu. He has no faith in his own ability, a very low level of concentration and an inability to keep his interest focused on any one thing for any extended period of time. Because of the development of relatively high academic goals (due to his early conditioning) and the desire to perform well to please his father, his self-esteem has been further lowered.

Two forms of compensatory behavior have developed which have allowed Tom to function on a marginal level. One, because of a very high frustration level, he has resorted to an aggressive impulsivity accompanied by a major loss of control, which has resulted in a rather consistent destruction of property. When he became extremely frustrated, Tom would throw and smash things as a way of releasing his tremendous inner turmoil. These episodes were frequently grossly out of proportion to the psychosocial stressor and happened very frequently, sometimes as often as twice a week. This behavior began in high school and continued through the first two years of college. Between these episodes, there was no indication of any generalized impulsivity or aggressiveness; he appears to be a mild, easygoing young man. It should be noted that Tom had begun to fear that these episodes of uncontrolled behavior might eventually be directed towards a human being rather than mere property.

A second mechanism for dealing with these feelings of worthlessness was Tom's development of a rather active sexual life, in which he was able to internalize the "macho" image. His sexual activity began at an early age and he was very successful in his rather superficial sexual encounters through high school and into college. His sexual behavior served two functions: (a) this was an area in which he was successful, which gave him a rather superficial feeling of worth; and (b), it became a mechanism of communication. Because of the low self-esteem Tom never developed an ability to communicate on a deep intimate level with anyone of either sex. Thus, the behavioral mechanism became a means of communication but never served a deeper, inner purpose and further left him feeling inadequate.

It is important to realize that Tom's self-esteem was low on all three levels which have been posited in this theoretical framework. On the mental level his low self-concept was shown by his feeling of being intellectually inadequate, on the physical level his low self- image was revealed by his feeling of being unattractive, and on the cultural level, his low social concept was shown by the fact that sex was used as a means of communication rather than having deeper inner meaning.

Within the theoretical framework presented, it was necessary to first work with Tom on the level of self-esteem, which I did through hypno-therapy. Tom proved to be a good hypnotic subject and I was able to work on the deeper levels of the unconscious. We began by emphasizing the feelings of self-worth and concentrating on the academic problems since this was the area that he originally expressed as being of major concern. We stressed interest, concentration and relaxation. Tom, because of this impulsivity and low frustration tolerance, could not study for any protracted periods of time. Because of the tenseness and anxiety, he would fail examinations, and he commented frequently on the fact that his memory was good for past events but very poor for the more recent. This we can interpret as follows: since he is very intelligent and perceptive, he is acutely aware of things happening and can remember these. However, when it comes to studying, his memory is short-lived for two reasons: (a) he has very poor reading ability as a result of being forced to read at a very early age and (b) his resulting comprehension is very low. His memory for past events is fine because these events happen on the social level on which he is not under the stress of having to remember for an immediate response. His comprehension is low when anxiety causes mental blocks for immediate material. By emphasizing the interest in his academic subject matter and an increased ability for concentration and relaxation, we were able to show a rather marked improvement. In the area of the mental, we were able to show improvement in self-esteem from the second session.

We worked therapeutically from 1½ to 3 hours per week for two months, resulting in marked improvement. After several weeks of hypno therapy Tom made reference to the fact that there was something he wanted to tell me, something that was bothering him but which he never could seem to remember when he came to the office. The second time this was mentioned, I decided to use a dream technique in hypnotherapy to see if we could get at the underlying problem which was bothering him. This technique consisted of putting Tom into a hypnotic trance and then making the suggestion that at the count of three he would have a dream. In the dream the problem bothering him would present itself and he would wake up after the dream (which was manifested by REM activity). After about five minutes he awakened, saying that he was well aware of the things that were now bothering him. First, it became apparent that Tom wished to change his major and that the major he wished to enter would pose a problem because of his low academic performance and because it was in an area that could present a type of competition with his father. (It is important to realize that this can definitely be worked out through the therapeutic setting to allay the conflict of competition.) The second important area was what he expressed in the words "would this immediate situation have a good ending?" He seemed to be asking whether I would eventually reject him as he felt others in the past had. The third area was simply expressed as "that of girls," which involved interpersonal relations. On this level, he had a girlfriend who he thought had rejected him, a situation that further caused him anxiety. It is important to note that the area of interpersonal relations concerned his relationships with both men and women. These three concerns represented areas of tremendous anxiety which was evident in the session. Although it was necessary to see Tom again that evening because of the anxiety, this session was extremely valuable in that it brought into focus the three most important areas of concern for him and we were able to get them out into the open in one session rather than painfully bringing each one out through a nondirective, analytic technique.

I also used the deeper hypnotic technique of the suspension of the ego in an attempt to develop a foundation of a feeling of spiritual acceptance and worthfulness. Because Tom is a relatively good hypnotic subject, we were able to work on the deeper level from the second session on. It is important to note Tom's comment that after two sessions of hypnotherapy, we had accomplished more on the etiological level than the previous years of supportive counseling. However, this is not to minimize the importance of the supportive counseling because Tom never could have sustained himself in the college milieu without the support system.

From the time therapy began, Tom's aggressive, destructive behavior was held in check for eight weeks and during this time he did not engage in any destructive behavior. Just before the exam period I received a phone call in which he was extremely agitated and had just engaged in a violent outburst of behavior. It is important to realize, however, that this first manifestation of uncontrolled impulsivity had a dimension of control inherent within it. Although he was tremendously agitated and frustrated, he was able to ask rationally, "What can I throw and destroy which will not be too costly or too important?" The answer was a plastic jar full of pennies, and well constructed chairs which would not break. His behavior did not result in the destruction of anything important such as the hi-fi or the windows, but merely made a tremendous mess on the floor, and he was able to release a vast amount of pent-up anxiety. One can clearly see that this last form of destructive behavior had a dimension of the

Gestalt in it, in that it served the purpose of immediately releasing some of his frustration which needed to be released. The follow-up session was valuable in quieting him and bringing back into focus the values toward which we had been working.

As indicated, we made progress on the mental level from the second session. The next area in which progress was made was the cultural. The need for immediate sexual release became less important and the ability to communicate with both men and women became more apparent. This was partly expressed by Tom's commenting, "I don't feel as 'horny' as I used to, and it is more important to be able to talk to someone on an intellectual level."

The physical level was the last to show improvement. He would not even look in a mirror: when he shaved, he would actually only see the razor on one small portion of his face, indicating how low he was in this area. We started working on this area by looking at various parts of his body in perspective. He didn't like his nose, didn't like his teeth, and so on, but he did agree that his hair was "a good color." So we began to work with points: the hair is good, the eyes are bright and "a good color," his legs are good from jogging. As we put the pieces together, he could see that as a single package, it was "quite acceptable." In fact, others see him as handsome young man. So we see that in building self-esteem through our hypnotherapeutic technique, we are actually dealing on two levels, the situational and the spiritual: situational being the immediate physical level and the spiritual, the inner, deeper transcendental level. Within the situational context, we need to deal with the mental, physical and social aspects of self-esteem. These do not develop equally or at the same pace, and improvements may well be made in one area before the other two show any improvement.

This case history represents a classical example of what psychiatrists call adjustment disorder with disturbance of conduct, more explicitly the "intermittent explosive disorder." Further, it is a classic example of the benefits which can be accrued through hypnotherapy in the building of self-esteem and represents the author's contention that most of the major areas of deviance are the result of feelings of low self-esteem in which the individual turns to inappropriate behavior as a last resort to maintain a modicum of self-esteem. While therapy has not been terminated, it is important to realize that tremendous improvement has been made and is continuing to be made.

Gail Gleason Milgram, Ed.D.

Director of Education/Associate Professor
Center of Alcohol Studies
Rutgers University

10
TEENAGE DRINKING AND SELF-ESTEEM

The U.S.A is a drinking society; alcohol is a socially accepted legal substance which is consumed by approximately 70% of the adult population. The majority of those who drink do so for non-problematic reasons: as a beverage, as a relaxer, as a mood-modifier at a social gathering, etc. The occasions and situations of use reflect the variety of motivations and patterns of use: a family meal, a wedding, a visit at a tavern, a religious ceremony, a celebraton, etc. The consumption of alcohol for many individuals is part of their life-style.

There are also individuals who consume alcohol for problematic reasons (e.g., to escape); their consumption patterns or quantity consumed may create problems for themselves and others. Statistics (Keller and Gurioli, 1976) indicate that there are five and three- fourths million alcoholics in the U.S.A. today, and approximately four million problem drinkers. That is, close to 10 million individuals are experiencing a problem with their use of alcohol and it is estimated that each individual with an alcohol problem directly affects the lives of at least three other individuals (e.g., spouse, children, parents, friend, co-worker, etc.).

Though the U.S.A. is an alcohol-consuming society in which the majority of drinkers do not have problems with that use, it is an extremely ambivalent and uninformed society with respect to the use of alcohol. Many individuals do not know that a 12-ounce can of beer, a 5-ounce glass of wine, and 1½ ounces of distilled spirits all contain approximately the same amount of alcohol. Alcohol's effects on the human body are most often not considered in terms of body weight, food in the stomach, feelings, experience, duration of drinking, etc. It should therefore not be surprising that so may myths related to alcohol (e.g. coffee will sober up an intoxicated individual, someone can't be an alcoholic because he only drinks beer, etc.) are still believed. Ambivalence regarding "drinking" abounds also; individuals who consume alcohol are reluctant to label themselves drinkers because the word drinker is interpreted to mean heavy drinker, alcoholic drinker, abusive drinker, etc. Ambivalence is also evident in the philosophy that "a drinker is a drinker is a drinker." This philosophy assumes that because one consumes beverage alcohol, that is the only type of drink that will be taken if available. Often parties are arranged without providing alternative non-alcoholic beverages because of this philosophy and attitude. Societal ambivalence also surrounds the disease of alcoholism.

Alcoholics are often protected, hidden or covered up in the family, social or work environment due to misinformation, misguided helping, and the ambivalence and misinformation surrounding this disease.

Teen-agers are part of this society. They are raised in a culture where alcohol use is accepted, where the same use of alcohol is clouded by ambivalence, and where misinformation about alcohol is passed from one generation to another. It should not surprise adults that teen-agers consume alcohol for much the same reasons and in similar usage patterns as society. Most young people have their initial drinking experience in the home with parents or other adult authority figures between the ages of 10 and 13. When the non-problem reasons (e.g., as beverage) for alcohol use are considered, it seems natural that the family acculturation/socialization process would include alcohol. Harrison, Bennett, and Globetti's (1970) data indicate that pre-adolescents are being socialized into the use of alcoholic beverages by their parents in the home, "where one would expect an atmosphere of control and propriety." It also follows that a higher proportion of children will be drinkers if either the mother or father is a drinker (Forslund and Gustafson, 1970).

Teen-age drinking may therefore be viewed as a social act and a learned behavior (Maddox and McCall, 1964). For the majority of the young, it is not initiated by rebellion, experimentation, or peer pressure. These variables play a role as the teen-ager matures and drinking occurs more frequently outside of the home setting with the peer group. It is not uncommon for an adolescent in this setting to experiment with different types of alcoholic beverages and even purposely differ from the drinking norm set by parents. This phenomenon is most easily understood when one thinks of early college drinking or the drinking of young military recruits. The norm in this setting might be to become "intoxicated" on Friday night; this norm might be accepted and adhered to for a time by children of light or moderate drinkers whose parents are opposed to intoxication. Maturation allows those individuals who are not experiencing alcohol problems to outgrow the norm of intoxication and return to habits, patterns and attitudes toward alcohol similar to those of their parents.

The discussion of teen-age drinking as a learned social act has dealt primarily with children of non-problem drinking parents. There are children of two other groups which need to be considered: non-drinkers and alcoholics. Children of non-drinkers do not grow up with the use of alcohol as part of their family life. Their parents have chosen to be non-drinkers and therefore do not introduce their children to alcohol. There are many reasons for the non-use of alcohol by approximately 30% of our adult population. Religious tenet, dislike of taste, discomfort with the effects, recovered alcoholic parent, child from an alcohol problem family, etc., are some of the motivations for non-use of alcohol. The children of non-drinking parents who accept the rationale for non-drinking as their own will most likely remain non-drinkers. However, there are children from this type of family orientation who do not accept the non-use of alcohol tenet. For these young people who choose to drink, the process involves a higher risk for two apparent reasons. The individual consumes alcohol at a later age and usually in circumstances or situations separated from the family (e.g., college). Initial drinking at this time is complicated by the fact that drinking norms in late adolescents do not necessarily reflect the range of choices available in society; Friday night intoxication might be an accepted norm in a campus setting but not for society as a whole. Another source of increased risk is the guilt that may be associated with drinking.

Children of alcoholics grow up in a family system which often revolves around the disease of alcoholism itself. Parent-to-parent as well as parent-to-child communication is often difficult. Many different emotions are aroused by the distress surrounding alcoholism as well as the unpleasant realities often faced (e.g. financial problems, parental discord, etc.). Bosma (1975) has reported a direct correlation between parental alcoholism and childhood and adolescent disturbances, and suggests that children of alcoholics are the group most likely to develop drinking problems.

The parental drinking pattern for most adolescents is the determinant of drinking behavior (Bosma, 1975). The peer group is also a factor when adolescent drinking is viewed in specific time frames. Jessor and Jessor (1975) examined parents, peers, and society, and concluded that becoming a drinker is an integral aspect of adolescent development. A brief review of six studies of teenage drinking conducted in the 1960's and 1970's supports this concept.

Comparison of Six Studies of Teenage Drinking

Survey	Sample	% Drinkers	
		Boys	Girls
Mandell et al. (1962) New York State	751 High School Students (x age = 17)	81	66
Demone (1966) Oregon	18 High Schools	88	84
Kimes et al. (1969) South Carolina	13,000 Students, Grade 12	88	75
Blackford (1975) San Mateo County, CA	Grades 7-12	82	80
Lee et al. (1975) New York City	1,513 Students, Grades 11 and 12	80	75
Rachal et al. (1975) USA, nationwide	13,122 Students Grades 7-12	77	69

It is clear that a large percent of our adolescent population drinks. The question which then comes to mind is: What percent of these drinkers are having problems related to their use of alcohol, or are having alcohol problems? This statement may appear to some as splitting hairs; having an alcohol problem or one related to alcohol are often considered one and the same thing. Though this may possibly be the case with an adult population, it is not true of adolescents. The act of consuming alcohol for an eighteen year old at a beach party in a state where the legal drinking age is twenty-one may cause a problem related to alcohol if the youth is discovered by legal authorities, parents, etc. Another youth, of the same age at the same party may be having an alcohol problem if he consumes as much as possible, as frequently as possible, with negative consequences. A youth may also become intoxicated and appear at a high school dance; she may be escorted home and face school and parental consequences. She is dealing with a problem related to alcohol and not an alcohol problem per se.

The New York State study (Mandell, Cooper, Silberstein, Novick and Koloski, 1962) found 20% of boys and 10% of girls to be heavy drinkers based on the fact that they consumed seven or more drinks per week. Quantity alone was considered in this study; in fact a youth who consumed beverage alcohol every evening during a family meal would be in the heavy drinking population reported. Also, size of drink was not requested of the respondents — a very important consideration when the youth population is being studied. Adolescents do not always drink standard size drinks (i.e., 12 oz. beer, 5 oz. wine, 1½ oz. distilled spirits), sometimes they drink smaller portions and sometimes larger ones. Knowing that an adolescent has consumed seven drinks does not provide information on the amount of absolute alcohol consumed; information on body weight and length of time drinking is also missing as are the related consequences (e.g. intoxication) following drinking. Though it is useful that the percent of the population consuming seven drinks a week is known, it is necessary to tread carefully with these data.

The Oregon study listed in the brief review did not provide problem drinking data, nor did the survey in San Mateo County California. However, the South Carolina study (Kimes, Smith and Maher, 1969) found 4.8% of the drinkers self-rated themselves as problem drinkers. This appears to be a percent of the population that is having alcohol problems per se or at least severe enough problems related to alcohol to be concerned. The U.S.A. nationwide study also found a self-rated serious problem drinking percentage; 2.5% of the total placed themselves in this category (Rachal, Williams, Brehm, Cavanaugh, Moore and Eckerman, 1975). However, 28% of the total population in this study was labeled problem drinkers because it represented those who had been drunk four or more times the previous year and/or had experienced two or more negative consequences of drinking in various life areas. Though being intoxicated is dangerous, high-risk behavior for adolescents, a large part of the group had problems and consequences related to the use of alcohol and were not problem drinkers.

A similar lack of distinction between these two categories occurred in the New York City Study (Lee, Fishman and Shimmel, 1975). This study found 12% of the total sample to be problem drinkers due to an unhealthy attitude toward and use of alcohol and one of the following:

> drink more than once/week;
> drink 5 or more drinks/occasion;
> blackouts;
> trouble because of drinking;
> drink more than friends;
> drink to get drunk;
> drink before or during school.

These criteria need to be analyzed, at least briefly. "Drink more than once/week" may be answered affirmatively by an individual who celebrates a religious ritual of which wine is an integral part, an individual who has one drink at each of two parties, etc. "Drinks 5 or more drinks per occasion" may indicate an adolescent who is having an alcohol problem; however, it would also include an individual who has five drinks (size unknown) at one drinking occasion per week or per month, or per year. An affirmative answer to "five drinks per occasion" also does not provide information on the duration of drinking occasion or body weight. Time and body size directly relate to the effects alcohol has on the body and are significant if alcohol problems are to be discussed.

"Blackouts," the next category, is clearly one of the symptoms of alcoholism and is identified as occurring in stage two of the disease (Jellinek, 1960). It may also be true that trouble because of drinking indicates a problem drinker. However, as discussed earlier it may also be due to the act of drinking, the circumstances, and the consequences. "Drink more than friends" is another criterion that could be interpreted in two ways. If an adolescent always drinks as much as possible and this is always more than friends, an alcohol problem may be present. It also could be true that an individual has one or two drinks per drinking occasion and that is more that his/her friends.

If the adult population was being studied, "drink to get drunk" would have meaning as an indicator of an alcohol problem. Unfortunately when the population is adolescents, it does not have the same meaning. Drinking to get drunk is a norm of drinking for certain populations (e.g. Friday night intoxication at college or a military base, etc.). Though getting intoxicated even occasionally is high-risk behavior, it is not viewed as a severe problem by those in the stage of late adolescence. "Drink before or during school" for most would denote an alcohol problem if the activity occurs on a regular basis. If it is a one time prank to see if it can be pulled off, it would provide a potential for a problem related to alcohol use, but not an alcohol problem; if the activity were part of coping with nervousness, worry over a test, etc., it would be categorized as a alcohol problem.

The scrutiny applied to the studies presented was provided as a basis for understanding the wide range of percentages used to label our "problem drinking" teen-age population: 2.5%, 4.8%, 12%, 28%. All the percents are based on criteria that vary widely and each has found youthful problem drinkers, "but the actual part of the percent given that would clearly be real problem drinkers is concealed" (Milgram, 1977). It is important to understand the nature and extend of teen-age drinking and related problems prior to a discussion of teen-age drinking and self-esteem.

The relationship between personality variables and adolescent alcohol use has been investigated by researchers; these variables include alienation, self-esteem and variables related to self-esteem (i.e. self-concept, self-rejection, pessimism, happiness, feeling of pressure, perceived personal problem, need satisfaction, and drinking patterns). Some studies focused primarily on one variable's relationship to alcohol |and drug| use, while others investigated alcohol use and its relationship to a combination of variables.

Blane, Hill and Brown (1968) analyzed the relationship of alienation, self-esteem and attitudes toward drinking in high school students. It was found that favorability of attitudes toward irresponsible use of alcohol was positively associated with alienation but not with self-esteem. Powerlessness and normlessness, two alienation subscales, were related to attitudes toward irresponsible use, but social isolation, the third subscale, was not. Also, alienation and self-esteem were negatively related. Smart and Fejer (1971) using the same measure of alienation (i.e. Dean Alienation Scale) found that, among Canadian students, alcohol use was positively related to social isolation and powerlessness.

In a study of high school and junior high school students, Wechsler and Thum (1973) found that, of all the students, the heavier drinkers were more likely to report illicit drug use and delinquent activities (including shoplifting and property damage, and involvement with the police); and also felt more alienation from their parents, had more personal problems that their peers, and had lower grades in school. Alienation, delinquency, and patterns of drug use were also investigated by Steffenhagen, Polich and Lash (1978). Alienation, measured by the Nettler Alienation Scale, and delinquency, measured by the Short Delinquency Scale, significantly correlated with drug use in 458 high school students from affluent suburban school systems. The correlation between alcohol use and alienation was .224, and that between alcohol use and delinquency was .527. Similar relationships were obtained for the other drugs; the correlation between alienation and delinquency was .329. These studies suggest a positive relationship between alienation and attitudes toward and use of alcohol.

The relationship of self-esteem to the disease of alcoholism in the adult population has been investigated in two pertinent studies. Nocks and Bradley (1969) determined the self-esteem of 61 hospitalized alcoholics by means of structured interviews. Their findings indicated a trend toward lower self-esteem with increased duration of a drinking problem and duration of awareness of the problem. Self-esteem in alcoholics and non-alcoholics was also determined by Charalampous, Ford and Skinner (1976), using the Rosenberg Scale (a 10-item test of self-esteem); alcoholics scored significantly lower than the nonalcoholics (p < .01). Studies of adolescent alcohol use and its relationship to self-esteem have not been as conclusive. Schaeffer, Schuckit and Morrissey (1976), in their study of students living in a co-ed dorm, found that heavy alcohol use was related to self-esteem (the Coppersmith Self-esteem Inventory), though no relationship could be established between self- esteem and drug use. The results also suggested the existence of a continuum with heavy drug or alcohol users showing the most pathology, and moderate-to-light drinkers and marijuana users exhibiting little or no pathology. Galli's (1972) study of attitudes toward drugs among school children and their parents also showed a relationship between self-esteem and alcohol use; sense of personal worth was related to the use of wine but not to other beverages.

However, in Blane et al.'s (1968) study, using the Janis and Field Personality Questionnaire to measure self-esteem, a positive relationship was not found between positive attitudes toward irresponsible alcohol use and self-esteem. Self-esteem was also not found to relate to alcohol use in Wroten and Safyan's (1975) study of high school students. Blane and Hewitt (1977) conclude a review of self-esteem and alcohol use by saying that "little evidence for a positive relationship between the personality variable of self-esteem and alcohol use exists, although very few studies to date have directly measured this variable."

Variables related to self-esteem have also been investigated in the literature. Ferguson, Freedman, and Ferguson (1977) correlated adjective pair-comparisons as a measurement of self-concept with those of a self-report drug-use scale. It was found that the overall scores predicted the use of beer and wine, distilled spirits, and cigarettes among both sexes and of marijuana and lysergic acid in boys, suggesting that the pair-comparison inventory could potentially be used to identify students needing counseling.

Self-concepts of college problem drinkers were investigated by Williams (1965) in an attempt to distinguish between personality characteristics which precede the development of alcoholism and those which result primarily from the social and psychological consequences of loss of control over drinking. Self-descriptions completed by 68 college problem drinkers from four fraternities at a New England college were compared to those of alcoholics investigated by Connor (1962). Williams, using the Gough Adjective Checklist, which was also used by Connor, found that college problem drinkers have low self-evaluation, indicating that this personality characteristic precedes the development of alcoholism. Williams also noted that if low self-evaluation does precede alcoholism, it may be a contributing factor to an individual's drinking to excess and eventually having alcohol problems.

Pessimism, another variable related to self-esteem, was investigated by Globetti and Windham (1967) in a study of high school students in a rural

Mississippi community. A significantly higher percentage of problem drinkers scored high on a deviant behavior index (p < .001) and problem drinkers scored slightly higher on an index of pessimism, derived from the Minnesota Survey of Opinion.

Happiness, as it related to alcohol use, was investigated by Demone (1966), feelings of pressure by McLeod and McGuire (1975), and perceived personal problems by Adler and Lotecka (1973). Greater use of alcohol was found to be related to unhappiness, feelings of pressure, and more personal problems. Jessor, Carman and Grossman (1968) investigated the hypothesis that alcohol use may serve as an alternative behavior for unattainable goals or for coping with the failure to attain valued goals. Sophomore-level volunteer psychology students from the University of Colorado participated in this study, which linked low expectation of need satifaction to patterns of drinking behavior.

Two studies by Globetti (1967, 1972) conducted in abstinent communities focused on the relationships among personality and environmental factors and teen-age drinking. In studying the use of alcohol by high school students, Globetti (1967) found that drinkers were more likely than non-drinkers to participate in mild forms of deviant behavior (p < .001), to be pessimistic, and to reject middle-class values. Drinkers also appeared to be more estranged from family, church, school, and community and their drinking appeared to be an expression of rebellion toward community authority. Globetti's study of problem and non-problem drinking, also in high school students, indicates that drinking under conditions of illegality and social taboos insulates drinking practices from social controls and leads to risks in the pattern of alcohol use (1972). To further explore the role of additional factors in youth drinking, Miraglia (1975) studied the relationships among social background, attitudes toward women's roles, sex-role conflict, and alcohol use in a female undergraduate volunteer population. Fear of success and sex-role ambivalence were found to positively correlate with drinking measures, and alcohol use among friends was identified as the most significant predictor of drinking.

Prendergast and Schaefer's (1974) study of correlates of drinking and drunkenness among high school students showed that frequency of drinking was significantly correlated with lax maternal control, perceived rejection by either the mother or the father, and psychological tension in the relationship with either the father or the mother. Frequency of drunkenness correlated significantly with lax maternal control and parental rejection. Dalzell-Ward (1973) studied separate areas of behavioral research (teen-age alcohol use, juvenile smoking, sexual activities, and student drug use) and found that they arrived independently at the same conclusion: the common factor among the young people studied was a desire for a self-image of toughness and rebellion. In accordance with this, Davies and Stacey (1972) found that heavier drinkers perceived themselves as more tough and rebellious than other groups of teen-agers (i.e., light-to-moderate drinkers, abstainers).

As stated by Steffenhagen in the Introduction, theories of drug dependence

The self-esteem theory postulates that the reactions of individuals to their social environment are mediated by a common factor: self-esteem. The self-esteem theory has not been supported or discounted by the review of the literature on personality variables related to adolescent alcohol use. This is due to the fact that social situations and drug use patterns have not both been related to self-esteem. The typology needed to be tested by research methodology is the one presented in Chapter 4.

Self-Esteem	Social Situation	Drug Pattern
Low	No pressure to use drugs	Non-use
	Pressure to use drugs	abuse
High	No pressure to use drugs	Non-use
	Pressure to use drugs	Drug use but not abuse.

The paradigm (in Chapter 4) which posits self-esteem as the foundation of the personality, can also be illustrated as follows:

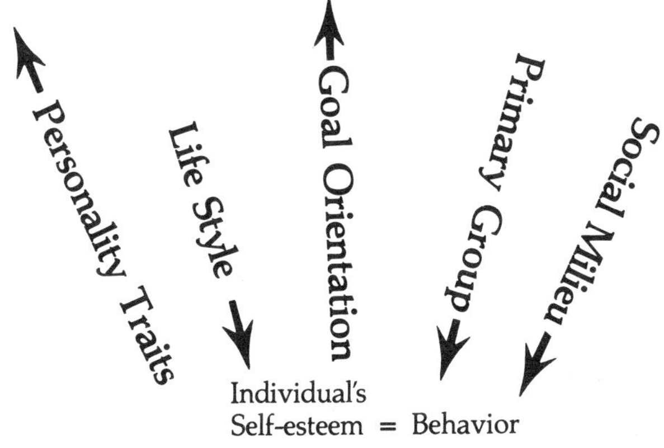

In the above illustration, the individual's self-esteem is the foundation, with personality traits and goal orientation being projected from this base. Life style, primary group, and social milieu are depicted as impacting on the individual's self-esteem; behavior arises as the consequence of the interaction of all the factors. The figure above illustrates that alcohol use and attitudes toward that use are related to the individual's personality traits and goal orientation. Life style, primary group, and social milieu are the factors that affect alcohol use in specific situations and regulate the drinking (i.e. quantity, frequency, consequences) that occurs. When the individual's self-esteem is considered the foundation from which these factors arise, the self-esteem theory becomes significant with respect to the habits, patterns, and attitudes regarding alcohol of the adolescent population.

This chapter has provided an overview of societal alcohol use including ambivalence and misinformation, adolescent drinking and alcohol problems, and a review of the literature on teenage alcohol use and personality variables. It was further suggested that these areas may be related to self-esteem among adolescents. The need for research in the area of self-esteem theory as related to teenage drinking is clear. Such investigation might prove valuable in explaining patterns of teenage drinking and might further provide a basis for predicting alcohol problem behavior.

Aside from the research necessary to explore the descriptive and predictive validity of the self-esteem theory, the theory, in its present form, has some implications worth noting. This primary focus of this theory is individual self-esteem. Raising an individual's self-esteem becomes more than a nice thing to do; it becomes a necessary strategy for primary prevention.[1] Since life experiences are related to the individual's self-esteem, it becomes important to train in behavioral competency those persons significant in the life of a child. That is, parents need to be aware of their role in developing a child's sense of competence, belongingness, usefulness, and personal potency. The role of educators is also a significant one: "Teachers need to learn to raise self-esteem in children and to help maintain the integrity of each student with the school system" (Owen, 1976).

Knowing more about the relationship between self-esteem and alcohol use might also affect societal responses to alcoholism. The results of dealing with alcohol in an honest and informed fashion might include motivation to use alcohol in a responsible manner, comfort in being a non-user of alcohol, use of techniques for lowering risks related to drinking, refusal to accept inappropriate or offensive behavior related to alcohol use, the recognition that alcoholism is a disease, the awareness that alcoholism is treatable, and, hopefully, earlier detection and treatment for people having alcohol problems.

The educational system is also an area significantly affected by the self-esteem theory. The heightening of an individual's self-esteem by educators in this context has already been mentioned. However, the implications are more far-reaching and necessitate provisions of a non-threatening, open, and honest atmosphere. Objective content material designed to meet the interests and needs of students (e.g., what is alcohol and why do people drink, for an elementary school audience; the effects of alcohol on the human body, for a junior high audience, etc.) becomes vital to the young person's growth and development. Values-clarification techniques, the development of coping skills, the ability to use the decision-making process, the use of assertiveness training to enable individuals to act on decisions and choose responsible behaviors, all become part of the educational process for growth and development which can aid the individual's self-concept.

The peer group, a strong influence on an individual's self-esteem must also be considered. In the educational process described, the peer group becomes a

---

[1]Primary prevention is defined here as the prevention of the occurrence of an illness and incorporates a broad range of activities and resources to enable people not to be patients.

source of positive reinforcement. As techniques or strategies to build self-esteem are incorporated into the educational system, peers are affected and also encouraged to respond. An example of this might be helpful. If, in conducting the values-clarification exercise of role playing, two adolescents are requested to deal with the situation of one being intoxicated and the other attempting to refuse a ride with the intoxicated driver, the benefits of the approach are many: the students immediately realize that they are dealing with reality; the students are motivated to seek alternatives; and the peer group provides reaction, additional alternatives, and, in general, becomes a significant factor in the learning process. The instructor is no longer putting forth rules; the group is analyzing, discussing and responding to a situation and providing a framework for responsible behavior.

The inherent benefit of the self-esteem theory is that it focuses on the worth of each individual and the subsequent heightening of each person's self-esteem. The self-esteem theory's explanation of teen-age alcohol use, alcohol problems, and prediction of behavior could profitably be tested by research. Investigations of the social context of drinking and peer pressure could lead to a clearer distinction between drinking experiences and problem drinking experiences on the part of the adolescent drinker.

REFERENCES

Adler, P. and Lotecka, L. Drug Use Among High School Students: Patterns and Correlates. *International Journal of Addictions*, Vol 8 (No. 3), 1973.

Blackford, St. Clair, L. Student Drug Use Surveys—San Mateo County, California, 1968-1975. San Mateo County Department of Public Health and Welfare, 1975.

Blance, H.T. and Hewitt, L.E. *Alcohol and Youth: An Analysis of the Literature, 1960-75.* Rockville, Maryland: National Institute on Alcohol Abuse and Alcoholism, 1977.

Blane, H.T., Hill, M.J. and Brown, E. Alienation, Self-esteem, and Attitudes Toward Drinking in High School Students. *Quarterly Journal of Studies on Alcohol*, Vol. 29, 1968.

Bosma, W.G.A. Alcoholism and Teenagers. *Maryland State Medical Journal*, Vol. 24 (No. 6), 1975.

Charalampous, K.D., Ford, B.K. and Skinner, T.J. Self-esteem in Alcoholics and Nonalcoholics. *Journal of Studies on Alcohol*, Vol. 37, 1976.

Connor, R.G. The Self-Concepts of Alcoholics. In: Pittman, D. J. and Snyder, C.R. (Eds.) *Society, Culture, and Drinking Patterns*, New York: Wiley, 1962.

Dalzell-Ward, A.J. Health Education. *Journal of Alcoholism*, Vol. 8 (No. 2), 1973.

Davies, J. and Stacey, B. TEEN-AGERS AND ALCOHOL: A DEVELOPMENTAL STUDY in Glasgow. London: Her Majesty's Stationery Office, 1972.

Demone, H.W., Jr. Drinking Attitudes and Practices of Male Adolescents. Ph.D. Dissertation, Brandeis University, 1966. (University Micro-films No. 66-13637).

Ferguson, L.W., Freedman, M. and Ferguson, E.P. Developmental Self-concept and (self-reported) Drug Use. *Psychological Reports*, Vol. 41, 1977.

Forslund, M.A. and Gustafson, T.J. Influence of Peers and Parents and Sex Differences in Drinking by High School Students. *Quarterly Journal of Studies on Alcohol*, Vol. 31, 1970.

Galli, N.A. A Comparative Analysis of the Attitudes and Behaviors of School Children and Their Parents Toward Drugs. Ph.D. Dissertation. University of Illinois, 1972 (University Microfilms No. 73-17,211).

Globetti, G. Teenage Drinking in an Abstinence Setting. *Kansas Journal of Sociology*, Vol. 3, 1967.

__________, Problem and Non-problem Drinking Among High School Students in Abstinence Communities. *International Journal of Addictions*, Vol. 7, 1972.

Globetti, G. and Windham G.O. The Social Adjustment of High School Students and the Use of Beverage Alcohol. *Sociology and Social Research*, Vol. 51, 1967.

Harrison, D.E., Bennet, W.H., and Globetti, G. Factors Related to Alcohol Use Among Pre-adolescents. *Journal of Alcohol Education*, Vol. 15 (no. 2), 1970.

Jellinek, E.M. *The Disease Concept of Alcoholism*. New Haven, Conn.: College and University Press, 1960.

Jessor, R., Carman, R.S. and Grossman, P.H. Expectations of Need Satisfaction and Drinking Patterns of College Students. *Quarterly Journal of Studies on Alcohol*, Vol. 29, 1968.

Jessor, R. and Jessor, S.L. Adolescent Development and the Onset of Drinking: A Longitudinal Study. *Journal of Studies on Alcohol*, Vol. 36, 1975.

Keller, M. and Gurioli, C. *Statistics on Consumption of Alcohol and Alcoholism*, 1976 Edition. New Brunswick, NJ: Rutgers Center on Alcohol Studies, 1976.

Kimes, W.T., Smith, S.C. and Maher, R.E. Alcohol and Drug Abuse in South Carolina High Schools. Columbia, S.C.: Department of Education, 1969.

Lee, E.E., Fishman, R. and Shimel, G.M. Emerging Trends of Alcohol Use and Abuse Among Urban Teen-agers. Paper presented at Annual Converence of the National Council on Alcoholism, Milwaukee, Wisconsin, April, 1975.

Maddox, G.L. and McCall, B.C. *Drinking Among Teenagers*. New Brunswick, N.J.: Rutgers Center of Alcohol Studies, 1964.

Mandell, W., Cooper, A., Silberstein, R.M., Novick, J. and Koloski, E. *Youthful Drinking: New York State*. A Report to the Joint Legislative Committee on the Alcoholic Beverage Control Law of the New York State

Legislature. Staten Island, N.Y.: Wakoff Research Center, 1962.

McLeod, J.H. and McGuire, J.D. Alcohol and Other Drug Usage Among Junior and Senior High School Students in Charlotte-Mecklenburg: A Comparison of Three Surveys. Charlotte, NC: Charlotte Drug Education Center, 1975.

Miraglia, P.J. Selected Correlates of Self-reported Alcohol Use in Catholic College Women. Ph.D. Dissertation: University of Pennsylvania, (University Microfilms No. 76-3203), 1975.

Milgram, G.G. Comment on problem drinking among American youth in *Defining Alcohol Use: Implications for a Definition of Adolescent Alcohol Use.* New York: National Council on Alcoholism, 1977.

Nocks, J.J. and Bradley, D.L. Self-esteem in an alcoholic population. *Diseases of the Nervous System*, Vol. 30, 1969. Owen, R.D. Prevention of Alcoholism with Implication for Elementary and Secondary School Education. Ph.D. Dissertation, University of Oregon (University Microfilms No. 77-4749), 1976.

Prendergast, T.J., Jr. and Schaefer, E.S. Correlates of drinking and drunkenness among high school students. *Quarterly Journal of Studies on Alcohol*, Vol. 35, 1974.

Rachal, J.V., Williams, J.R., Brehm, M.L., Cavanaugh, B., Moore, R.P. and Eckerman, W.C. *A National Study of Adolescent Drinking Behavior, Attitudes and Correlates.* Research Triangle Park, NC; Research Triangle Institute, Center for Study of Social Behavior, 1975.

Schaeffer, Garry M., Schuckit, M.A., and Morrissey, E.R. Correlation Between Two Measures of Self-esteem and Drug Use in a College Sample. *Psychological Reports*, Vol. 39, 1976.

Smart, R.G. and Fejer, D. Recent Trends in Illicit Drug Use Among Adolescents. Canada: Mental Health Division Department of National Health and Welfare, 1971.

Steffenhagen, R.A., Polich, J.M. and Lash, S. Alienation, Delinquency and Patterns of Drug Use. *International Journal of Social Psychiatry.* Vol. 24, 1978.

Wechsler, H. and Thum, D. Teen-age Drinking, Drug Use and Social Correlates. *Quarterly Journal of Studies on Alcohol*, Vol. 34, 1973. Williams, A.F. Self-Concepts of College Problem Drinkers: A Comparison with Alcoholics, *Quarterly Journal of Studies on Alcohol*, Vol. 26, 1965.

Wroten, J.D. and Safyan, P. Prevalence of Drug Use Among Adolescent Students in Forsyth County North Carolina Schools. Unpublished manuscript, 1975.

A CASE HISTORY: ALCOHOLISM AND SELF-ESTEEM
R. A. Steffenhagen

This case history deals with the problem of alcoholism and self-esteem and provides some background information followed by a testimony of the client.

Tony is thirty years of age, has a medical diagnosis of alcoholism and has been a heavy drinker for the past 18 years. His discharge from the army related to drug abuse and he has been unable to hold jobs for any protracted period of time. His history also includes other drug use, and he has had headaches and blackouts associated with this. This is the first time he had actively sought help; he had been through detoxification and had been following several treatment modalities before coming to me. This behavior is consistent with that of many alcoholics.

Tony first came to me in the winter of 1979 indicating that he had heard about my theory of self-esteem, that he was in the process of being rehabilitated, and was considering making a career in the human service area with a specialty in alcohol rehabilitation. He indicated that he was returning to college, was going to prepare himself academically for a profession, and that he wanted to work under someone who could serve as his mentor. We spent an hour discussing the possibilities and I suggested hypnotizing him, if he wished, so he would have an understanding of my therapeutic technique. I had not considered Tony a client in any way, but rather, I thought of him as a student who occasionally might call or ask for help. I had given him some of my material to read and suggested we might work more closely as he became more prepared academically. We made an appointment for the following week.

The next week, Tony came in and I hypnotized him taking him to a deep level with incredible results. Without question he manifested all the dynamics of low self-esteem—mentally, physically and socially. Mentally, Tony never considered himself a superior human being although he has a very high IQ and is an extremely capable young man. Physically, he never considered himself handsome, although certainly other people have and do. Socially, his relationships have always been rather tenuous and of a superficial nature.

After three sessions, Tony almost lost all desire to drink. I saw him weekly for approximately five weeks and from that time on it has been occasional and our meetings have been as much academic as they have been therapeutic. We discussed the relative merits of AA and Tony is one of the people to whom AA has absolutely no appeal and to whom he could not relate. By April, Tony had his drinking totally under control; he had lost all desire to drink and, emotionally, was in total control of himself. Before Easter, under a rather pressured situation, he had indulged in a beer while at home and had related to me that even though he had been depressed and feeling lonely as a result of not seeing his children (he is divorced and the children live with their mother), the beer had no effect and he had no craving though the refrigerator had contained a six-pack that belonged to his roommate—he had only the one.

The second time Tony drank, it was upon meeting friends and they pressured him to stop and "have a beer with them." He agreed, had two beers and said that was it; his third would be a coke. Even though they pressured him to 'have another,' he was in total control and in fact gave them more grief than they did him. From this point on, Tony became a social drinker. He is in total control, has never drunk more than two, and even under highly pressured, tense situations, he is able to maintain his equilibrium without difficulty.

This case exemplifies the theoretical position of this book that if good self-esteem is developed, the individual feels good about himself, and he is then in control and can handle "the winds of adversity." If alcoholism is a symptom of low self-esteem, then by building self-esteem, we can produce a 'cure' which means an individual can go from total lack of control of his alcohol consumption to full control. I would further like to comment that, since April, Tony has done a relatively small amount of social drinking on different occasions; he has been in one or two situations where past friends have deliberately tried to get him loaded and under no circumstances has he lost control. A rather unusual development has come about and that is that Tony has commented that his unconscious has built a protective mechanism whereby his body will *absolutely* not tolerate more than two beers, and that even if he were to attempt physically to drink more than two, he seems unable to do so, almost a modified antiabuse factor. I do not wish to elaborate on this since I do not know whether it is something that would be a by-product of self-esteem therapy.

Part 2 of this case history is Tony's autobiographical sketch of himself in the process. It is now nine months since I first saw him and he is doing great.

Testimonial

I met Dr. Steffenhagen about a month ago. I went to see him after hearing that he was studying drug abuse, which was the field in which I had chosen to continue my academic studies, and also that he was using hypnotherapy, which I was very interested in, as a possible curative measure for substance abuse.

Before I continue I would like to give you a general background on myself, with respect to my personal addiction to alcohol.

I started drinking alcohol experimentally when I was 9 years old. This experimentation continued in a moderate sense until I was 17 and went into the service, at which point my intake of alcohol increased to the point of blacking out and delirium tremens. At the time, being an inexperienced drinker, I figured this is what social drinking was all about. That was 18 years ago, and I have been drinking in excess for these 18 years, to the point where my liver is elongated and I have an extreme chemical deposit from the liquor and beer. I have been evaluated medically as an acute alcoholic.

Not until November of last year (1979) would I admit in any way that I had an alcohol problem, even though I had lost a business, a family, and every friend I had through alcohol abuse.

Over this period of eighteen years I had my ups and downs with drinking and life in general. After a period of ten years, the latter ten years of my life I noticed little differences in my life patterns, such as insomnia, forgetfulness, shakes every now and then. I attributed these conditions to being overtired, pressure, nervous conditions due to business, not realizing to what stage my alcoholism was advancing. At times life just didn't seem worth living, but these feelings came and went on a periodic basis, so I didn't think much about it. This continued on for eight years with things going from bad to worse and the feelings becoming more and more frequent and lasting for a longer duration. Two years ago I had progressed to drinking a fifth of liquor a day, drinking morning, noon and night and making excuses why I had to have a drink. I couldn't sleep, nothing seemed right. I was in the middle of a divorce that was tearing me up inside. I was about to lose my children whom I loved very much. The pain was intolerable, so I drank to the point of oblivion and would pass out. This went on for two years; hiding liquor, losing jobs or just quitting the jobs because I felt no reason to continue living. My whole purpose and goals were completely shattered into non-existence.

This brings us to the point of where I was before seeking help two and one half months ago. At this time I had lost my ability to think, reason, or judge anything correctly. I was constantly dropping things, stumbling up stairways, falling down at different times, I knew what the cause was, drinking to excess, but didn't care. My children and my ex-wife, after putting up with it for eight years, finally had enough of my drinking and unemployment. In the last month of this acute alcoholism I started to have violent tendencies, which were the "straw that broke the camel's back." She told me I had to get out. I had no place to go, very little money, and was hurting like hell inside. The pain was so intense I couldn't bear to live without my children. I decided to kill myself, so I bought five fifths of liquor and a couple of beers and proceded to drink them figuring I would drink myself to death and that would be that. But as you can see from this documentation, I failed, thank God.

It took me five days to consume the spirits I had bought, plus what I was drinking at various bars. On the fifth day, I woke up in Utica, New York, and had absolutely no recollection of how I got there. Strange things were happening to me. It was about twelve o'clock at night and I seemed to have just opened my eyes from some type of sleep. My last recollection was sitting in Rutland, Vermont and talking to my ex-boss, but that was two days previous. Out of nowhere I started hearing music, so I tried to turn the radio off and to my surprise found it wasn't on. The music and voices were very persistent. I tried every method I knew to mentally block them, but it was to no avail; they continued.

Now the horror show started. I began feeling my skin crawl; my scalp seemed to be moving; I was having muscle spasms and couldn't control my breathing. It seemed like someone was trying to suffocate me, and I kept sucking for air. Getting out of the car seemed to help this. I was paranoid to a point beyond belief; I couldn't look anyone in the eyes. Every time I saw a police car,

I was so scared I had to stop the car at the next rest area and relieve myself. By this time I was on my way back to Vermont. I had no idea why I was doing this: maybe it was the familiarity and I figured that whatever was happening would stop, but it didn't. I had all sorts of visualizations in the process of returning to Vermont; trucks on the wrong side of the road coming at me, people along the road that would disappear after I went by them, people with no faces and a hand growing out of the top of their heads. At this point I had to have been completely insane. My body was numb, I felt cold sweat running down my back and I couldn't think. My mind wouldn't let me think of anything but my children not being with me ever again. My life was absolutely worthless and so was I. I had failed at absolutely everything and I wanted to die now like I never had before. As scared as I was, I had one spark of my own inner being that was still kindled, and with this spark of life, I cried out to God for his help and cried in the car knowing if I stopped thinking of God, there was no hope left. So I hung on by praying for guidance all the way back to Burlington.

When I arrived in Burlington, I finally had a decision to make. Somewhere, as I look at it now, God had intervened and given me the answer I needed; call someone for help or I wouldn't last a day. My mind was going in and out of reality and reason at a rapid rate. I made phone calls to any number that I came to in the phone book which dealt with alcohol, and one was an alcohol information referral service. I didn't know what it was, but it sounded right.

They referred me to another agency which dealt with detoxification. Not knowing what this was all about, I agreed to go there regardless of what they were going to do to me. The state of mind I was in had to be dealt with. I couldn't do it myself, and was willing to go to any length to stop it.

Needless to say, the detoxification center did an excellent job of getting me through the crisis period, which took seven days. Upon completion of their program, they asked me if I would consider going to a farm for recovering alcoholics, and I consented to do it for another twenty-eight days. This gave me time to think, to evaluate my position in a protected environment that was absolutely alcohol free, and to physically and mentally re-nourish myself. I thank everyone involved at Maple Leaf for their understanding and patience with me. I left there feeling physically a hundred percent better but I still had no purpose in life. I started thinking about what to do with my life and decided after the treatment I had received from the different agencies that what I wanted to do was help other people in the same condition to restructure their lives in a more purposeful way.

This was when I was introduced to Dr. Steffenhagen's theory of hypnotic therapy for deviance abuse by one of his research workers that I had the pleasure of meeting while going through the detoxification period. I figured if I wished to continue in the field of substance abuse, I would need an authority in the field who could answer the multitude of questions I had about alcohol and drugs. Steffenhagen's method of dealing with alcohol and drug and self-esteem seemed very logical and practical to me as a possibility for treatment. So I called his office at the University and made an appointment to speak to him about his research and working with him.

Upon arriving at his office a few days later, we discussed the possibilities of hypnotherapy, the probabilities of its success, and the results he had accomplished in a very few sessions with clients. One thing led to another and I consented to try hypnotherapy. We started working on a problem I had had for some years; insomnia. Using hypnosis he relaxed me as I had not been relaxed in many years. All the tension and pressure seemed to drain out of me, and I felt really good about myself in contact with reality once again, with an awareness of my physical and mental feelings. I felt what I would consider my inner self being released or relieved of a great burden that had been with me most of my life, an uncomfortable feeling that had been with me for so long. I never knew I was supposed to feel anything else but constant pressure and inadequacy of being less than other people.

I felt so good before I left his office that I asked him if I could continue with the therapy and see if somehow we could get a handle on my drinking problem, and he agreed to see me again. On my second visit we went through basically the same process, only this time working on the alcohol problem and building my values in life and my feelings about myself and the world around me. After leaving his office, good things started happening to me. I was aware, for the first time in many years that I was somebody and had a right to stand next to anyone of my choosing or reject anyone I wished to. I looked into a mirror and saw a stranger staring back at me, a person whom I had never seen before, *me*. I liked what I saw. I don't remember the last time I had looked into my own eyes while I was shaving and could actually face myself until a few weeks ago. That man in the mirror just smiled back at me, with an inner contentment.

The weeks followed, and in the process I decided to return to college and get my bachelors degree in transpersonal psychology. Everything else seems to be falling in place for me. At this point in my life I have a sense of being' once again, and of an inner knowledge of myself (self-actualization).

My craving for alcohol is almost non-existent, and in time I have no doubt that it will cease to exist altogether. I am in the first ninety days of sobriety in the last eighteen years, which is a very critical point as far as recurrent drinking. I am confident in every way that every day life is getting better, and I no longer need, or want, to use alcohol or any other drug as a crutch or stimulant to maintain or deal with my problems. I am fully capable at this time of managing and controlling my own life, without the use of deviant means. To substantiate this I have recently taken the SUIB-SCII profile test, and in the area of self-esteem I scored a 71. The normal or average score is 50.

If I were to write an analysis of Dr. Steffenhagen's work, my personal evaluation of his methods and theories of deviance abuse and self-esteem is, put simply: "If we take the man and rebuild his values, goal structure, and inner being, we will rebuild the man and the world will fall in place for him."

Walter O'Connell Ph.D.
Veterans Administration Glass Ark
Drug Treatment Center
Houston, Texas

11

THE IMPOSSIBLE DREAM: INSTITUTIONALIZED ACTUALIZATION OF SELF-ESTEEM & BELONGING

"Life is a purpose to be fulfilled not a problem to be solved"
(see Szasz, 1976. Pp. 120, 129).

INTRODUCTION

This paper is a brief report on my odyssey of seven years within the Alice-in-Wonderland world of drug addicts and their otherwise addicted keepers, the bureaucratic medical-model healers. It goes without saying that my expressed views are not intended, in any shape, form, or manner, to reflect the official views of the Veterans Administration and/or any of the half-dozen institutions with which I am presently affiliated.

The tenor of the paper is that there is no concerted effort to understand or therapize drug addiciton. In fact, the very boundaries of the problem are mind-boggling to our extraverted ego-oriented and punishmentprone society. (How many Diogenes would be needed to find a score of persons not addicted to external goals, roles, and controls for "proof" of a sense of significance, worth, power, and esteem?)

The reason for writing this paper is to externalize and share inner experiences. In my estimation, feelings and intuitions are often more valuable for recording than many "objective" studies, reporting minor observations with equally imperfect measures. One premise of this paper, gleaned from 30 years experience in mental hospitals is that we have a very long way to go before we can teach patients, in particular drug addicts, the "hows" and "whys" of humorous, socially-responsible living. A major, grossly-overlooked, blocking influence is the ego-addiction fostered by institutions. The institutional ego is simply a large scale ego-addiction. Roles, goals, and controls become attachments for power-seeking in the external world (O'Connell, 1979a). Growth involvement and deep self-esteem are entirely missing in such extraverted ego-graspings.

Courage and/or craziness is required to write this chapter. Its constant, unpopular cry is that self-esteem is possible only by advancing beyond the ego-esteem gained by the addicted elite in the orthodox, institutionalized model of

163

personhood. The ego-addictions and subsequent needs for ego-esteem fostered by institutions are, as a rule, both tenacious and nonconscious. It is assumed need for ego-esteem and direct interpersonal power that keep puzzlement about the explicit goals and ways of development at a minimum.

What follows is a brief account of the vagaries involved in establishing an actualization program aimed at self-direction for esteem (SE) and belonging (SI) within the powerful field of the institutional ego. As a case in point, the misadventures inherent in establishing a treatment approach for drug and methadone addiction (beyond simplistic narcissistic gimmicks) are discussed.

Power Through Strength or Seduction?

The theme of this chapter is that drug-addiction, like other forms of ego-induced misery, is a learned style of human incompetence. Addiction is one effect of the concerted yet unwitting constriction of the ego-identitites of victims and victimizers, whose roles become interchangeable. The ideal treatment of choice would be to train addicts (ego — as well as drug-) to become active agents in learning about their constrictive mistakes, as well as mastering a guiding theory such as the practice of the natural high (O'Connell, 1975; 1979a, 1980). By becoming active agents in the expansion of self-esteem (SE) and social interest (SI), addicts, who demand immediate and total gratification of psychic needs from external sources, may become true artists. By this approach, "passive" victims (who are in reality nonconsciously active) become masters of competency, molding their own fun and flow, while indirectly contributing to the SE and SI growth of others by practicing the concrete steps of natural high growth.

Blocking the way to such novel yet practical healing of addictions is the popular professionalized way of doing things. One thesis of this chapter is that there will be only unsuccessful "quietment," instead of self- actualizing treament for addiction, until institutionalized inanities are pared away from an authentic, healing, medical practice. Institutional addiction is a type of ego-addiction on a large scale — hence, the zealous tenacity which motivates the unawareness of (and adherence to) the quietment-of-victims model from which world-image institutional addicts faithfully derive power.

All narcotizing addictions grow from discouragement. Discouragenic attitudes and movements carry the implicit message of an unchanging unworthiness. "I am no good...you are no good...life is no good and cannot change" is the lugubrious litany of discouragement. Paradoxically, people get power (or influence) from such a constricted world-view: all find stability of roles, goals, and controls in what they see as this certitude of "human nature." In this discouragenic doctrine, there is non-productive power for all. Those at the apex of influential success are esteemed highly by most. Weak (low SE and narrow SI) forms are relegated to the bottom of the power base; those with high nuisance-value, are esteemed or deemed negatively. As Kurt Adler has said on many occasions, the privileged at the top must keep the perennial peasants at the bottom, beating their breasts, through ego-induced degradation ceremonials, else they will "wise-up" and beat the heads of the so-called masters. The hidden catch in this nonconscious, soul-sapping game is that it is addictive by definition. Both the "successes" at the top and the "failures" at the bottom are hyperdependent upon the permanence of the dyadic, slave-master, gruesome-twosome. Therefore, all such game-players are clinging to external roles, goals, and controls in time. Even those rebels fighting their ego-casting, their primal definitions from others, have limited them selves by negative obedience, donning the roles, goals, and controls of chronic opposition. Moreover, rigidity of attitudes and actions is the very essence of all ego-addictions, of which substance-abuse is the most accepted example (Beecher & Beecher, 1971). When the participants in this deadly drama see their institutionalized reasons for stable existence falling away, they experience all the bodily and psychic symptoms of panic portrayed by withdrawal reactions of junkies.

Directly opposed to the institutional game is the God head game of instrumental change. Natural high therapy is the game-of-games, performed by inner and outer movements on three levels, giving each person skills in the art of expanding SI and SI on inner (level I), interpersonal (level II), and transpersonal (level III) dimensions. The interloper who labels the institutional game gets the full fury that therapists experience by telling patients of their responsibilities before the trusting, cooperation-as-equals is established. Moreover, the critic of institutional constrictions is apt to receive the blast by an overwhelming number of elite citizens who feel as if the very source of their being is buffeted. If you can recall the innocent debunker in the tale of the emperor's new clothes, you might remember that no one thanked the boy for his courageous, incisive insights. Such heretics are no longer burned physically. But mentally they can be subjected to the pernicious labeling of stupid, masochistic, hostile and/or mentally ill. A very incisive autocratic thrust is to interpret criticism as an unconscious projection of the revoluntionary's (or evolutionary's) power-strivings upon the normal (meaning here "more numerous") of society's time-honored rationalities. Once the critic is labeled with egregious terms, the traditionalist can provoke craziness in weak (inadequate SI and SE) antagonists or selectively ferret out anomalies for labeling. Any threat to external power can be reframed as hostility from the other. Such powerful ploys hide the behavioral contributions of the elite to the madness of the world and obliterate the real purpose of the revolutionary's feedback and self-disclosure. Here we have a thumb-nail sketch of how unsuccessful education and quietment is maintained and why deep and broad humanistic changes are not forthcoming.

For critics to weather the discouragenic drama, they must embody the prototype of the natural high life style. Constant attention to the sense of humor (O'Connell, 1979b) based upon a loving acceptance of a paradoxical world, devotion to the expansion of SE and SI, and the seeking and developing of an encouragenic support group are necessities for the contemporary critics' actualization and survival. What might be simply stated is difficult to be heard within the institutional quietment. Once more to reiterate the premises: healing of substance abuse is most profitably conducted by teaching all persons to be responsible for their own actualization while contributing to growth of others. This view is not one of new narcissism. Other people are not seen as "objects": a route is offered to loving concern (i.e., compassionate neutrality) toward others. An incalculable savings of money and environmental resources will be realized when we stop demanding from professions and natural resources a magic, immediate route toward expansive states of belonging. Self-esteem and synergic power can be truly reached by dedicate personal practice with the contribution of an authentic support group. A second tenet is that the natural-high pioneering pilgrim will be the recipient of unending ire from those who see their present power-position threatened by mature independence, be they professional or peon.

To survive entrapments from orthodox ego-addicts, developers of actualizing approaches must "be as wise as serpents and as harmless as doves." Unfortunately, innovators of alternative perceptions to the mechanical and diminuting models cannot develop the deep trusting relationship of the wise therapist before specifying mistaken certainties which need changing. The pillars of institutionalization seldom come for feedback as curious clients. The pioneers of hopeful theories are not in the enviable position of teachers from other disiplines (physics, physiology, biology, Eastern religions) who go about giving workshops, teaching the abstract concepts of psychospiritual syntheses. These intellectual entertainers, however, laudable their efforts, are not in the lion's mouth. They are not working for the non-jolly giant in his own house and talking the absolute necessity of behavior change for all. Actualizers, to remain as such, will not react in destructive, defensive ways when the angry antagonist does or does not change. A further obstacle to taking the actualizer seriously, one which does not have the venom of invidious labeling yet effectively silences the sounds of growth, is by slavishly pointing out the need for research before action. One cannot deplore the value of research efforts, only the purpose when the theme is used to halt moves toward thoughful theory-building. Institutional pundits guard research funds and cautious CWAMAs (count-weigh-and measurement addicts) make value-judgment on what efforts are crucial (O'Connell, 1979a). Without material resources and decision-making powers of implementation, innovators must be content with mini-studies, clinical and anecdotal studies, while assiduously working on their own SE and SI. Then there is the crowning koan of them all: How can the powerful ego-addict happily embrace any study of his own constrictions? One needs self-esteem to look warily and humorously upon the diseases of ego-esteem. Nevertheless, the theory of the natural high calls for democratic cooperation-as-equals as the essential condition of real treatment, self-actualization for all. Natural high is psychospiritual, dealing with instrumental means in psychology and religion for self-realization (O'Connell, 1979c). Human goals of growth and constriction are not hidden behind obfuscating abstractions. Goals are concretized. The sense of humor, traditionally studied seriously but not with gravity, is a criterion of actualization. All of these premises are beyond the ken of one who diagnoses the other (without treating), a common movement of institutionalization.

Ego-actualization precedes self-actualization. We live in the "daze" of the constricted ego, looking with paranoid blinders, for easy, sudden, external cures. Harbingers of the world of interacting deep psyche, an inner relativity replacing the fixed machine theory, are not celebrated as yet. Has anyone ever heard of an institutional course called Creative Dissent, taught with a here-and-now accepting puzzlement? Not yet. Such a sad state might explain the transformation of the liberal students into cynical conservatives. Having no practical theory for self-growth and no support group for actualization, they are soon swallowed up into ego-perpetuating routines and their soul (spirit, self) is stillborn. And so it goes.

Natural High Therapy: For Drug- and Other Addictions

Natural High (NH) Therapy is an optimistic, action-oriented approach to living in the here-and-now which stresses the response-ability of each person for the creation of one's own state of self-actualization. This theory and therapy is the only psychological system which focuses directly upon the sense of humor, in all its ramifications, as the essential movement of the actualization process. The sense of humor is the end-result of self-training for the expansion of one's sense of worth and feelings of universal belongings, plus the development of an appreciation for the basic pardoxes of the human condition. All techniques of inner and outer change, both individual and group, are used to encourage persons to become active agents in the game-of-games, the actualization through training and practice on self-esteem (SE) and social interest (SI).

Natural high therapy can be considered a branch of holistic health, with its emphasis on the acquisition of skills of true artistry, self-development. The theory is holistic in its psychospiritual emphasis, focusing upon the instrumental elements of "The Perennial Philosophy" (Huxley, 1972) as a wonderful way toward *SE* and *SI* development. Institutional rituals, with their hidden subtle ways of granting power (interpersonal influence) to the elite, are viewed as disease agents, and totally irrelevant to the practice of natural high.

Natural high practice is a didactic-experiential adventure, each "pilgrim" or patient being a student of his/her own existence. These students learn the theory and techniques of the three levels of the natural high while observing, without blame, habitual idiosyncratic mistakes which unconsciously constrict SE and SI. Level I, the machinations of inner ego constructions, is the cornerstone of the whole actualization approach; Level II, encouragement, gives the ideal movements of active social interest; the transpersonal dimension, Level III, has as its goal further enhancement of SE and SI by transcending ego-addictions and experiencing the timeless, eternal self. The super-natural high is similar to the natural high in feelings of unconditional worth and basic similarity and belonging. Moreover, this numinous state is produced under "marketplace" situations of severe stress and is the affective counterpart of the congnitive-perceptual sense of humor.

The time of therapy is not restricted to the therapist's office in natural high therapy. Any moment can be used for recording the constrictions of ego-induced unnatural lows and isolations, then sharing and celebrating these creative acts. Above all, there is no place for blame and punishment in this democratic practice.

Natural High Therapy has profited, paradoxically, from a seven-year exposure to the adverse conditions of a methadone-maintenance, outpatient drug dependency treatment center (DDTC). Centers such as the Glass Ark, mushroomed almost overnight ten years ago. Their inherent, unexamined conditions spawn a discouragenesis usually associated with state hospital back wards. Once the drug clinics are moved away from the hospital base, the condition becomes one of "out-of-sight, out-of-mind". Funding can get diverted and the quality and quantity of personnel are subject to deterioration. Drug programs, originally developed on a store-front model with untrained ex-addicts as counselors, gradually and silently changed into medical models under the tremendous pressure to meet Joint Commission for Accreditation of Hospitals (JCAH) standards (Dorkens & Morrison, 1976). Time is spent in filling folders with unreliable data (often of non-existent activities). Such peripheral data as recreational activities and job histories are gleaned from patients, while strangely enough in other contexts the patients' words are otherwise discounted. The move toward documentation, rightfully motivated by goals of expanded treatment, can readily be subverted into a reason for not relating to patients at all. And lastly, the patients' life styles are a contributor to discouragement. Hundreds of Glass Ark MMPI's indicate severe psychopathology. Almost without exception, all clients have elevated psychopathic-deviate clinical scales, with the majority having, in addition, pathological schizophrenia and manic scales. The mixture of the discouraged personnel, trained (if formally trained at all) in the autocratic-healer and compliant-patient ("talking about symptoms-and-childhood") model with the authority-avoiding, instant-esteem-through-chemistry patient, has been devastating to the function of isolated DDTCs.

Even more unfortunate is the absence of any official attention (other than to blame) for the discouraged personnel and client potentiation. On a national level, a phenomenon called "the Vietnam Syndrome" is blamed on the aftermath of a nonglorious war and public hero blindness. It is being regarded as a new kind of disease to be "treated" by (discouraged) personnel, without an attractive theory for the authority-mistrusting consumer, the Vietnam veteran. Natural high therapy regards the particular plight of the latest veteran to be a psychosocial phenomenon germane to the times. Devious uses of power are being more closely examined since the 60's especially by our youth. But the treatment industry has not examined its own use and misuse of power. Natural high therapy has made formidable strides in that direction, the whole thrust being the expansion of personal strength through development of self-worth and universal belonging. In such a state of being, one is neither addicted to (nor victimized by) ego-strivings which are merely poor substitutes for the true strength of self-actualization.

Chronic drug addicts, almost all of the Vietnam era have, for the most part, been attracted to natural high therapy, if they are open to therapy at all. Natural high is not based upon any "close" subservient relationship with the healer. In fact, the therapist must be an authentic model and reinforcer in action before trust is given. The therapist must be able to share ego-constricton, hopes, and goals, as a living example of self-disclosure (O'Connell, 1975). The giving and requesting of authentic verbal feedback is a well-practiced art, part of the natural high life style. Therefore, it is no wonder that the bureaucratic-autocrat, of no matter what the status, equates this theory with a probable irreversible ego defeat, to be avoided at all costs.

In 1976 O'Connell began natural high therapy in earnest both as a treatment and research method for outpatient addicts and as a way of interacting and program problem-solving for the clinic staff (O'Connell, 1976a; O'Connell & Bright, 1978' O'Connell, Bright, & Grossman, 1978). Instead of the disastrous autocratic shoving and/or multiple rivalries stimulated by previous directors, the steps of level II (encouragement) were presented to staff at development sessions. The Glass Ark personnel, in this model, were seen as a system of interacting influences, responsible for becoming aware of self- and other-encouragenic and/or discouragenic actions and reactions. Self-disclosure, feedback, and a search for similarities (while not ignoring differences) are the salient steps of this treatment ritual. Feelings are stated loud and clear, without blame. Help is requested in the spirit of the Adlerian question, "What can we do together, as equal-status persons, to solve this problem?"

While this approach often prospered with drug patients, the opposite was true with the staff. The results were not much better than the autocratic failures of previous directors. In essence, the staff, for the most part, clung to their discouragements based upon certainties of unchangeable worthlessness of patients, theories, techniques, and even life itself. The staff, like the patients, harbored deep discouragements. Isolated from hospital support and without having authority over personnel, (since each worker had his own service chief), an out-patient director has little control over the consequences of non-cooperative staff behaviors. In truth, it would be better to call such non-democratic behavior cooperation-as-unequals. Some staff members passively refused to attend mutual problem-solving sessions. Others took any feedback, no matter how gentle and specific as racial attack. A few, with medical ego-addictions, wanted to view any insistence on a system for consistent and reliable medical decisions on methadone as a forbidden practice of medicine by ancillary personnel. The parent organization, having great fears of any inroads into the domain of medicine, listened to and reinforced rumors about the closed "family meetings." Eventually this writer with his own stupid demands for a therapeutic community, violated the tenets of natural high therapy. The autocratic approach that all directors grasped eventually contributed to the demise of this program as a therapeutic community.

After demanding that which can be given only spontaneously (e.g., love, encouragement) eventuated in the death of the Dreikurs (1971) approach with staff, this situation itself became an opportunity for the growth of level III with patients. Patients were no longer protected from discouragement movements of anyone, as they would be in an ideal democratic program. So all staff frailties were then openly acknowledged without rationalization. The main discovery of the death and transformation labs (O'Connell & Bright, 1977) were incorporated into natural high training for drug patients. In effect, no matter how discouragenic the contributions of others, the crucial matter of one's own state of self-esteem and social interest is the personal responsibility throughout life. Honoring the words of Adler, everything can be anything else. Perceptions, affects, memories are effects of one's state of actualization, the quality of self-worth and belonging. Only those who believe they have control, do have control; SE and SI are the only phenomena under complete personal control. No other person or event of life can be in one's charge, although individuals frustrate themselves into insanity in droves attempting to master that which they cannot absolutely control.

Natural high therapy for addiction has entered another stage, one which addicts appreciate and practice much more. They learn to meditate and clear the mind of ego-noise, together in groups. At the same time, they start to treat themselves gently, perhaps for the first time. When the mind wanders, they bring the mind (the focus of attention) back to breath-counting (feeling the breath at the top of the nostrils). When patients can one-point (do one thing at a time completely with relaxed alertness), they are ready to concentrate and contemplate. Starting at five-minute periods per day, they concentrate or focus fully on a segment of natural high theory (e.g., self-esteem, social interest). Then may come contemplation, letting the symbols unfold without diagnosing, judging, or interpreting. Even if the mind wanders, the addict's reactions or even the contents of the wanderings are a projective test of where one is on the actualization pilgrimage. Addicts, as a rule, hate to write, so they are not pressured to record these personal experiences. "Straights" (non-drug addicts in private practice) record these adventures for discussion with the therapist. Any patient may focus, on the elements of encouragement and practice, for example, looking for similarities with others. Even more important is familiarity and acceptance of the "space between thoughts" which may have commonality with the Jungian self, spirit, or soul and with right-brain speculation (Watzlawick, 1978). Whenever patients feel level I ego-constrictions taking place, they can one-point, clear the mind and so avoid the aftermath of ego-induced frustrations, the chemical fix.

Deep Discouragement

The identification of heroes and villains is not the intent of this paper. All persons are responsible for their states of actualization and contributing encouragenic and discouragenic acts toward others. Blame, punishment, and pampering is counter-productive, leading directly to rigidity of SE and SI constrictions. In natural high theory, the sharable secret is to honor the here-and-now creative constrictions (of SE and SI) of all. The focus is on blameless feedback and disclosures of self- (and other-) defeating behaviors.

An occasion for natural low lamentation is the ever-present autocratic system which has been successful in thwarting the practice of the ideals of both democratic, spiritual living. Autocratic, bureaucratic, institutionalization survives by being low-key and out of the public eye. When attacked, it has an effective way of silencing through the degradation of labeling which only the most motivated actualizer can parry. Institutionalization lives on the art of image-creating, giving the illusion of performing instrumental acts through words and proclamations. The responsibility of modeling and reinforcing encouragenic behaviors is shunned like one would avoid untreatable lepers. It almost seems that despite our lack of shared knowledge on encouragement, institutional gamesters intuitively know what encouragement is, for they are so adroit at movements in the opposite direction. Above all institutionalization quietly fosters ego-addictions: miscasting, defining, validating, and invalidating *people* (not simply behaviors) on the basis of thoughts, words, and deeds. Invalidated persons squander life in a mad pursuit of external signs of approval or in a much more mad and equally rigid reflexive opposition to rules and regulations. Institutions, with their unwritten laws, enforce a focus on the past, and a diminution of the powers of persons in the here-and-now. Days of celebration are delimited by assigning set times when we can talk about universal love and compassion (e.g. Christmas, Easter, Independence Day). The struggle for creation and freedom is fixed in the past. The anticipation of low (e.g., death and dying) in any form is often labeled as masochism, sadism, depression or as some form of disease to be entrusted to institutionalized non-dynamic experts. In any ruling, defining system of home, church, and state, the delusion to be perpetuated is that of an automatized happiness. Paradoxically, even orthodox psychoanalysis assumes the ultimate motive is to return to the inorganic. This belief in itself would guarantee depression for the majority of humans.

However, no malice toward institutions is intended, since we all, by our blind compliance and equally short-sighted violence against them, merely fuel their powers. Furthermore, an integral part of all of us is our own small-scale model of institutionalization, our ego-addictions, directing our demands for compliance to and from others. Every characteristic mentioned for universal institutions is faithfully reflected in addiction to ego-esteem. Tragicomically, we diminish ourselves and others through discouragement (as institutions so perfectly taught us). Then we strive unwittingly to over-compensate for ego-induced constrictions (level I), quite unsuccessfully.

If all of this is true, it is impossible to continue a program based on dyadic responsibility in an institutional setting. The average drug dependency treatment center (DDTC) is doomed to failure, judged from an actualization standard. Inherent contradictions in staffing, training, financing and goals render the DDTCs dangerously impotent by *any* standards. DDTCs were created in the image of the autocratic-bureaucratic model apply, compounded by the political expediencies of the 60's. The reader is referred to the comments of expert psychiatrists on the drug treatment dilemmas (Adam, 1978; Dennard, et al., 1972; Szasz, 1974; 1976; Torrey, 1975; Weill, 1972; Wurmser, 1973). Even the Veterans Administration reports are critical of the lack of training and profusion of institutional neglect for DDTCs (Baker, et al., 1975).

In seven years, at an outpatient drug clinic, the author never witnessed a discussion, instigated by anyone else, concerned with treatment as a *dyadic* responsibility. In contrast, for NH treatment is a serious game in which healers try to contribute behaviors which will assist the clients in expanding SE and SI, and to guess, often aloud, as how the other will resist encouragenic efforts. No negative judgments are made of patients. In fact they are regarded as creative, not "sick," in "efforts" to resist. Such defensive maneuvering is interpreted in NH as cooperation with treatment, (albeit not cooperation-as-equals), and "expected" phenomenon not to be marred by depreciation of self and others. Persons can stay in a behavioral plateau forever, so long as they do not overtly or covertly blame and punish self, others, or life. While this premise is readily acceptable to the NH therapist, that tutor also has faith, buoyed by clinical evidence, that the therapist's persistent pressure to have the client focus, within and out of the therapy session, on constrictions and expansions of SE and SI and on mistaken certainties toward life tasks, will eventually lead to improvement, enroute to cooperation-as-equals.

The client's change is both rapid and striking, as a rule, with private, pay-as-you-go persons. The more discouraged the individual, the greater the likelihood of institutionalization. In this situation, the NH therapist needs the assistance of other clinical personnel who perhaps have much more power (influence) than does the therapist. The therapist can have all the truth in the world, but be impotent because of others' unexamined litanies of discouragement which very effectively block all new learning. Unfortunately, bureaucratic institutions seem to perceive all persons as alike within categories, the classifications being the permanent labeling of personnel (as well as patients) within "disciplines". Once a schizophrenic, addict, etc., always a schizophrenic, addict; once a psychiatrist, always a psychiatrist. As labeling of persons becomes an institutional rite, words transcend reality (as with the chronic schizophrenic). Patients are given "treatment." The staff's word, and not the patient's experience, is the recorded reality.

Behavior itself is seldom examined in its complexity. Concentration upon *dyadic* responsibility is the unpardonable sin in institutions. Moreover, natural high therapists believe that this one observation — whether staff and patients are allowed to focus upon how each person contributes to discouragement of others — is the prime interaction that separates institutional from instrumental settings. The constant dyadic quality of the interactional human system is totally ignored, suppressed, or repressed by the institutional mind. Therefore, the past is given selective attention at the price of the present. The defined "defect" is seen in the other, never the helper, and becomes an unfolding or "maturation" of some unknown genetic and/or biological taint or the residual of early psychic traumata.

Imbued with such a static non-interactional model of disease, professionals subtly cherish and seek decision-making powers to most effectively invalidate the psychiatric patient as helpless and hopeless. Often there is intense rivalry among the siblings in the professional house for ultimate skill and power in performing degradation ceremonies. At times, the elder pundits of institutional psychiatry sharpened their skills by provoking the signs of behavioral defects of chronic schizophrenics in an uneven game called "staffing". But they were never available for contributing to the ego-development (and possible self-development) of the "captive". Dyadic therapy was conveniently ruled out because the patient was "unmotivated...and inaccessible to psychotherapy." Of course, the dyadic responsibility of the helper is saved from the light of consciousness by such verbal cleverness. Laing, Szasz, and Haley have well-commented on such ego-addictions of the helpers, disguised under the static mores of institutions, and were summarily discounted as crazy heretics by those offended (O'Connell, 1975; 1979a). *Ark Archives*

The rarefied atmosphere of the isolated DDTCs seems to stimulate something in the psyches of the staff which preclude the creation and maintenance of an actualizing community. Glass Ark Clinic directors seemed to perceive the clinic as a personal *causa-sui* project, a narrow means to ego-power. Their sense of worth and belonging was sharply focused, contingent upon successful performance, as judged by their own standards. This pathologizing state of affairs was partly the effect of a pervasive leadership vacuum on national and local levels. Decision-makers felt free to concern themselves with quietly allocating funds. The unwritten law from above seemed to be quietment at all costs, whether from patients or personnel. It is needless here to detail the complete disparity of actualizing and institutionalizing promises and purposes (O'Connell, 1979a).

Onto the physical and psychological conditions of isolation, the clinic directors projected their own power ploys. The first two outpatient DDTC directors did not survive long enough to make the move out of the hospital to the outskirts of downtown. Overall there have been six out-patient directors in less than eight years. As time goes by, negative certainties about drug patients increase, yet only the patients themselves share an awareness of chronicity and regression in staff functioning, which parallels their own process of discouragement.

Each tragicomic chain of events was simply one of the scores of common incidents, all pointing to chronic indirection and open-decision avoidance from Washington to Houston. Whatever vague directives appeared followed an obsessive-compulsive meandering over peripheral issues concerning control of patients, seen invariably (but never officially) as intractable criminals. Trust only movement, according to Adler.

This DDTC outpatient setting which I served for seven years never, in movement, accepted the natural high therapy premise that there is a constant dyadic responsibility between patient and staff behaviors. Therefore, in my views, DDTCs continue to be grounds for an eventual scandal. The Ark is a hidden Hell where patients are addicted to methadone and then pressured (not therapized) toward giving up their subsequent methadone addiction. Since therapy is never discussed in such an officially sanctioned, burned-out setting, there is no "therapy" except in word only. Meaningless abstractions are substituted for compassionate sharing and seeking of knowledge in such hellish quietment centers.

Remarkably the Ark embarked upon a nine month period of relative tranquility (O'Connell, Bright, & Grossman, 1978). Unfulfilled promises and induced rivalries disappeared as the program followed the Adlerian democratic format (Dreikurs, 1971) of open meetings with feedback and self-disclosure for all. The patients' pleas for tranquilizers and methadone changes sharply decreased since no physician was available, except on weekly visits. The emphasis shifted from staff bickerings on methadone quantities to developing with patients a workable system of rules and regulations relatively acceptable to all. The idyllic period ended with the eruption of my ego-needs and the pressing institutional needs to have physicians available.

No one would argue that the DDTCs receive the best of personnel. DDTCs have a way of getting rid of undesirable addicts and personnel when they are far away from the hospital. DDTCs also stimulate ego-needs of clinic directors, away from rules and regulations. Clinic directors are not trained and are unsupervised in their arbitrary decisions. For the most part, directors of the Ark have articulated no theory of behavior change and seem to be looking for none. Whatever theory of treatment, it seems consonant with the unshared life style of the current director. In actual practice, clinic affairs rock on to the tune of staff-patient persistent power ploys. Due to another silent, undiscussed turn of events, the personnel at the clinic are over 90% black, with female leaders. There will be more uniformity for a while: but against whom or what? For what purpose? Will the ensuing goal-direction be for authenticity, knowledge and practice to cooperate-as-equals with chemically-addicted discouraged veterans of an unpopular war in a joint effort at actualization? No way, as long as institutionalization of the mind with its quietment disguised as treatment numbs the psyche.

Personal Premises

Even before I became the first college student and first "Yankee" attendant at a Texas mental hospital, I must have had a strong sense of what mental hospitals and treatment relationships should be like. For as soon as I could walk, I visited relatives in mental hospitals. I also accompanied my father, a disabled WWI veteran, on his outpatient trips to the Veterans Bureau. A curious puzzlement was always with me about what transpired between people and for what purpose. Fortunately, for the eventual actualization of ego and the self, I have experienced chronic conflicts with institutional ego-addicts about the following premises, centered in my experience with staff and patients, as to what are right and wrong (unpopular words) interactions and transactions. Some of the conflictual premises are:

(1) The prime purpose of hospitalization is to help patients experience and change their troublesome self-defeating mistaken-certainties. Institutional rituals of living and recording are completely ancillary to this instrumental tutoring for changing attitudes, feelings, and movements.

(2) Patients should not be discouragenically labeled, either descriptively or through avoidance, as untreatable. Professionals are employed to discover novel attempts at treatment and to test such theories and techniques via clinical and experimental research.

(3) Mental health professionals have easy recourse to narrow ways of conceptualizing problems of living. Viewing present behaviors as "nothing-but" manifestations of insidious disease processes determined fully by unknown organic and/or early psychic traumata is often an excuse for useless power and laziness on the part of patients and personnel.

(4) Closely allied to the above observation is the all-too-standard practice of judging patients by abstract diagnoses which often have a discouraging ego-fulfilling effect upon staff and patients. Differences rather than similarities are high-lighted, culminating in the paranoid- like stance of perceiving the human environment in "We vs. them" war-like terms.

(5) Psychological treatment, rather than quietment malpractice, rests upon the state of actualization of worth and belonging of the healers, along with their knowledge of theory and concrete techniques. Since no one is entirely free from the intrusion of childhood constrictions, therapists must constantly learn and practice their own sense of humor and ways of creating and maintaining strong support groups. The latter, gently-but-firmly, give feedback and self-disclosure; and are the perennial practice field for the constantly-evolving therapist or healer.

(6) The treatment should not be worse than the disease. All drastic intervention "works;" that is, the patient can be overwhelmed easily by "quietment." The crucial issue is what this interaction does to the patients' faith in their own significance and belonging as persons.

Methadone maintanance programs are subject to serious scandals on the foregoing issues. One way of avoiding life-style tutoring is through sinister staff semantics. Rather than press for leadership in creating new theories and techniques, institutionalized "healers," professional and otherwise, seek evidence that nothing can be done. If patients do not quickly "heal" through desultory rituals, they are isolated into an incurable category, releasing the healer from effort and guilt. In my experience, drug patients suffer the most from the staff search-and-stimulation of discouragement, due to staff negative omnipotence. Curiosity, puzzlement, and an eagerness to learn and discover new therapeutic approaches quickly evaporate when negative insight overwhelms the encouragenic orientation. The appearance of disabling discouragement in the field of addiction is much more tragicomic than its counterpart in the mental hospital. For the average addict is much more alive and moving than the typical mental hospital inmate (O'Connell, Bright, & Grossman, 1978). Even more puzzling is the very sudden appearance of discouragement in drug addiction treatment, a state which tells much about our lack of resourcefulness and the sterility of psychotherapeutic theories and techniques.

The Awe-full Aftermath

The way is difficult for an optimistic behaviorally-oriented treatment group existing in a discouragenic setting controlled by callous, bureaucratic complacency. In living situations with degrees of freedom, members of such growth groups could learn to react with humor rather than with negative nonsense to the de-humanistic certainties of controlling others. But total institutions mean that direct pressure is brought to bear upon patients by personnel (e.g., amount of methadone, pick-up schedule, or even existence as a patient). Such conditions drastically deepen the discouragenic dramas within DDTCs.

When patients feel trapped by demands of helpers, they react in kind with their particular useless power (influence) ploys, mainly power struggles, revenge, and displays of disability (O'Connell, 1975). Illustrative hidden themes are: "You can't tell me what to do," "Now I'll hurt you," and "I'm just a hopeless victim" (Dreikurs, 1971). When staff and patient transactions are used to destroy mutually any social interest (similarity, belonging), authentic treatment cannot operate. Once the participants stabilize negative perceptions and reject the idea that their acts contribute to others' discouragement, instant hell is truly upon us. Cooperative efforts at treatment evaporate and projection of negative qualities goes on, wholly unexamined. When patients acquire all the negative labels, any staff is very reluctant to change, since the very meaning of their avoidance and isolation is dependent upon constantly confirming these negative qualities.

For example, EF spent almost two years in the natural high group, meeting two hours a week. Over the years he was openly angry at what he considered neglect by staff. His anger extended even to any interruption in group when he was talking. With 25 patients in the group, EF spent his early months fuming and impulsively running out of the group. As EF began to understand the theory and techniques of the natural high experientially, his demanding behavior diminished markedly. When EF became a natural high devotee—

watching, sharing, and even celebrating on occasion, ego-induced constrictions — he began to regard the staff's unchanging negative perceptions of him in a humorous light. Even though the failure to communicate among staff members brought further stress, EF did not use such happenings to indulge in power struggles, revenge, or dis-ability reactions on the useless side of life.

EF was one of numerous U.B.s (urine balker) noted at the DDTC. Since the staff's *causa-sui* project has been primarily control of the urine-methadone exchange, staff anxiety was always high when patients would not give urine upon demand. Rather than focus upon the discouraged purpose of maladaptive interactions, staff took the urine balkers' withholding as personal insults to their weak institutionalized egos (e.g., "We are worthless unless we can force those bastards to give urine on demand"). Even though for considerable periods of time, the hospital lab was "too shorthanded" to analyze DDTC urine; even though it was common knowledge, commonly suppressed, that there was marketing in the sale of urine results, the staff electively focused on the U.B.s' resistance-to-rules.

EF was a U.B. for years, one behavior guaranteed to suddenly stabilize a helpless-hopeless image. But contrary to staff's negative certainties, the typical U.B., motivated to resist rigid unilateral demands, had more favorable prognosis than did hyper-dependent patients — those who would slavishly allow staff biding, no matter how contradictory or infantilizing the directives (O'Connell, Bright, & Grossman, 1978). Most of the U.B.s I have known have had good initiative, if not quashed by staff.

EF eventually found his own job as a high school vocational teacher. Since his negative image was so stabilized, most staff were not informed of the patient's employment until EF told his supervisor that he was a methadone-maintenance patient. During the interim, staff negative certainties about EF still abounded. Staff solidarity was based on unacknowledged self-discouragement. EF, on the other hand, was selected for his teaching position, because he verbalized well the encouragenic premises of natural high therapy. This reversal of textbook staff-and-patient attitudes is the raw material of comedy (as well as the stuff of tragedy). Those U.B.s who work-play at ego-and-self understanding can use their urge for freedom to overcome, by meditation and humor, their own inner constrictions. Other angry U.B.s simply resist natural high practice as they resist all of their life tasks, and so enter chronicity by mindless oppositions.

And so ends the saga of the fool who would attempt to push discouraged personnel into being instruments of encouragenesis. Such unwanted endings as the failure of personnel to accept a doctrine of change give credence to the axiom of behavior modification that one who pioneers encouragement must have positive power or influence over even the hirings and firings of staff. People do not change simply by pointing out the goals of misbehavior. Patients who continue the natural high approach (albeit for "underground") at the Glass Ark know this truth. Staff and institutional leaders are not so concerned with the knowledge of responsible personal change. Their goal is rather the communication of the image of competence and concern, which masks the main motivation of control.

About a year after my directorship, I was nominated for the Director's Certificate of Commendation. When the hospital director rejected that request, the Chief of Psychiatry followed with a quality-increase suggestion. But within a year the tenor of the report, seen below, changed from admiration to administrative anger.

> Dr. O'Connell's outstanding performance as Director of the Glass Ark has resulted in significantly improved staff morale, introduction of effective new treatment techniques, improved patient compliance with the treatment regimen, institution of program evaluation and in-service staff training programs, and elimination of criminal and counter-therapeutic activities involving both patients and staff. These remarkable accomplishments have been performed despite virtually constant adversity. Staff ceiling at the Glass Ark has been diminished by four positions while the patient load has increased to over 300 during Dr. O'Connell's tenure as Director. Both Central Office and the Psychiatry Service Administration are aware that the productivity of the Glass Ark warrants additional staff according to published standards but budgetary constraints have kept the staff below acceptable levels. Nevertheless, Dr. O'Connell has maintained a high level of patient care at the Glass Ark. I believe that Dr. O'Connell's administrative and clinical accomplishments under the conditions he faces have been genuinely remarkable (Fann, 1976).

"Whistle Blowers" (Simon, 1978) and lads who question the emperor's new clothes will never be successful in the world of ego and institutional-addicts. To demand such approval would be damned discouragenic!

In final summation, one point emerges. Natural high therapy sounds like a theory with techniques for actualization perfectly suited for hospice work with terminal clients (Stoddard, 1978). No doubt it is; natural high embraces psychologies, psychiatries, religions, and thanatologies which precipitate psycho-spiritual happiness through expanded thoughts and feelings of inherent self-worth and innate belonging. Ego-addicts can find no solace face-to-face with dying patients, unless they possess an ego-charisma like an Elizabeth Kubler-Ross. So more than an ego-psychology, which emphasizes success in the external world, is needed. Work in thanatology must be psychospiritual, leading to a self-esteem, with the "self" synonymous with "spirit" or "soul" (O'Connell, 1979a). The hyper-physics of Teilhard de Chardin (O'Connell, 1975) takes soul-making seriously. Therein, humankind is not an accidental accretion, but is actively creating through love the radial energy necessary to power universal evolution. If people believe this premise (through experience, not merely memorization), depression would go out of style. Likewise, so would paranoia, if persons practiced the social interest to see others also in this light. Metanoia — not paranoia — is a goal of natural high. Drug addicts and institutionalized schizophrenics are our modern lepers. Level II steps of encouragement (O'Connell & Bright, 1977) are not profitable in terms of external rewards for the psychotherapist. To reward such interactions, a theory of faith is necessary which goes far beyond the graspings, greeds, and attachments of ego-addictions and institutional material gains. Therefore, the real lesson of my Glass Ark experience is this: The world of treatment needs psychospiritual practice. Otherwise, those with high social nuisance value will forever be duped, dumped, miscast, and projected upon as hopeless, helpless, and subtly but utterly forever damned. The big business of madness makes materialistic monopolies, as the psychiatric pariah, Thomas Szasz (1974; 1976) solemnly states.

REFERENCES

ADAMS, J. *Psychoanalysis of Drug Dependence: The Understanding and Treatment of a Particular Form of Pathological Narcissism.* New York: Grune and Stratton, 1978.

Baker, S., Diduff, M., Thorsland, E., and Tribble, C. *A Review of the Role of Automated Data Processing in V.A. Drug Dependence Treatment Centers Using Methadone Modality.* Washington, D.C.: V.A. Health Care Review Service Report, February, 1975.

Beecher, W., and Beecher, M. *The Mark of Cain: An Anatomy of Jealousy.* New York: Harper and Row, 1971.

Dorken, H., and Morrison, D. JCAH Standards for Accreditation of Psychiatric Facilities: Implications for the Practice of Clinical Psychology. *American Psychologist*, 1976, *31*, 774-784.

Dreikurs, R. *Social Equality: The Challenge of Today.* Chicago: Regnery, 1971.

Fann, E. *Quality Increase.* Houston: V.A. Hospital, December 20, 1976.

Huxley, A. Introduction. In Prabhavananda, S., and Isherwood, C., *The Song of God: Bhagavad-Gita.* New York: American Library, 1972.

Lennard, H., Epstein, L, Bernstein, A., and Ransom, D. *Mystification and Drug Misuse: Hazards in Using Psycho-Drugs.* New York: Harper-Row Perennial, 1972.

O'Connell, W. *Action Therapy and Adlerian Theory.* Chicago: Alfred Adler Institute, 1975.

O'Connell, W. *Super Natural Highs.* Chicago: North American Graphics, 1979a.

O'Connell, W. The Sense of Humor: A Neglected Source of Energy. *Individual Psychologist*, 1979, *16* (b).

O'Connell, W. Natural High Therapy: A Psychospiritual Pilgrimage. *Medical Surgical Journal*, 1979, *14* (c).

O'Connell, W. Natural High Therapy. In Corsini, R. (Ed), *Innovative Psychotherapies.* New York: Wiley, 1980 (In press).

O'Connell, W., and Bright, M. *Natural High Primer*. Houston: Natural High Associates, 1977.

O'Connell, W., and Bright, M., Natural High Therapy: Encouragement Out of Despair. *The Individual Psychologist*, 1978, *15*, 36-40.

O'Connell, W., Bright, M., and Grossman, S. Negative Nonsense and Drug Addiction. *Rational Living*, 1978, *13* (l), 19-24.

Simon, G. The Psychologist as Whistle Blower: A Case Study. *Professional Psychology*, 1978, *9*, 322-340.

Stoddard, S. *The Hospice Movement: A Better Way of Caring for the Dying*. New York: Random Vintage, 1978.

Szasz, T. *Ceremonial Chemistry*. Garden City, New York: Doubleday Anchor, 1974.

Szasz, T. *Heresies*. Garden City, New York: Doubleday Anchor, 1976.

Torrey, E. *The Death of Psychiatry*. New York: Penguin, 1975. Watzlawick, D. *The Language of Change: Elements of Therapeutic Communication*. New York: Basic Books, 1978.

Weill, A. *The Natural Mind*. Boston: Houghton Mifflin, 1972. Wurmser, L. Unpolitical Thoughts about the Politics of Drug Issues. *Journal of Drug Issues*, 1973, *3*, 178-184.

CASE HISTORY: POLY DRUG ABUSE AND SELF-ESTEEM
R. A. Steffenhagen

The following case history is a classic example of poly drug abuse resulting from low self-esteem.

Jim came in my office for the first time in February of 1978 with the complaint of poly drug abuse and depression. He is a middle- class, white college male, age 19, who had been doing drugs for the past seven years. He began with alcohol, then pot, and then began doing harder drugs, all before high school. It should be noted that within the framework of the theory presented, the initiation into drugs was totally a social condition and that the search for drugs was not occasioned by an attempt to escape reality; however, it began to serve this function very early. Jim is a freshman at the University of Vermont and is a tall, handsome young man of rather slight build. The girls find him quite attractive and he finds no difficulty socializing with members of the opposite sex. I suspect his relationship with his peers is better with women than with men. The reason for this will become apparent as we develop his case history.

Jim came to me for the first time in a state of deep depression and with the complaint that "I'm probably like many of your other clients; my problem is one of poly drug abuse." Then he went on to indicate that he was in the state of prolonged deep depression and that he was constantly medicating himself with drugs to cope with this depression. He further commented on the fact that he was beginning to think in terms of suicide in that he was wondering, "What it would be like to stick a shotgun to his chest and blow himself away." He said, "Eventually I got to where I knew things had to change, or for one moment I might decide to use that gun. I knew I needed a psychiatrist but I hated the thought of going to a shrink. A friend suggested that I see a hypnotist to see if that would help any." And it was at this point that Jim came to see me. He further commented on the fact that his drug use had probably peaked at this particular point and that although he wasn't using the gun he was destroying himself both physically and mentally with the excessive use of drugs.

Jim is a native Vermonter surrounded by the beauty of Vermont, but a beauty which had little effect upon making his childhood happy. Jim's parents, like so many other parents, got married, had children and then found that they did not love one another. Because of religious or cultural conditioning, they felt the need to stay together for the sake of the children — a condition which probably was more detrimental for the psychic well-being of the children than divorce would have been. It should be noted that Jim commented on the fact that he never really felt loved. As he says, "In my mind I have a very small sense of love which I can share with anyone due to my father's example while I was young and impressionable." He commented on the fact that his father definitely tried to make their life happy but that this was impossible. He further comments on the fact that while his father was living at home he was in love with another woman and that he felt unloved and unwanted. The tensions in the household proved more than Jim could handle and he couldn't get along with his mother or brother for more than five minutes at a time. In order to cope with this, he made friends with a neighbor boy his same age and he dealt with his own unhappiness by spending as much time as possible with his friend and his friend's family. It should be noted that in many ways his friend, Carl, the friend's mother and father were in reality Jim's brother and his mother and father.

This type of compensatory mechanism probably would have helped Jim to cope with his own needs for love except for a very traumatic unexpected event. One morning Jim woke up to find the fire truck at the neighbor's farm and saw the house in a state of smoking ruin. When asked what happened, his mother told him that a fire had started during the night in the neighbor's house and that the whole family had died in the fire. As he says, "I couldn't understand how something like this could happen and as far as I was concerned, it didn't really happen and that was it. From then on people were always saying that everyone in the house was dead and so forth, but I would just let it pass through my head with as little contemplation as possible." This type of trauma is extremely devastating, for someone of his age, especially when the death involves one's own family, and in this instance they were his adopted parents. Working through bereavement is difficult at best, but when the individual has extremely low self-esteem, has suffered feelings of being unloved, the problem of bereavement becomes much more severe. In his own mind, for a year, he had entirely shut out the death of his friend Carl and his "adopted parents." He would not face the issue, he would not deal with the reality but kept believing that Carl would come over and they would play together as always, and that he would be able to go over and eat and sleep at their house. However, in his dreams he was always with Carl. Then one night, a year later, he woke up at the end of the dream in which he had said, "Carl, where are you, where are you?" and when Carl wasn't there as he always was in the dream, Jim then realized that he was dead and cried for the first time since the death of his friend.

The trauma of the death was further complicated by feelings of guilt over an incident which happened between himself and the neighbor's youngest daughter. One day while they were talking she commented on the fact that God was with her and that when she died she would go to heaven. Because of his rather secular upbringing, and the unhappiness occasioned by the lack of love he had turned from God and commented to her that there was no God, there was no heaven, and that when you die that is the end. She could not accept this and ran in the house crying. In reflecting upon this, he commented that he doesn't know how he could have attempted to change someone's attitude and that he was glad that she believed in herself and not in him. But it is apparent that in order for this realization to take place today, many years later, he must have internalized a feeling of guilt when she died.

Although he accepted the death, cried and dealt with the loss of his friend, this did not in any way resolve the problems at that time. He met another friend several years older who was beginning high school at that time. He identified with this older male Kurt, who began to function as an ego ideal since his father never functioned in that particular capacity. This particular friend for whatever reason was getting into drugs and this, of course, became the right thing to do for Jim. He began experimenting with drugs at this time, at age 12, he began with alcohol, then tried pot, and then moved on to harder drugs at this young impressionable age. This experimentation was seen as a change for the better; he was meeting new people, and probably feeling wanted and liked for the first time. He was meeting girls, he was having a lot of fun and school came last. It is important at this point, to emphasize the fact that the drug subculture does provide the emotional support of a primary group and that since he didn't feel loved at home, the drug subculture played a vital part in meeting his needs at this particular time.

When he started high school, he was well into the drug scene and tried almost every drug available. He experimented with downers, speed, opium, PCP and LSD. His comment was at that time, "it didn't really matter what you were taking as long as you got off." He began to differentiate between what students call "clean" and "dirty" drugs and he began to limit his consumption largely to cocaine and LSD. He estimates in his senior year in high school he dropped acid approximately 40 times. He comments, "It seemed that LSD in the long run had almost changed the way I thought in one way or another. My thinking was not in parallel with reality. My drug use was becoming a major problem along with one other thing, which proved in the end to be the more dangerous." He commented that his father once said that when parents were not around to offer the needed support, children would frequently become dependent on members of the opposite sex earlier in their adolescent years than would kids coming from happier or well-adjusted families. This then led into the second problem which was the fact that he became deeply and emotionally attached to a girl at age 15; his comment, when I first saw him, was "married at 15; divorced at 19," and, of course, what he meant was that for four years he was totally dependent upon her for emotional support; she became a 'Linus' blanket."

After four years of this deep emotional involvement which proved to be sexually but not emotionally satisfying, the relationship ended; this led to the deep depression that was referred to earlier in the history. He began to go out with what he called "sleazy girls" in an attempt to satisfy his physical needs and did more and more drugs in an attempt to satisfy his emotional needs. He says, "It seemed that if I wasn't dependent upon something, a parent that wasn't there, a girl, or drugs, I would for the most part be unhappy. When each one in its own separate place caught up with me, it always left me devastated. In the end, when I had nothing left to turn to, I would always turn to drugs. It was the one escape that I could always take for granted. With my ego in the condition it was, drugs could only make it worse. It seemed to increase my paranoia and ill-feelings." He also referred to the fact that it seemed he was beginning to lose his mind, and at this point he began to think of suicide. He had commented on the fact that the more depressed he seemed to become the more drugs he took, and "the combination of depression and drugs was slowly killing me mentally and physically."

At the point that Jim came in he stated his problem as being one of depression, drugs and nightmares and he stated very honestly that if something wasn't done to help he would eventually commit suicide. I began seeing him twice a week for about five weeks and some of these sessions ran as long as 2½ hours. One day Jim asked whether he was becoming addicted to hypnosis and to me, whether he was merely changing one addiction for another, and what would he do if I weren't there? I assured him that the dependency he was developing upon the hypnosis and upon me would be very short-lived and that transference would not take place and would not have to be worked out. I began to work with Jim with my usual hypnotic technique in which I constantly attempted to reinforce the feeling of self-worth and to develop a spiritual baseline for self-esteem. In this regard, it should be noted that because of his past unhappiness he took a dim view of spirituality and questioned whether he would be able to accept a spiritual baseline for developing self-esteem. Using the hypnotic technique one reaches deeper through the unconscious and it is not necessary to deal with this on a conscious rational level. I reassured him that his spiritual development would take place but that it was not related to any orthodox religion and would merely be seen by him as the feeling of self-worth, a belief in himself.

We discussed his early socialization process, his feelings of inadequacy, his feelings of not being loved, his drug abuse patterns and the feelings of hate that he has held for his ex-girlfriend. Over the five-week period, the hatred began to phase out; he has totally stopped all heavy drug abuse and is beginning to feel like a fine, worthwhile human being. It should be noted that after the initial dramatic improvement, there was a period in which everything seemed to reach a very low point, a condition which almost always occurs in therapy. He came in one day commenting that it looked as though everything was falling apart, and the signs of improvement were only transitory, and he had lost faith. I listened to him and spent a great deal of time pointing out that as one gets better, even minor setbacks are viewed as being of major proportion because they are then seen in relation to a very positive improvement and thus, even though they may be minor, they may seem much worse than even the original condition. I commented that this, in essence, was a good sign and that he should not worry, that he would soon feel better again. Early in therapy I had commented in reference to his statement *that he could not continue living like this*, that we would succeed, that he would become happy and there was no question in my mind about helping him. His comment on this low point was, "What a bullshitter, telling me that this low point is a good sign. Within a week I was feeling wonderful, my whole outlook on life began to change from negative to positive. I did not allow negative thoughts to enter my mind; if I did, I would replace it with an optimistic thought. Soon I began to think that life is short, that I had better get on the ball if I want to catch the train. From there on I would always try to make the best of a bad situation."

It should be noted that as Jim's self-esteem began to develop, his need for drugs began to diminish dramatically, his feelings of self-worth began to increase and the depression began to disappear like a morning mist. He is now enjoying school, his relationships with girls are beginning to improve dramatically, he is not merely content with "jumping in the sack" but is more concerned with making close emotional relationships.

As was stated, his poly drug abuse has totally disappeared. When I asked him about his consumption of marijuana, he commented that it was still very high and I became a bit concerned and began to probe, as I felt that the amount of consumption would begin to decrease with the development of a better self-esteem. Here again, we get into the situational context and must always look at the patterns of drug use in relationship to the social milieu. He commented that his particular room in the dorm was nicknamed the toking room in that even when he and his roommate weren't there other students would frequently be in there toking. Toking has become for him a social condition which is part of his environment and a part that is now different from the original context in which he was using drugs. He tokes for enjoyment and it is as a social condition rather than a need to escape reality; he is not using it as a crutch. I would hypothesize that the amount he smokes will be only in relationship to the social situation.

Jim is very fortunate in being a very intelligent young man with a good physical body or he might not have survived so successfully the drug abuse period. As might be predicted by the theory of self-esteem, we begin to see a major increase in the mental component when he began to feel better about himself. We begin to see an increase in the cultural dimension, as his relationship to other members in his peer group became closer, rather than merely using sex as a means of communication. For Jim the physical has never been a major problem. He has been able to accept his body without much deliberation and we have seen the development of self-esteem take place on the mental and cultural level. His final comment was, "I can't thank Dr. Steffenhagen enough for his devoted time he spent changing my negative attitudes on life, ie. How can you pay a person for giving you happiness?, you can't, all you can say is "thanks a lot for changing my life"."

Joseph Harry, Ph.D.
Department of Sociology
Northern Illinois University

12
SELF-ESTEEM AND THE EVOLUTION
OF EFFEMINACY IN GAY MEN

There now exist a number of studies comparing the self-esteem of gay and heterosexual men (Bell and Weinber, 1978; Siegelman, 1972; Saghir and Robins, 1973; Spence and Helmreich, 1978; Hart et al., 1978). These studies typically show either no differences in self- esteem between gay and non-gay males or show only very modest differences. What differences are found seem to be due to the low self-esteem of that minority of gay men who are effeminate. Siegelman (1972) found that it seemed to be effeminacy rather than sexual orientation which was associated with low self-esteem. Saghir and Robins (1973) also found that it was the effeminates among gay men who disporportionately reported certain types of psychiatric disorders and that such disorders were related to a history of childhood effeminacy among his gay respondents. Weinberg and Williams (1974) also found that effeminate gay men have more psychological problems than non-effeminate gays. In the light of these findings it is reasonable to infer that effeminacy or femininity is a significant source of low self-esteem.

The interpretation of the association between femininity and low self-esteem is not immediately apparent since there seems to be nothing intrinsic to femininity per se which should be conducive to low self-esteem. Recent research dealing with the concept of androgyny has shown that it may be necessary to distinguish between gender-role (cultural) femininity and psychological femininity (Bem, 1974; Spence and Helmreich, 1978). The former is manifested by an interest in activities and objects typically culturally defined as appropriate for the female gender. The MMPI uses items measuring femininity in this manner. The latter is viewed as psychological affiliativeness or expressiveness and in recent years has been often measured by the femininity scales of Bem (1974) or Spence and Helmreich (1978) which ask the respondent about the applicability of a number of psychologically feminine traits to themselves. Various researchers have found the correlations between the cultural femininity scales and the psychological femininity ones to be either small or non-existent (cf Spence and Helmreich, 1978). Hence, it appears that the two types of scales may not be viewed as alternative ways of measuring a single concept. We are then left with the problem that, although femininity in gay men has been reliably shown to be related to lower self-esteem, we do not know whether that femininity is psychological, cultural-role, or some other gender-related concept.

The problem of the meaning of femininity (or effeminacy) in the studies of gay men is further clouded by findings of *positive* relationships between self-esteem and psychological femininity. Spence and Helmreich (1978) found a correlation of .34 between these two measures in a sample of 56 male homosexuals. In our data below we also find a significant .17 correlation between these two measures (N#1525) in a sample of gay men. Hence, it appears that psychological femininity is a positive correlate of self-esteem while the measures of "femininity" in the studies of gay men cited above are negative correlates. Since the Siegelman (1972) study used the MMPI Mf Scale, a principally cultural measure, it may be that it is cultural or gender-role femininity which is negatively related to self-esteem. Both the studies by Weinberg and Williams (1974) and Saghir and Robins (1973) employed measures of respondent self-assessed femininity and hence it is impossible to determine which form of femininity they were actually measuring. From these studies it seems clear that the femininity concept negatively related to self-esteem is not that of psychological femininity since the latter is positively related to self-esteem, at least at the zero-order level. Since no studies of gay men to date have included both cultural and psychological measures of femininity, we do not know what the relationship between these two forms of femininity may be. In the data below we explore the relationships of self-esteem with psychological and cultural femininity separately.

The effeminacy exhibited by a number of gay men appears to have its origins early in their lives. A variety of researchers have found that a large majority of gay men were effeminate during childhood. Whitam (1977), comparing 206 homosexual men with 78 hetrosexual males, found that 94 percent of the former versus 26 percent of the latter exhibited at least one of six cross-gender characteristics during childhood as measured by adult recall of childhood. These characteristics included having wanted to be a girl, having preferred to play with girls, being considered a sissy during childhood, cross- dressing, and preferring female sex-typed toys such as dolls. Whitam (1979) has subsequently replicated these findings on Brazilian homosexual and heterosexual men. Similar large differences during childhood between gay and heterosexual men have been reported by Saghir and Robins (1973). Sixty-seven percent of their male homosexual respondents versus three percent of male heterosexual respondents were found to display a girl-like syndrome during childhood. Freund (1974) has also found pre-adult differences between gay and heterosexual men on cross-gender behaviors and interests. Hence, the differences in cross-gender characteristics between gay and heterosexual men during childhood appear to be both large and well-documented, whatever the remaining differences during adulthood.

The differences in femininity between gay and heterosexual men reported for their respective childhoods appear to be very largely cultural differences in sex-typed activities and interests rather than differences in psychological femininity. Hence, it cannot be determined from the presently published literature whether such cultural differences during childhood were accompanied by comparable differences in psychological femininity. It would be hazardous to assume the existence of a parallel set of differences in psychological femininity for childhood since, to the extent that psychological masculinity and femininity may be learned phenomena, as are their cultural counterparts, childhood configurations among such psychological measures need not (yet) parallel the adult configuration.

A related line of research has been in the study of effeminate boys and comparisons of them with conventional boys. The differences between these two types of boys are strikingly similar to those between the recalled childhoods of gay and heterosexual men, although it does not immediately follow that effeminate boys would grow up to be gay. However, Green (1974), Zuger (1966) and Lebovitz (1972) have restudied small numbers of effeminate boys during their adolescence whom they had studied as children. They found that the majority of these boys had grown up to be homosexuals, trans-sexuals, or transvestites. Homosexuality was found to be much more common among them than transvestism or trans-sexualism. Hence, such studies of effeminate boys may be potentially informative about homosexuality.

Green (1976), Green and Money (1966), Zuger (1966) and Bates and Bentler (1973) have been the principal students of boys exhibiting cross-gendering. Such boys have typically been found to prefer the games, toys, and company of girls. They differ on all of the items on which Whitam (1977; 1979) found gay and heterosexual men to have differed. They are intensely indifferent to sports, particularly the rougher sports involving direct body contact or team sports. Parallel differences have been reported by Bell and Weinberg (1978) and Saghir and Robins (1973) between gay and heterosexual adult males in interests in sports. In experimental studies the two types of boys have been found to differ in expectable directions in choices of masculine versus feminine toys (Green, 1974).

Another reliable, but not so readily comprehensible, difference between effeminate boys and conventional ones is that a sizable majority of the former seem to have an intense interest in the arts, decorating, and particularly in play-acting (Green and Money, 1966; Stoller, 1968). They found that an interest in play-acting was true of 75% of the feminine boys evaluated while none were totally devoid of such interest. In their factor analytic study of the characteristics of effeminate and conventional boys, Bates et al. (1973) found the item "He play-acts, puts on little dramas" to be part of a feminine behavior factor. Whitam (1979) has also found that a childhood interest in being an actor, entertainer, or movie star is both associated with childhood effeminacy and a significantly distinguishing characteristic of gay versus heterosexual adult men. Also, Bell and Weinberg (1978) and Saghir and Robins (1973) have found heterosexual and gay males to differ in the extent of their interest in the theater.

The childhood interest in the arts and play-acting common among effeminate boys may minimally be interpreted as an aspect of cultural femininity. Stein and Smithells (1969) have reported that during childhood the arts are typically defined as "sissy stuff" by other boys and are permissible only for girls. For effeminate boys such play activities may constitute alternative avenues of expressiveness since they appear to have little interest in the activities culturally made available for expressiveness among boys, e.g., sports. Since play acting and creative activities also often bring rewards from adults and teachers such activities may also develop into avenues of achievement for effeminate boys and be elaborated into either avocational or vocational adult interests. Hence, artistic interests may simultaneously serve both expressive and instrumental needs among effeminate boys. Whether they have meanings beyond being an elaboration of a component of cultural femininity for such boys or whether they have some causal status within the childhood cross-gendering complex we cannot assay.

Like the studies comparing the recalled childhoods of gay and heterosexual adults, those of effeminate and conventional boys do not permit one to determine whether the cross-gender characteristics of effeminate boys are to be interpreted as cultural femininity, as psychological femininity, as both, or as some other gender-related phenomenon. All of the measures employed in the studies of such boys have been cultural ones rather than psychological. In developing their scale of Feminine Gender Identity, Freund et al. (1974; 1977) have suggested that the childhood possession of cross-gender characteristics among males is an indicator of a feminine gender identity. In their studies it has been found that adult trans-sexuals differ greatly with no overlap from heterosexual males in the extent to which they exhibited cross-gender characteristics during childhood, adolescence, and adulthood combined. Homosexuals were located between the two on the feminine gender identity scale but with considerable overlap with both trans-sexuals and heterosexuals. Hence, it was inferred that, at least to some degree, the childhood cross-gendering of adult gay men may be interpreted as a feminine gender identity.

For several reasons we take issue with the proposition of childhood cross-gendering as an indicator of the possession of a feminine gender identity. First, the possession of a considerable degree of childhood cross-gendering cannot in itself distinguish between trans-sexuals and homosexuals. Second, while both trans-sexuals and homosexuals may have, or have had during childhood, a considerable interest in the cultural components of the feminine gender-role the former have had a continuing belief that they in fact are in some sense women—or very much want to be physically women—while the very large majority of the latter have no interest in being women. Third, Freund et al. (1977) have found in their revised FGI Scale, those items which best distinguish between trans-sexuals and homosexuals are the ones (Part B of the FGI Scale) dealing with how and to whom the trans-sexual wants to relate sexually. They found that the large majority of trans-sexuals prefer to assume quite "passive" roles in sexual activities and to relate sexually to heterosexual rather than to homosexual males. Since heterosexual males are, by presumption, principally or only interested in relating sexually to women, the inference for the trans-sexual is that he is thereby in fact a woman. Thus, the heterosexual male's attentions directed toward him validates his identity as a woman, whereas the homosexual male has little or no need to have such an identity validated since he has no such identity. Fourth, trans-sexualism appears to be associated with cultural cross-gendering which is persistent from childhood to adulthood, whereas such cross-gendering may or may not be persistent in homosexuals. Presumably, a feminine gender identity is one basis for such persistent cross-gendering.

In the light of the above it would appear that the presence of cross-gendering during childhood may be a necessary but not sufficient indicator of a feminine gender identity. Hence, one may not securely label such cross-gendering as feminine gender identity. An interpretation which makes a more minimal assumption is that such cross-gendering is indicative of a feminine gender-role preference, whether accompanied or not by a feminine gender identity. As used below, we define feminine gender-role preference as a preference for the activities and interests culturally defined as appropriate for women. Whether feminine gender-role preference is accompanied by psychological femininity among homosexual males is an empirical question and cannot be answered solely from measures of cultural interests.

Whitam (1977) has speculated that a large, although unknown, percentage of gay men undergo a defeminization process between early childhood and adulthood whereby they lose most of their effeminacy. Green and Money (1966) report having observed a tendency for effeminate boys to replace their more obvious forms of cross-gendering with more subtle, and therefore more acceptable, ones. For example, rather than dressing up in their sister's clothes, they help her with her wardrobe and hair; rather than putting on their mother's makeup, they help her with her makeup or resort to painting pictures of beautifully adorned women. Alternatively, they may simply be eager to help with the housework. Such a transformation of the effeminate boys' preferred activities seems certain to have a survival value at an age when his conventional peers have strong aversions to such "sissy stuff."

If a large percentage of pre-gay children undergo a defeminization process from childhood to adulthood, one must ask why such an early and enthusiastic interest in cultural femininity either vanishes or becomes so muted in its manifestations. The most compelling answer is that they learn that such interests on the part of a boy are quite negatively sanctioned and that many of the rewards available to boys arise out of activities culturally defined as appropriate for boys, e.g., sports and delinquency. The negative sanctions against a boy engaging in cross-gender activities seem to be strong and vigorously applied during childhood. Many boys quite gleefully label their less aggressive or effeminate peers as "sissies." The label "sissy" appears to be the childhood equivalent of "faggot," although it lacks the sexual implications of the latter. Whitam (1977; 1979) and Freund et al. (1974) have reported that a considerably larger percentage of gay than heterosexual men recall having been considered "sissies" during childhood. These authors also report a similar difference in the extent to which gay versus heterosexual men were "loners" during childhood. Having observed the play behavior of four-year-olds, Fagot (1977) has reported that feminine boys play alone three times as much as other boys, apparently being considered undesirable or unworthy playmates. Because of these negative sanctions for their cross-gendering, pre-gay children seem to face a reward structure demanding that they defeminize.

In the light of the above cited earlier research we undertook a study of adult gay men designed to answer a number of questions. Is there a defeminization process operative in the pre-adulthoods of gay men? Is effeminacy in childhood or adulthood related to lower self-esteem? Does the interest in arts and play-acting observed in effeminate boys persist into adulthood? Does such an interest have implications for adult self-esteem? Do psychological and cultural femininity have differing implications for adult self-esteem? These questions are explored in an analysis of 1,556 gay men from the Chicago area.

Research Methods and Measures

As all students of homosexuality concede (Bell and Weinberg, 1978), it is impossible to obtain representative samples of homosexuals. Given the frequent reluctance of such individuals to be identified as homosexuals, researchers must accept samples of respondents which are to varying degrees self-selected. The implications of this state of affairs are that, to a greater degree than in research areas where representative sampling is possible, the accumulation of reliable information rests substantially on replication of findings and the use of alternative sampling strategies so that, across time and studies, there may be multimethod convergence of findings. This state of affairs must be accepted by the rsearcher studying homosexual persons, who must always be sensitive to the existence of findings which arise due to sampling procedures.

Our set of respondents are 1,556 gay men from the Chicago area. The principal method adopted for sampling was to have questionnaires distributed throughout the Chicago area by *Gay Life*, the major Chicago area gay publication. This newspaper is a giveaway shopper rather than a subscription publication. It has a circulation of approximately 18,000 and is distributed at nearly all of the area gay establishments. During the month of questionnaire distribution, November, 1978, there were 104 establishments at which both *Gay Life* and our questionnaire were distributed. Of these establishments, 54 percent were gay bars with the others being gay organizations (5), steam baths (7), gay hotels (2), adult bookstores and arcades (17), restaurants (17), a moviehouse (1), and a medical clinic (1).

Each week stacks of *Gay Life* papers are placed in these establishments, usually near the door. During two weeks of November stacks of both *Gay Life* and our questionnaires were so placed. Each copy of the questionnaire had stamped on the cover in red or lavender ink the title, "Lifestyle Study of Gay Men." A total of 17,600 were so distributed. It was hoped that distributions through *Gay Life* would produce a somewhat more heterogeneous set of respondents than the usually highly educated samples obtained through subscription readership surveys. Also, the diversity of the set of establishments at which the questionnaires were distributed was intended to increase heterogeneity. We estimate that this diverse set of establishments is rather comparable to the set of locales used in the Bell and Weinberg study to acquire volunteers. It is certainly a more diverse set of locales than the bars and gay organizations used to recruit respondents employed in the Weinberg and Williams or the Saghir and Robins studies.

It was anticipated that the respondents obtained through *Gay Life* would under-represent the older. Such under-representation of the older has occurred in all studies of gay men except, perhaps, in the Bell and Weinberg (1978) study in which long lists of volunteers were first obtained and then the older were disproportionately sampled from these lists. In order to offset this anticipated deficiency it was planned to send questionnaires to the membership of Maturity, a Chicago area organizatin of gay men over forty with a claimed membership of 275. Felicitously, before we contacted Maturity they had become aware of our *Gay Life* distributions and contacted us to request that they be included. Questionnaires and return envelopes in the number of 275 were mailed to their membership. While we are not certain, we suspect that their actual membership may be considerably less than the claimed 275 due to their keeping on their mailing lists persons who have long since discontinued activity in the organization or paid dues.

One thousand, seven hundred, and seventy questionnaires were returned. We excluded 214 because they did not meet one or more of several predetermined criteria: not living in Chicago and suburbs (116); incomplete response (21); responded after cutoff date (48); were not gay or did not indicate sexual orientation (23).

While ten percent of the questionnaires distributed were returned, it is not possible to calculate a traditional response rate because of the methods of distribution. It is unknown how many questionnaires ever got into the hands or eyesight of potential respondents. Some may have been thrown away by owners or managers of the recipient establishments who may not have wanted the questionnaires present. Some may have sat for a few days and then been thrown away. A few may have been destroyed by gays opposed to surveys. For example, seven of the questionnaires can be accounted for by one person having returned to the researcher, not questionnaires, but miscellaneous advertisements in our pre-paid envelope. For these reasons one may only conclude that the actual response rate is higher than ten percent by an unknown amount.

The demographic characteristic of our respondents are similar to those found in other major studies of gay men. The deficiencies in our sample, shared by all other major studies of gay men, are the under-representation of black gays, of the less educated—although we have elsewhere argued (Harry and DeVall, 1978: 155-159) that to some considerable degree the apparent excess education of studied gay men is real and not an artifact of sampling—and, despite our compensatory efforts, of truly older—over 60—gay men.

Measures

Because the characteristics of the cross-gendering scales to be used in the analyses below are of considerable substantive, rather than only methodological, significance, we defer their cosideration to the section on results. Here we briefly describe the other multi-item scales employed.

1. Psychological Femininity and Masculinity. We here adopted the measures of psychological masculinity and femininity developed by Spence and Helmreich (1978). Since the recent researches of Bem (1974) and of Spence and Helmreich (1978), it has been recognized that psychological masculinity and femininity are not the polar opposites of single dimension which earlier reearchers had assumed and built into a single scale of cultural masculinity-femininity. Rather, the two traits have variously been found to be either unrelated or modestly positively related among heterosexual respondents. Among our Chicago respondents, the femininity scale had a standardized item alpha-reliability of .77; it contains eight adjective self-rating items. The comparable coefficient for masculinity is .76.

2. Self-Esteem. This three-item scale includes, "On the whole I am quite a happy person," "I take a very positive attitude toward myself," and "On the whole I am satisfied with myself." Its standardized item alpha reliability is .81. We note that this scale should be interpreted more as "self-acceptance" rather than self-esteem in the sense of dominance or superiority which other researchers often employ.

RESULTS

Defeminization

The scales measuring cross-gendering were based on a block of six items asking the respondents, "Were you regarded as a sissy?" "Did you want to be a moviestar, actor, or entertainer?" "Were you usually a loner?" "Did you ever wish you had been a girl rather than a boy?" "Did you prefer playing or associating with girls rather than boys?" and "Did you ever dress up in female clothes (drag)?" These questions were asked of respondents for each of the three time periods, Childhood—"Before Age 13," Adolescence—"Ages 13 through 17," and Adulthood—"18 Years and Over." By asking these same questions for the three time periods, our intent was to be able to follow cross-gendering from childhood to adulthood. The response categories provided for each of these items were, "Yes," "No," and "Don't Know." Following Freund et al's (1974) practice, these respective responses were scored 2, 0, and 1 when they are used in multiple-item scales. In tabular presentations below, the "Don't Know" responses have been merged with the "Nos."

Figure 1 presents the percentages responding affirmatively to each of these six items for each of the three time periods asked about. Delaying consideration of the loner and actor items, it is apparent that the other four show sharp declines in frequency between childhood and adulthood. These four items appear to measure cross-gendering more immediately than do the actor and loner items

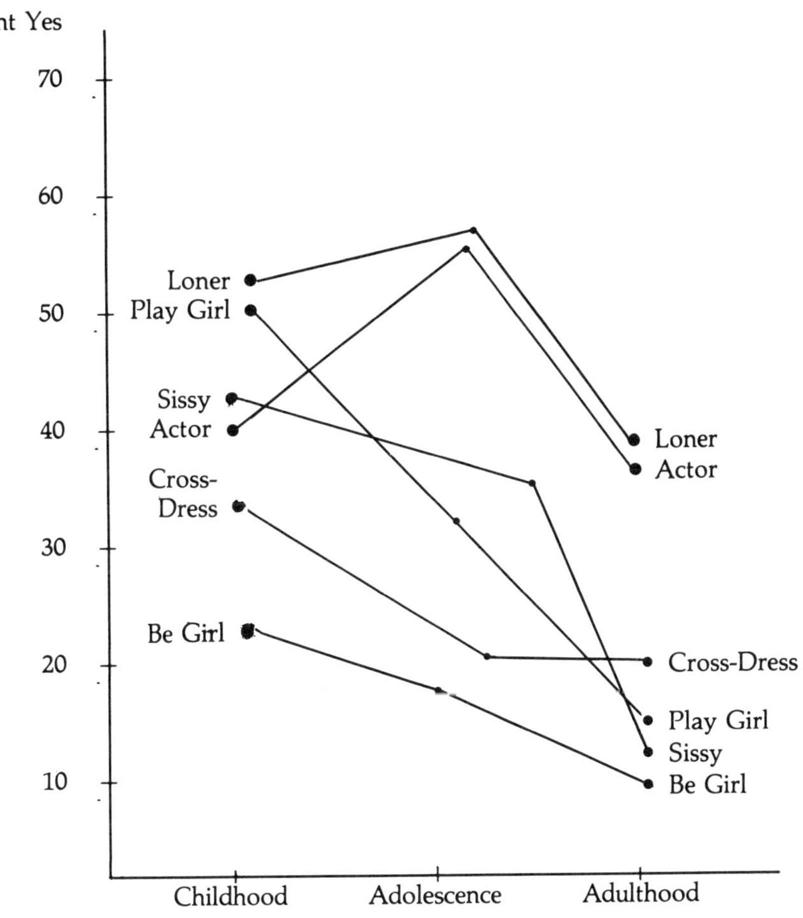

FIGURE I

CROSS-GENDERING ITEMS FOR THREE TIME-PERIODS (Percent Yes)

and provide rather direct and strong evidence in favor of the hypothesis of cultural defeminization. The item of cross-dressing differs slightly from the other declining items in that there is no further decline beyond adolescence. We interpret this non-change as being due to the fact that, once a young man has entered the gay world there are provided for him some opportunities to cross-dress in selected circles or on selected occasions. Hence, he no longer faces an environment which uniformly disapproves of such behaviors. In support of this point, we report that adult cross-dressing, but none of the other adult cross-gendering items, is significantly related to having mostly homosexual rather than heterosexual friends ($X^2 = 15.70$, df = 2, p < .001, gamma = .24).

We also calculated percentages for each of the six childhood items by the same item for adulthood. For all six items a majority of those possessing a given trait during adulthood also possessed it during childhood. This implies that the acquisition of cross-gendering during adulthood is less likely and that by far the most common pattern is for early acquisition of that trait whether or not it persists into adulthood. For each of the four direct cross-gendering items the relationships between the corresponding childhood and adult measures were quite asymmetrical. This means that although a child possessing a given trait during childhood may or may not possess it during adulthood, if he possessed it during adulthood he was very likely to have also possessed it during childhood. In contrast, the items on acting interest and being a loner showed considerable and symmetric persistence into adulthood. We offer that the greater social acceptability of the latter traits may permit more persistence.

The items shown in Figure 1 serve as the basis for constructing several scales. A childhood cross-gender role preference scale was created out of the four childhood items of "sissy," "be girl," "play with girls," and "cross-dressing" (standardized alpha-reliability = .65). The corresponding items for adulthood were used to create an adult cross-gender role-preference measure (standardized alpha-reliability = .45). Another scale measuring a persistent acting interest across time was created out of the three actor items (standardized alpha-reliability = .76). A final scale of persistent loner across time was created (standardized alpha-reliability = .72). These constitute our measures of the principal independent variables. We validated our measure of adult cross-gendering by relating it to the respondent's self-reported masculinity/femininity in appearance. Trichotomizing both we found a very strong association between the two ($X^2 = 160.80$, df = 4, p. < .001, gamma = .54).

To examine the extent to which childhood cross-gendering persists into adulthood we present Table 1.

TABLE I

CHILDHOOD CROSS-GENDERING BY ADULT CROSS-GENDERING*

ADULT Cross-Gendering	CHILDHOOD CROSS-GENDERING			
	None	Some	High	N(100%)
None	87(28)	64(55)	45(17)	983
Some	11(9)	25(57)	34(34)	372
High	2(3)	11(53)	21(44)	177
N(100%)	316	845	370	
$X^2 = 139.47$	df = 4	p < .001	Gamma = 0.49	

*Row percentages in parentheses.

While there is a strong association between these two measures, that association is also asymmetrical. Extremely few respondents who were not cross-gendered during childhood later acquired any cross-gendering. Also, the large majority of those highly cross-gendered during childhood defeminized to some degree. Also, the very large majority of those cross-gendering during adulthood were also cross gendered during childhood. Indeed, childhood cross-gendering seems to be a virtually necessary, but not sufficient, condition for adult cross-gendering.

Cross-Gendering and Self-Esteem

Table 2 presents the relationships of both childhood and adult cross-gendering with adult self-esteem, psychological masculinity, and psychological femininity. We see that both childhood and adult cross-gendering are negatively associated with self-esteem and masculinity, and psychological femininity. We see that both childhood and adult cross-gendering are negatively associated with self-esteem and masculinity. Those most cross-gendered are fairly low on these two measures. It is interesting to note that femininity has only a quite weak association with childhood cross-gendering and none at all with adult cross-gendering. This implies that cultural femininity should not be taken to imply psychological femininity. Cultural interests and psychological traits may not correspond very well.

In order to explore whether it is childhood versus adult cross-gendering which is most associated with the adult measures of psychological well-being Table 3 presents self-esteem, masculinity, and femininity by both childhood and adult cross-gendering simultaneously. In this table the cross-gendering measures have been dichotomized at "any" versus "none." The resultant four

Table II

ADULT PSYCHOLOGICAL MEASURES BY CHILDHOOD AND ADULT CROSS-GENDERING (Percent)

Adult Psychological Measures

Childhood Cross-Gendering	Self-Esteem				Masculinity				Femininity			
	Low	Med	High	N(100%)	Low	Med	High	N(100%)	Low	Med	High	N(100%)
None	18	50	32	314	24	37	40	309	39	38	23	310
Some	31	43	26	852	28	42	29	843	36	34	31	845
High	35	46	19	377	34	46	20	369	31	36	33	373

$X^2 = 34.57$, df $= 4$, p $< .001$, gamma $= 0.20$ $X^2 = 31.83$, df $= 4$, p $< .001$, gamma $= 0.19$ $X^2 = 10.80$, df $= 4$, p $< .03$, gamma $= 0.10$

Childhood Cross-Gendering	Self-Esteem				Masculinity				Femininity			
	Low	Med	High	N(100%)	Low	Med	High	N(100%)	Low	Med	High	N(100%)
None	24	46	29	983	25	41	33	971	36	36	28	976
Some	36	45	20	368	32	45	23	369	33	37	30	369
High	43	39	18	174	41	39	20	164	33	29	38	167

$X^2 = 42.16$, df $= 4$, p $< .001$, gamma $= 0.25$ $X^2 = 30.46$, df $= 4$, p $< .001$, gamma $= 0.21$ $X^2 = 8.05$, df $= 4$, p $=$ ns, gamma $= 0.07$

types of respondents are collectively referred to as "Defeminization Status." We see that adult cross-gendering appears to be a more important variable affecting self-esteem since the defeminized approximate the never-cross-gendered in their self-esteem. Similar relationships hold in the case of masculinity with the adult cross-gendered being lower than the defeminized who in turn are somewhat lower than the never-effeminate. Femininity again displays no marked associations with adult cross-gendering, although there is a modest significant difference between the never-effeminate and the other three groups combined ($X^2 = 7.87$, df $= 1$, p. $< .01$; gamma $= .22$).

Table III

ADULT PSYCHOLOGICAL MEASURES BY DEFEMINIZATION STATUS
(Percent)

Adult Psychological Measures	Defeminization Status			
	Always Effeminate	Newly Effeminate	Defeminized	Never Effeminate
Self-Esteem				
Low	39	23	27	17
Med	42	62	46	49
High	19	15	28	34
N(100%)	499	39	706	273

$X^2 = 56.02$, df $= 6$, p $< .001$

Adult Psychological Measures	Always Effeminate	Newly Effeminate	Defeminized	Never Effeminate
Masculinity				
Low	35	32	27	22
Med	43	48	43	35
High	22	20	30	42
N(100%)	490	40	700	267

$X^2 = 41.87$, df $= 6$, p $< .001$

Adult Psychological Measures	Always Effeminate	Newly Effeminate	Defeminized	Never Effeminate
Femininity				
Low	33	30	35	40
Med	34	40	35	38
High	32	30	31	22
N(100%)	496	37	702	271

$X^2 = 9.56$, df $= 6$, p $= ns$

The Interaction of Adult Cross-Gendering and Persistent Acting Interests

Turning to an exploration of the possible adult consequences of a persistent acting interest we found that a persistent acting interest was fairly strongly related to defeminization status ($X^2 = 95.12$, df $= 6$, p $< .001$). Of the always-effeminate, 25 percent had never had acting interests versus 50 percent of the newly effeminate, 38 percent of the defeminized, and 55 percent of the never-effeminate. These data revealed that cross-gendering, both childhood and adult, were significantly associated with a persistent acting interest. These data replicate for adulthood what Green and Money (1966) found among boys. However, the data also show that persistent acting interest is associated with a persistent cross-gendering. In attempting to explain this curious linkage we entertained the hypothesis that cross-gendering might be a vehicle for the expression of achievement motivations. Under this interpretation the portrayal of the feminine role serves as a means of acquiring recognition or, more primitively, of attention-getting, despite its often negative feedback consequences. As Whiting and Edwards (1973:180) have observed in their cross-cultural studies of the behavior of children, that attention seeking seems to be both a 'masculine' form of dependency and a measure of competitiveness in a self-arrogating aspects. However, this interpretation seems to imply an association of persistent acting interests with masculinity or competitiveness.

TABLE 4

LIKELIHOOD RATIO ANALYSIS OF MASCULINITY BY PERSISTENT ACTING INTEREST BY ADULT CROSS-GENDERING

Partial (1st-order) Associations				Marginal (0-order) Associations	
Effect	df	LR Chi-Sq.	p	LR Chi-Sq.	p
MT	2	0.30	0.862	1.80	0.407
MA	2	26.24	0.000	27.74	0.000
TA	1	38.03	0.000	39.53	0.000
MTA	2	16.53	0.000		

Adult Cross-Gendering (A)	Persistent Actor (T)	Masculinity (M) Percentages				
		Low	Med	High	N(100%)	Gamma
Some	Low	43	44	13	140	
	High	32	43	25	388	.25
None	Low	22	40	37	414	
	High	28	42	30	553	-.13

Given that adult cross-gendering is negatively associated with self-esteem and masculinity and that persistent acting interest is fairly strongly positively associated with adult cross-gendering, our hypothesis of a link between masculinity and acting interest seemed unlikely. However, we proceeded to analyze self-esteem, masculinity, and femininity by persistent acting interest with adult cross-gendering controlled. Table 4 presents masculinity by persistent acting interest by adult cross-gendering.

In the symbolism of this table each variable is referred to by a letter — M for masculinity, A for adult cross-gendering, and T for persistent acting interest. The significant interaction effect found in these data shows that the association between masculinity and a persistent acting interest depends on whether the persons are cross-gendered or not. Among the cross-gendered, masculinity is positively associated with acting interest while among the non-cross-gendered, it is slightly negatively associated. Hence, when combined with cross-gendering, persistent acting interests seem expressive of masculinity. We also found this same interaction effect using dependent measures of dominance, competitiveness, and being a persistent loner. Those both cross-gendered as adults and actorized were higher on competitiveness and on dominance and were less likely to have been persistent loners. The interaction effect for self-esteem was a borderline one of .051 significance. A parallel analysis of femininity found that only acting interest, and adult cross-gendering, were positively related to femininity. These interactions appeared only when we used the adult cross-gendering measure but not when we used the childhood one.

These data reveal that the persistent acting interest appears to provide for the cross-gendered individual a good measure of psychological strength in the form of self-esteem and the masculine virtues. These associated virtues clearly appear to somewhat offset the liabilities of the cross-gendered adult gay person. It seems that a combination of cross-gendering and persistent acting interest have, at some stage in these gay men's lives, become vehicles for the expression of masculinity. Alternatively, a somewhat stagey, although effeminate, style of deportment is underpinned by a masculine aggressiveness. These data thus appear to document and partially explain the occasionally made observation that effeminate males are not really feminine because their presented selves are too aggressive and harsh and that, while trans-sexuals are often genuinely feminine, effeminate gay men are not (Tripp, 1975). The latter possess psychological strengths in their effeminacy. Differently put, persistent effeminacy takes guts.

It became apparent in the analysis of the relationships of the psychological measures with acting interests and cross-gendering that the adult effeminates are a psychologically very heterogeneous group. Those effeminates who had acting interests were fairly high on our various psychological measures while those cross-gendered but not actorized seemed very low. To further explore the sub-types among the effeminates we created a scale out of the items asking if the respondents had ever wanted to be a girl. This scale seems, in a rough way, to measure trans-sexual desires. We then looked at the psychological measures by acting interests and the trans-sexualism scale among the adult cross-gendered. The data revealed that trans-sexualism and acting interests, even though positively associated, had opposite relationships with self-esteem. While the actorized were found to be relatively high on self-esteem, the trans-sexualized seemed almost desperately low. It also seemed that it is the trans-sexualized — those with trans-sexual tendencies — who account for much of the lower self-esteem of the adult cross-gendered.

It appears that those cross-gendered as adults are a very psychologically heterogeneous group, consisting largely of the rather strong actorized effeminates and the very troubled trans-sexualized. While our data showed that both groups engage in considerable cross-dressing, all they seem to have in common is their dresses. For the actorized cross-dressing is both a form of achievement — as in drag shows — and a means of self-expressiveness. Hence, the association of femininity with only actorization rather than with cross-gendering. A different way of conceiving of the actorization measure is that it is an androgyny factor through which the individual combines both achievement and expressiveness. Given that it seems to satisfy multiple needs it thereby appears rather resistent to being changed just as trans-sexuals have been found extremely difficult to treat through psychotherapy.

As a final exploration of how differing forms of femininity may contribute to self-esteem we analyzed self-esteem by psychological femininity by adult cross-gendering (cultural-role femininity). We found that psychological femininity was positively correlated with self-esteem after controlling for adult cross-gendering and that adult cross-gendering was negatively correlated with self-esteem after controlling for psychological femininity. These first-order partial relationships were somewhat stronger than the relationships without the controls. Hence psychological and cultural femininity have opposite relationships with self-esteem despite the fact that the two forms of femininity are modestly positively associated. These data once more suggest that it is hazardous to equate psychological and cultural femininity. For some purposes the two may have opposite effects.

CONCLUSIONS

The above data have shown that there is widespread defeminization process in the histories of many gay men. We presume, but have not demonstrated, that ths process occurs due to the negative sanctioning of effeminate characteristics among pre-adult gays. Defeminization appears to be inhibited by either commitments to a feminine gender identity (trans-sexualism or quasi-trans-sexualism) or to the feminine gender-role. Gay youths with such commitments are considerably more likely to be effeminate as adults.

It was found, as others have reported, that those gay men who are effeminate have less psychological well-being than the masculine appearing. The latter, including both the defeminized and the never-effeminate, were found to have higher self-esteem and masculinity. However, adult effeminacy was found to be considerably more complex in its psychology than originally anticipated. Those men who were effeminate due to a preference for the feminine gender-role, but not a feminine gender-identity, were found to possess considerable psychological strengths and to be psychologically androgynous. For them the feminine gender-role appears to be a vehicle for the aggressive expression of femininity. In contrast, those whose adult effeminacy appeared to be based on a commitment to a feminine gender identity were found to have the least psychlogical well-being among the various groups explored.

We note that while cultural femininity and feminine gender identity have been important concepts in the analysis of the above data, psychological femininity has played only a limited role. The cross-gendered were found to differ little from the non-cross-gendered on psychological femininity. Hence, one may not infer psychological femininity from visible effeminacy. A persistent acting interest was the principal correlate of psychological femininity. This again suggests that creative interest, acting, and the arts may serve as important vehicles for the emotional expressiveness of gay men. We suggest, without evidence, that such expressiveness may take either of two forms. In some cases one's personal deportment may become the vehicle of expressiveness — the artistic medium. In these instances a stagey effeminacy results. In other cases artistic creativity results. The testing of these possibilities we leave to future research.

References

Bates, J.E., Bentler, P.M., and Thompson, S. Measurement of deviant gender development in boys. *Child Development*, 1973, 44:591-598.

Bell, A., and Weinberg, M. *Homosexualities*. New York: Simon and Schuster, 1975.

Bem, S.L. The measurement of psychological androgyny. *Journal of Consulting and Clinical Psychology*, 1974, 42:155-162.

Fagot, B. Consequences of moderate cross-gender behavior in pre-school children. *Child Development*, 1977, 48:902-907.

Freund, K. Male Homosexuality Pp. 25-81 in J.A. Lorraine, (ed.), *Understanding Homosexuality*. New York: American Elsevier, 1974.

Freund, K., Nagler, E., Langevin, R., Zajac, A., and Steiner, B. Measuring feminine gender identity in homosexual males. *Archives of Sexual Behavior*, 1974, 3:249-60.

Freund, K., Langevin, R., Satterberg, J., and Steiner, B. Extension of the gender identity scale for males. *Archives of Sexual Behavior*, 1977, 6:507-519.

Green, R. *Sexual Identity Conflict in Children and Adults*. New York: Basic Books, 1974.

Green, R., and Money, R. Stage-acting, role taking, and effeminate impersonation during boyhood. *Archives of General Psychiatry*, 1966, 15:535-538.

Harry, J., and DeVall, W. *The Social Organization of Gay Males*. New York: Praeger, 1978.

Hart, M., Roback, H., Tittler, B., Weitz, L., Walston, B., and McKee, E. Psychological adjustment of nonpatient homosexuals: critical review of the research literature. *Journal of Clinical Psychiatry*, 1978, 39:604-608.

Kelly, J., and Worell, J. New formulations of sex roles and androgyny: a critical review. *Journal of Consulting and Clinical Psychology*, 1977, 45-1101-1115.

Lebovitz, P.S. Feminine behavior in boys. *American Journal of Psychiatry*, 1972, 128, 10, 1283.

Saghir, M. and Robins, E. *Male and Female Homosexuality*. Baltimore: Williams and Wilkins, 1973.

Siegelman, M. Adjustment of male homosexuals and heterosexuals. *Archives of Sexual Behavior*, 1972, 2:9-25.

Spence, J.T., and Helmreich, R.L. *Masculinity and Femininity*. Austin, TX: University of Texas Press, 1978.

Stein, A., and J. Smithells Age and sex differences in children's sex-role standards about achievement. *Developmental Psychology*, 1969, 1:252-259.

Stephan, W. Parental relationships and early social experience of activist male homosexuals and male heterosexuals. *Journal of Abnormal Psychology*, 1973, 82:506-513.

Stoller, R. *Sex and Gender*. New York: Science House, 1968.

Tripp, C.A. *The Homosexual Matrix*. New York: New American Library, 1975.

Weinberg, M., and Williams, C. *Male Homosexuals*. New York: Oxford University Press, 1974.

Whitam, F. Childhood Indicators of male homosexuality. *Archives of Sexual Behavior*, 1977, 6:89-96. Occupational choice and sexual orientation in cross-cultural perspective. *International Journal of Modern Sociology* (in press), 1979.

Whiting, B., and Edwards, C. A cross-cultural analysis of sex differences in the behaviors of children aged three through eleven. *Journal of Social Psychology*, 1973, 91:171-188.

Zuger, B. The role of familial factors in persistent effeminate behavior in boys. *American Journal of Psychiatry*, 1970, 126:1167-1170.

CASE HISTORY: SELF-ESTEEM AND HOMOSEXUALITY
R. A. Steffenhagen

The following case history is that of a young gay male with suicidal thoughts and low self-esteem.

One day one of my students, an attractive young lady whom I had gotten to know quite well, came into my office and asked if she could talk to me. She knew that I did student counseling and asked if it weren't too much of a burden, would I be willing to see a friend of hers. She went on to state that recently she had learned that a close male friend was gay. They had been out together and he unburdened himself to her indicating how upset and depressed he was. She also indicated that he had commented on thoughts of suicide. We discussed her friend John for about an hour and although I had never previously worked with any gay males I agreed to see him and evaluate the situation and then possibly recommend further counseling. We set a time for the following Tuesday and John was at the office promptly at two o'clock. As one would anticipate he was a bit embarrassed even though Susan had laid the ground work for the first meeting. The first session was spent with John discussing his problem, commenting on the fact that he had relatively recently broken up with his lover and was feeling extremely distraught and at odds with himself.

John is a white Anglo-Saxon male, age twenty, upper middle-class background, coming from a very pampered life-style. The mother is the domineering figure in the family controlling both the husband and her two sons. John appeared to have a relatively normal childhood, successful in high school and doing excellently in college. We discussed his feelings about himself and it was clear that he had extremely low self-esteem. The brother is successful heterosexually and John had no indication of himself being gay until his third year in college. John's sexual orientation during his first two years in college was heterosexual; in fact he was rather promiscuous and had a very close and very active sexual relationship with one girl for an entire year before the reversal in sexual interest.

As was stated we discussed his problem, his depression, his agitation, and his low self-esteem. John indicated that if possible he would like to continue working with me and, although I had questions about working in this area since I had not worked with gays in the past, I indicated I would be willing to try and that after a month we would assess our progress and if necessary make a recommendation for additional counseling at that time. It should be noted that John was very comfortable discussing emotional problems with me and that I felt at ease in working with him. An immediate rapport developed and our counseling relationship went well.

John's first homosexual encounter came at the end of his sophomore year in college. It seems that late one night in the dorm a male approached John sexually. He had recently broken off with his girl and the sexual drive was strong. Although he didn't think consciously that he was interested, he found himself submitting passively to the encounter. It was several weeks later before he had his second encounter and then gradually he began to develop an active sexual relationship with men. We began to work with hypnosis; John was an excellent hypnotic subject and I began working on the development of self-esteem.

Within my theoretical framework it was evident that John's self-esteem had never been extremely good although it was not low enough to cause him any major problems through his first two years in college. Early in the therapeutic process I stressed the need for John to use the term bi-sexual rather than homosexual or gay or queer. It is interesting to note that after about a year of homosexual relationships, he had developed the gay jargon and thought himself as being totally gay. While I did not attempt to alter his sexual preference I felt that it was very important to allow for sexual interest to be developed in both directions and the ultimate decision, of course, must be his.

As stated before, John was an extremely good hypnotic subject and enjoyed the relaxation aspect of the hypnosis as well as the intellectual ability to explore his own motives through the hypnotic process. While I had him in a deep session one day, I questioned him as to his first few experiences and asked explicitly whether he enjoyed them. He emphatically stated that he did not enjoy his first homosexual experience, he did not enjoy his second, he did not enjoy his third, or his fourth encounter — he was literally raped and this was extremely unpleasant and yet he continued in this direction.

In an attempt to understand the dynamics of the behavior, we decided upon doing a reincarnation regression and it appeared that John was a member of His Majesty's Navy during the early 1800's. He took on the characterization of a cabin boy aboard a sailing ship and it appeared that the captain was inclined to "like young boys." It appeared that in a very passive way, the captain had used him sexually although he had never himself engaged in an active homosexual experience. The meaning of this is totally unclear except that the desire to do a reincarnation regression was based on the assumption that certain unconscious hidden material might lie there which would give us an indication of what was occurring. Certainly this was not extremely illuminating although seemingly indicated a type of passive interest.

After the first four or five sessions, John began to use the term bi-sexual and began to think of himself in this way.

At the point at which I began working with John, his self-esteem was extremely low and he was harboring suicidal thoughts. Our whole therapeutic regime was based on building self-esteem and we were able to accomplish this successfully after about three months of therapy. John's depression and anxiety abated, and at the end of his college career, he was a very happy young man. His self-esteem developed, and without question, he had very good self-esteem at this time. Towards the end of the school year, we got together occasionally and John indicated that his sexual interest was beginning to go in both directions and he was turned on by both men and women. At this point I offered the suggestion that since he was such an extremely amenable hypnotic subject, we could begin to use hypnosis in a behavior modification technique and possibly begin to build an aversion to the nude male and a very strong attraction to the nude female. John had indicated earlier in therapy that he had the desire to ultimately become heterosexual and that he wanted the stability and security of a family and children. However, when asked if he wanted to use hypnosis in this way, he responded after a relatively brief pause; "No not at this time. I'm having too much fun the way it is — being bi-sexual."

This case history is particularly interesting because it is a prime example of how culture creates self-esteem problems for the gay male. The pressures in our culture against homosexuality are such that it is very difficult for many men to maintain feelings of self-worth, self-confidence, self-acceptance. Homosexuality has been considered anywhere from deviance to absolute psychopathology and with such values and attitudes permeating the culture, it certainly makes it difficult for the gay male to feel good about himself.

As was stated, John developed a strong sense of self-esteem and felt really good about himself at the termination of hypno-therapy. This indicates that within the self-esteem theory of deviance, homosexuality is not deviance but rather sexual preference. Harry (Ch. 12) certainly speaks to the point: self-esteem varies within gay males, with some gays manifesting more self-esteem and some much less; further effeminacy in the young gay male is detrimental for developing a good sense of self-esteem. In this particular case, we see good self-esteem and homosexual interest. If our theory is correct, and we go from low self-esteem to good self-esteem, then we should reverse 'the form of deviance.' We have seen in the other case histories that when self-esteem develops, the problems abate, be they suicide, poly-drug abuse, intermittent explosive disorder, etc., whereas in this particular case, a gay interest remained.

There is another dimension to this problem that possibly has not previously been examined and that is that low self-esteem, for some individuals, might foster sexual inversion in that the male does not need the degree of self-confidence that he might need in approaching a female (i.e. it is easy for a male to be picked up by another male; he can play the passive role without an active participation on his part). In these cases it is possible that changing self-esteem might have an effect on changing the sexual direction. When the individual feels good about himself, he becomes more assertive and is able to direct his attention towards the female without worrying about being rebuffed.

I have had two additional student cases over the past couple of years in which a dramatic increase in self-esteem did precipitate a stronger female interest though it was difficult to determine whether it would eliminate the male interest. It may be that the norm is the bi-sexual, and individuals who've gotten over the cultural barrier surrounding the same sex interest are able to develop a broader perspective.

This case history illustrates how self-esteem affects behavior. It suggests strongly that sexual interest is strictly preferencial and that the cultural values and attitudes are largely responsible for the problems of self-esteem which surround many gay males.

APPENDICES

A TEST OF SELF-ESTEEM: A MODEL
R. A. Steffenhagen

The following test is provided as a model of a self-esteem test constructed in the framework of the theory presented in this text. Robinson & Shaver (1973; 45) comment that self-acceptance and self-regard correlate only at the .21 level and that self-regard is another term for self-esteem. It is this author's contention that there have been entirely too many synonyms for self-esteem and that these varied concepts are frequently not synonymous, may not even be self-esteem or at best only components of self-esteem.

Robinson & Shaver say further that self-esteem and self-acceptance are conceptually and empirically related and that self-acceptance is necessary for self-esteem; this latter idea is supported by author's case history material and further, self-acceptance has been presented as a component of the model. In the model, self-acceptance is an underlying component of the mental format and crucial to good self-esteem.

Robinson & Shaver (p. 47) suggest that we can tap self-esteem directly by asking people how much they like themselves. We would contend that questions of this nature do not really get at self-esteem. In a student transcript we have:

T. How do you feel about yourself now?
S. It doesn't really matter — laugh — it is just kind of stupid, when I used to think about self-esteem I thought it was just feeling really good about yourself — liking yourself — Now when I think of it, it's dumb to have to either like yourself or dislike yourself — because you just are anyway — whether you like it or not.
T. Quite a change in perception. You feel really good now.
S. I just feel so much more sensible. I used to picture people who really liked themselves as getting the biggest kick out of feeling better than someone else. That is what I associated self-esteem with.
T. That is just being egotistical.
S. Yeah, really you can't really feel better than someone else, etc.

Thus, we see that liking one's self while important to situational self-esteem isn't the foundation for good spiritual self-esteem as it may seem. Liking and truly accepting oneself are quite different.

We have empirically shown that ego strength and self-esteem are not the same — that a person with good ego strength may have very low self-esteem.

We are suggesting that many of the existing self-esteem tests and measures may further be merely individual components of self-esteem. We have indicated that self-concept, self-image and social concept are all components of self-esteem but not self-esteem as such. In our diagram of self-esteem we also suggest that self-esteem comprises status, courage, and flexibility. The former on the higher level of abstraction and the latter on the lower level. A self-esteem test will then have to include questions which tap these various components. The following test moves from the higher to the lower level of abstraction. The case history material shows how self-esteem does not develop *in toto* but that increases are accrued at differential rates and that the goal in therapy is to develop and strengthen all three components. We further hypothesize that all individuals will not be equally low in all areas.

The test construction is as follows:

		Questions
Self-concept (mental)	Flexibility	1–3
	Status	4–6
	Courage	7–9
Self-image (physical)	Flexibility	10–12
	Status	13–15
	Courage	16–18
Social concept (cultural)	Flexibility	19–21
	Status	22–24
	Courage	25–27

Table I includes the test-retest reliability measures. On the basis of these figures, items 3, 19, 20, 27 should be omitted as they provide too much variance.

The test shall ultimately be subjected to a clinic population of low self-esteem clients and then further re-administered after therapy for further refinement.

Scoring

The test can be scored in either of 2 methods:

1) scored by computing the score from responses underlined, each underlined response counting as 1; scores will range from 0 low to 27 high. (Higher score = H.S.E.)

2) scored from 1 to 5, using the underlined responses as the direction of (strongly agree or strongly disagree); scores will range from 27 low to 135 high. (Higher score = H.S.E.)

TABLE I

	Chi Sq.[1]	Pearsons R	Chi Sq.[2]
1.	.0000	.56	.008
2.	.0087	.68	.020
3.	.03	.65	.066
4.	.00001	.61	.175
5.	.00000	.66	.000
6.	.0005	.669	.013
7.	.003	.787	.000
8.	.00003	.772	.004
9.	.00000	.869	.000
10.	.00016	.756	.022
11.	.005	.805	.000
12.	.00012	.725	.122
13.	.00007	.815	.003
14.	.055	.509	
15.	.002	.785	.000
16.	.020	.490	
17.	.009	.374	.053
18.	.001	.706	.008
19.	.025	.618	.684
20.	.037	.671	.039
21.	.002	.498	.014
22.	.035	.745	.0002
23.	.003	.645	.005
24.	.069	.626	.003
25.	.003	.721	
26.	.00000	.799	.0002
27.	.037	.617	.123

1–5x5 cross tab.

2–2x2 cross tab.

SELF-ESTEEM TEST
R. A. Steffenhagen

Directions: Check the correct box for each question which best indicates the way you feel most of the time — try not to leave any blanks.

1. I enjoy new challenges.
    (X) Strongly Agree (X) Agree (__) Neutral (__) Disagree
    (__) Strongly Disagree

2. When things go wrong I become very discouraged.
    (__) Strongly Agree (__) Agree (__) Neutral (X) Disagree
    (X) Strongly Disagree

3. Once I make a decision I tend to stick to it.
    (X) Strongly Agree (X) Agree (__) Neutral (__) Disagree
    (__) Strongly Disagree

4. I feel I am as competent as the average person.
    (X) Strongly Agree (X) Agree (__) Neutral (__) Disagree
    (__) Strongly Disagree

5. When I contribute to group discussions I believe my contributions are as valuable as those of others.
    (X) Strongly Agree (X) Agree (__) Neutral (__) Disagree
    (__) Strongly Disagree

6. I will not hesitate to take control of a situation when asked to.
    (X) Strongly Agree (X) Agree (__) Neutral (__) Disagree
    (__) Strongly Disagree

7. I am likely to postpone uncomfortable tasks.
    (__) Strongly Agree (__) Agree (__) Neutral (X) Disagree
    (X) Strongly Disagree

8. I prefer to compromise rather than argue.
    (__) Strongly Agree (__) Agree (__) Neutral (X) Disagree
    (X) Strongly Disagree

9. I am intimidated by aggressive people.
    (__) Strongly Agree (__) Agree (__) Neutral (X) Disagree
    (X) Strongly Disagree

10. Maintaining a good physical condition is important to me.
    (X) Strongly Agree (X) Agree (__) Neutral (__) Disagree
    (__) Strongly Disagree

11. I enjoy wearing bright distinctive clothing.
     (X) Strongly Agree (X) Agree (__) Neutral (__) Disagree
     (__) Strongly Disagree

12. I like to participate in games even if I am mediocre.
     (X) Strongly Agree (X) Agree (__) Neutral (__) Disagree
     (__) Strongly Disagree

13. I do not like to look in a mirror.
     (__) Strongly Agree (__) Agree (__) Neutral (X) Disagree
     (X) Strongly Disagree

14. Other people think I am physically atractive.
     (X) Strongly Agree (X) Agree (__) Neutral (__) Disagree
     (__) Strongly Disagree

15. Dressing attractively is important to me.
     (X) Strongly Agree (X) Agree (__) Neutral (__) Disagree
     (__) Strongly Disagree

16. At times I enjoy being alone.
     (X) Strongly Agree (X) Agree (__) Neutral (__) Disagree
     (__) Strongly Disagree

17. I would rather watch social and sports events rather than participate.
     (__) Strongly Agree (__) Agree (__) Neutral (X) Disagree
     (X) Strongly Disagree

18. I would rather have a job I enjoyed than one which paid much more but
     I didn't enjoy.
     (X) Strongly Agree (X) Agree (__) Neutral (__) Disagree
     (__) Strongly Disagree

19. I enjoy being alone as well as being with friends.
     (X) Strongly Agree (X) Agree (__) Neutral (__) Disagree
     (__) Strongly Disagree

20. My inhibitions sometimes keep me from having a good time.
     (__) Strongly Agree (__) Agree (__) Neutral (X) Disagree
     (X) Strongly Disagree

21. The idea of moving to another part of the country frightens me.
     (__) Strongly Agree (__) Agree (__) Neutral (X) Disagree
     (X) Strongly Disagree

22. I tend to be self-confident.
    (X) Strongly Agree (X) Agree (__) Neutral (__) Disagree
    (__) Strongly Disagree

23. People respect me for the way I live.
    (X) Strongly Agree (X) Agree (__) Neutral (__) Disagree
    (__) Strongly Disagree

24. I often avoid doing things because of what others would say.
    (__) Strongly Agree (__) Agree (__) Neutral (X) Disagree
    (X) Strongly Disagree

25. I am willing to stand up for my beliefs.
    (X) Strongly Agree (X) Agree (__) Neutral (__) Disagree
    (__) Strongly Disagree

26. I would support the value system of my profession.
    (X) Strongly Agree (X) Agree (__) Neutral (__) Disagree
    (__) Strongly Disagree

27. I frequently call friends and suggest doing things socially.
    (X) Strongly Agree (X) Agree (__) Neutral (__) Disagree
    (__) Strongly Disagree

ANNOTATED BIBLIOGRAPHY
Mark Rainville, B.A.

Alcorn, H. G. The relationship between death anxiety and self-esteem. Unpublished dissertation, United States International University, 1976.
> Self-esteem is negatively related to anxiety toward death.

Allen, D. I. Student performance, attitude and self-esteem in open area and self-contained classrooms. *Alberta Journal of Education Research*, 1974, 20, 1-7.
> There were no differences in the self-esteem of students taught in the two learning environments.

Allen, J. A. The relationship of self-esteem to interpersonal perception and response. Unpublished dissertation, University of Missouri, Columbia, 1975.
> Subjects with low or defensive self-esteem would be more likely to respond reciprocally to accepting and rejecting stimulus others (than high self-esteem subjects).

Allen, L. R. Self-esteem of male alcoholics. *Psych. Record*, 1969, 19, 381-389.
> Lowered Cornell Personality Inventory scores for alcoholics who volunteered for treatment exemplified F.M. Pattison's existential guilt; guilt induced by a violation of social relationships and by the alcoholic's withdrawal from social situations.

Allen, R. S. The effects of Duso upon the reported self-esteem of selected fifth grade subjects. Unpublished dissertation, University of South Carolina, 1976.
> There was no significant relationship exhibited.

Aloia, A. F. Relationships between perceived privacy options, self-esteem and internal control among aged people. Unpublished dissertation, California School of Professional Psychology, Los Angeles, 1973.
> There is a significant relationship between perceived privacy options and self-esteem among the aged.

Altman, H. A. & Scollon, J. The influence of process variables on self-esteem. *Psych.*, 1973, 10, 37-43.
> Results indicate no significant self-esteem improvement among 4th graders when exposed to counselor-offered core conditions (e.g., empathy) in group role-playing and group discussion situations.

Anamerman, M. S. & Fryear, F. L. Photographic enhancement of children's self-esteem. *Psychology in the Schools*, 1975, 12, No. 3, 319-325.
> A significant increase in behavioral self-esteem, but no change in subjective self-esteem resulted from five weeks of self-photography sessions.

Anderson, N. R. Self-esteem manipulations as persuasive messages. Unpublished dissertation, University of Washington, 1972.

> Self-esteem was negatively related to yielding to, and positively related to reception of a persuasive message.

Apolonio, S. F. Preadolescent's self-esteem, sharing behavior and perceptions of parental behavior. Unpublished dissertation, Florida State University, 1974.

> The self-esteem of preadolescents is related to their perceptions of parental behavior.

Apperson, J. Sex, self-esteem and psychological motivation for sexual behavior. Unpublished dissertation, Michigan State University, 1973.

> In men, self-esteem is negatively related to the conscious sexual motive of dominance and positively related to the motive of affiliation; whereas among women self-esteem is negatively related to deference motives.

Arrowood, F. A. & Short, F. S. Agreement, attraction and self-esteem. *Canadian Journal of Behavioral Science*, 1973, *5*, No. 3, 242-252.

> No support was found concerning increased self-esteem as a determinant of interpersonal attraction.

Atkins, F. W. Delinquency as a function of self-esteem. Unpublished dissertation, University of Oregon, 1973.

> The tentative conclusions drawn are that delinquents have lower self-esteem than non-delinquents and that self-esteem is positively related to socio-economic status.

Averill, C. A. An examination of the relationship of self-esteem to parental support and control, internal-external locus of control and social desirability in parents from a low income multi-ethnic community. Unpublished dissertation, University of Missouri-Kansas City, 1977.

> Self-esteem is significantly related to parental support and control, internal-external locus of control and social desirability.

Balaief, L. Self-esteem and human equality. *Philosophy and Phenomenological Research*, 1975, *36*, No. 1, 25-43.

> Essay dealing with equality in the psychological dimension which proposes that self-esteem in America is largely based on work identity; hence results in devastating circumstances for the excluded.

Baran, S. F. The effects of prosocial and antiosocial television content on the modeling behavior of children with varying degrees of self-esteem. Unpublished dissertation, University of Massachusetts, 1973.

> Television viewing manifests in more aggressive modeling behavior in high self-esteem children and more prosocial modeling behavior in low self-esteem children.

Baron, P. H. Self-esteem, ingratiation, and evaluation of unknown others. *Journal of Personality and Social Psychology*, 1974, *30*, No. 1, 104-109.

> Manipulated self-esteem (high, low, control) was positively related to ratings of an unknown other; only high manipulated self-esteem subjects made more favorable ratings in the public condition (vs. private).

Baruch, G. H. Feminine self-esteem, self-rating of competence and maternal career commitment. *Journal of Counseling Psychology*, 1973, *20*, No. 5, 487-488.

> Among undergraduate females, a positive relationship was found between the three variables.

Beatty, R. W. Effect of basic education, job skill, and self-esteem on the job success of the hard-core unemployed. *Proceedings from the 81st Annual Convention of the American Psychological Association*, Montreal, Canada, 1973, Vol, *8*, 595-596.

> Significant improvements in basic education and job skill were not accompanied by a higher self-esteem.

Beckman, L. F. Self-esteem of women alcoholics. *Journal of Studies on Alcohol*, 1978, *39*, No. 3, 491-498.

> The self-esteem of female alcoholics is lower than that of male alcoholics.

Bedeian, A. G. The roles of self-esteem and n-achievement in aspiring to prestigious occupations. *Journal of Vocational Behavior*, 1977, *11*, No. 1, 109-119.

> The data indicates a positive relationship between self-esteem and the tendency to aspire to high prestige jobs.

Bennett, L. A. Self-esteem and parole adjustment. *Criminology: An Interdisciplinary Journal*, 1974, *12*, No. 3, 346-360.

> This longitudinal study shows a small, positive correlation between the self-esteem of institutionalized criminals just before release and while adjusting on parole.

Bennett, L. A. & Sorenson, D. D., & Forshay, H. The application of self-esteem measures in a correctional setting: reliability of the scale and relationship to other measures. *Journal of Research in Crime and Delinquency*, 1971, *8*, No. 1, 1-9.

> The self-esteem inventory is seen as an adequate tool for investigation in the correctional field.

Benson, P. & Spilka, B. God image as a function of self-esteem and locus of control. *Journal for the Scientific Study of Religion*, 1973, *12*, No. 3, 297-310.

> The self-esteem of male Catholics is positively related to loving-accepting God images and negatively related to rejecting images.

Berger, C. R. Attributional communication, situational involvement, self-esteem and interpersonal attraction. *Journal of Communication*, 1973, *23*, No. 3, 284-305.

> Subjects with extreme low or high self-esteem would be more defensive than moderate self-esteem subjects when receiving ego-threatening communications.

Berger, C. R. Sex differences related to self-esteem factor structure. *Journal of Consulting and Clinical Psychology*, 1968, *32*, 442-446.

> Self-esteem was statistically shown to be a multidimensional construct. Female's self-evaluation depends on their belief that others like them.

Berkowitz, A. H. The effect of transcendental meditation on trait anxiety and self-esteem. Unpublished dissertation, University of Colorado at Boulder, 1977.

> There was no measurable effect of T.M. on self-esteem over time (13.5 weeks).

Berman, F. & Osborn, D. Specific self-esteem and sexual permissiveness. *Psych. Reports*, 1975, *36*, No. 1, 323-326.

> For only males, a positive relationship exists between the variables.

Bewley, K. W. The effects of a modified Adlerian approach on the self-esteem of selected second and third grade students. Unpublished dissertation. Baylor University, 1974.

> Group counseling was successful in raising the self-esteem of the sample.

Binder, M. E. Sex guilt, self-esteem and the acquisition of sexual information. Unpublished dissertation, the University of Texas at Austin, 1976.

> Self-esteem is not related to the recall of sexual information.

Bingham, G. D. Career attitudes and self-esteem among boys with and without specific learning abilities. Unpublished dissertation, Rutgers University, 1974.

> For males with learning disabilities, a significant relationship exists between self-esteem and career attitudes in preadolescence, whereas the same relationship manifests in adolescence for males without learning disabilities.

Boags, R. S. The effects of self vs. ideological advocacy on the self-esteem and endorsement of Black power ideology of Black college students. Unpublished dissertation, the University of Southern California, 1975.*

Bridgette, R. E. Self-esteem in Negro and white southern adolescents. Unpublished dissertation, University of North Carolina at Chapel Hill, 1970.

> The research suggests that I.Q. and mother's education substantially contributed to racial differences in self-esteem.

Briggs, D. C. *Your Child's Self-esteem: The Key to Life.* Garden City, New York: Dolphin, 1975.

> A book suggesting methods of raising children's self-esteem.

Brissett, D. Toward a clarification of self-esteem. *Psychiatry,* 1972, *35,* No. 3, 255-263.

> The *phrase* self-esteem encompasses two basic, distinct, and ideally complementary socio-psychological processes, self-worth: an intrinsic personal feeling and self-evaluation: An extrinsic social behavior (role performance).

Bruch, M. A.; Kunce, J. T. & Eggerman, D. F. Parental devaluation: A protection of self-esteem. *Journal of Counseling Psychology,* 1972, *19,* No. 6, 555-558.

> The results were inconclusive concerning why inner-city high school seniors devaluated their fathers.

Brust, F. V. The relationship of individualized instruction in learning skills to self-esteem and achievement. Unpublished dissertation, Columbia University, 1972.

> Individual academic instruction had no influence on self-esteem.

Burbach, H. F. & Bridgeman, B. Relationship between self-esteem and locus of control in Black and White fifth grade students. *Child Study Journal,* 1976, *6,* No. 1, 33-37.

> Self-esteem was found to be significantly related, among all females and Black males, to taking credit for academic successes; while among White males, self-esteem was related to accepting blame for failure.

Burleigh, D. L. General self-esteem, self-perceived competence for task at hand, expectations of others and task performance. Unpublished dissertation, State University of New York at Buffalo, 1976.

> This study attempted to determine the interrelationships among general self-esteem, self-perceived competence and expectations of others in a task performance situation.

Bussanich, F. M. The influence of locus-of-control, self-esteem and success-failure feedback on attribution of responsibility. Unpublished dissertation, The University of Texas at Austin, 1976.

> Self-esteem was negatively related to internalizing responsibility for failure.

Calhoun, G. & Morse, W. C. Self-concept and self-esteem: another perspective. *Psychology in the Schools,* 1977, *14,* No. 3, 318-322.

> Self-esteem is defined as a person's satisfaction with his personal concept of self.

Calsyn, R. F. The causal relationship between self-esteem, locus of control and achievement: A cross-lagged panel analysis. Unpublished dissertation, Northwestern University, 1973.

> Initially increasing self-esteem, in attempting to increase the achievement level, is not aided by any naturally occurring causal pattern.

Campbell, R. N. Self-esteem and sense pleasure: the root motivations of human behavior. Unpublished dissertation, Graduate Theological Union, 1976.

> Proposes that the self-esteem drive is paramount as the motivator of all human behavior.

Carlson, R. On the structure of self-esteem. Comments on Ziller's formulation. *Journal of Consulting and Clinical Psych.*, 1970.

> Three limitations were noted concerning Ziller et al.'s measure of social self-esteem; implicit masculine and cultural bias and lack of a distinction between level and source of self-esteem.

Cashion, B. G. The relationship between family integration, self-esteem and social participation. Unpublished dissertation, University of Maryland, 1974.

> A positive relationship exists between family integration and social participation, and family integration and self-esteem.

Castner, A. E. The relationship between the process of keeping a journal and self-esteem using sixth grade students. Unpublished dissertation, University of Maryland, 1969.

> A relationship exists between the variables.

Chambliss, F.; Mailler, D.; Hulnick, R. & Wood, M. Relationships between self-concept, self-esteem, popularity and social judgements of junior high school students. *Journal of Psych.*, 1978, *98*, No. 1, 91-98.

> No evidence was found that self-esteem was related to social self-concept accuracy.

Charalanpous, K. D.; Ford, B.; Skinner, F. F. & Skinner, K. Self-esteem in alcoholics and nonalcoholics. *Journal of Studies on Alcohol*, 1978, *37*, No. 7, 990-994.

> Alcoholics have lowered self-esteem and those alcoholics with higher self-esteem are less likely to seek treatment.

Charley, M. D. The relationship between self-esteem and learning disabilities: A comparative cross-sectional developmental study of white middle class elementary school-aged children. Unpublished dissertation, Northwestern University, 1974.

> Although learning disabled children have lower self-esteem and are underachievers in comparison to normals, the self-esteem level cannot necessarily be related to the degree of the disability.

Chartier, M. R. & Golhner, L. A. Study of the relationship of parent-adolescent communication, self-esteem and God image. *Journal of Psychology and Theology*, 1976, 4 No. 3, 227-232.

> Significant relationships were found between self-esteem and parental communication and between self-esteem and God image.

Christian, K. W. A method of assessing self-esteem through numerical self-reports. Unpublished dissertation, University of California at Davis, 1972.

> Self-esteem is positively related to feelings of personal control.

Clark, W. Effects of self-esteem upon perception of the sick role in an urban, poor, minority group population. Unpublished dissertation, The University of Mississippi, 1975.

> The self-esteem of a patient contributed significantly to three dimensions; denial dependency, reciprocity, role performance of the perceived sick role.

Clarke, S. K. Self-esteem in men and women alcoholics. *Quarterly Journal of Studies on Alcohol*, 1974, *35*, No. 4, 1380-1381.

> The self-esteem of the female alcoholic is no lower than that of the male alcoholic.

Clayman, S. F. Locus of control, chronic self-esteem and recommendation relevance as determinants of acceptance of positive and negative self-evaluation feedback. Unpublished dissertation, University of Maine, 1974.

> Negative self-evaluative feedback was more effective in getting subjects to see a therapist than positive, or no feedback.

Clement, W. M. An investigation into possible relationships between values and self-esteem among a selected population of aged people.

> Unpublished dissertation, School of Theology at Claremont, 1972.

Concludes that further study is warranted in determining the contributing factors to self-esteem variability in relationship to value systems of the aged.

Cohen, R. S. & Lefkowitz, F. Self-esteem, locus of control and task difficulty as determinants of task performance. *Journal of Vocational Behavior*, 1977, *11*, No. 3, 314-321.

> Task-specific self-esteem was related to task performance.

Coleman, R. E. Manipulation of self-esteem as a determinant of mood of elated depressed women. *Journal of Abormal Psychology*, 1975, 84, No. 6, 693-700.

> The successful induction of positive vs. negative cognitive statements on determining depressions demonstrates a potentially useful technique for self-esteem enhancement.

Collett, P. Structure and content in cross-cultural studies of self-esteem. *International Journal of Psychology*, 1972, 7, No. 3, 169-179.

> Investigating structure, (rather than content) may be a preferable procedure for idiographic cross-cultural research.

Colletti, C. & Walsh, E. Social class psychological processing and self-esteem. Paper presented at the 1977 Meeting of the Penn. Sociological Society.

> Findings suggest that the variations in psychological processing within social categories, especially in middle to low occupational levels is important in determining the validity of a positive correlation between social class and self-esteem.

Colman, A. M. & Oliver, K. R. Reactions to flattery as a function of self-esteem: self-enhancement and cognitive consistency theories. *British Journal of Social and Clinical Psychology*, 1978, *17*, No. 1, 25-29.

> There is a positive relationship between self-esteem and the liking of a flattering evaluator.

Comstock, M. L. Effects of perceived parental behavior on self-esteem and adjustment. Unpublished dissertation. University of North Carolina at Chapel Hill, 1973.

> Perceived parental behavior influences the self-esteem of the child.

Crandall, R. On the relationship between self-esteem, coping and optimism. *Psychological Reports*, 1972, *30*, No. 2, 485-486.

> Discusses a recent article in which E. Levonian (see Psych. Abstracts, Vol, 45, 618b) concluded that self-esteem is negatively related to coping and optimism.

Cross, F. M. & Miller, D. B. Sex roles as related to self-esteem and internal-external control. Paper presented at the 40th meeting of the Southern Sociological Society.

> Early socialization processes explain the experimental findings that female undergraduates score higher than male undergraduates on the sex role scale, but lower on the self-esteem and internal-external control scales.

Crow, C. W. The effects of a vocational exploration group experience on control expectancy, self-esteem and vocational maturity of high school students. Unpublished dissertation, Arizona State University, 1973.

> The researcher concluded that the Vocational Exploration Group's potential for effecting positive personality change in high school students should be examined further.

Crown, S.; Lucas, C. J.; Stringer, P. & Supramanium, S. Personality correlates of study difficulty and academic performances in university students: 11. Conscience and self-esteem. *British Journal of Medical Psychology,*1977, *50*, No. 3, 275-281.

> Conscience and self-esteem were found to be inversely related to one another.

Cruz, M. D. Social factors and self-esteem among Puerto Rican and non-Puerto Rican students. Unpublished dissertation, University of Illinois at Urbana, Champaign, 1974.

> No racial differences in self-esteem were found.

Cruz, P. R. The effects of experimentally induced failure, self-esteem and sex on cognitive differentiation. *Journal of Abnormal Psychology*, 1973, *81*, No. 1, 74-79.

> Following experimentally induced failure, high self-esteem subjects worked slower on a cognitive differentiation test.

Dabbes, F. M. A view of Levonian's remarks on studies of self-esteem and persuasibility. *Psychological Reports*, 1970, *27*, No. 3, 854.

> Discusses confusion in sections of E. Levonian's criticism on self-esteem and persuasibility research studies.

Daly, F. D. Self-esteem achievement and related variables of inner-city college students. Unpublished dissertation, Illinois Institute of Technology, 1972.

> College academic achievement was found to be unrelated to self-esteem.

Dauw, D. C.; LaVan, H. & Fasieniecki, I. Influence of young executive's values and self-esteem on organizational behavior. Paper presented at the 1977 meeting of the Illinois Sociological Society.

> The results suggested that there are similar values and levels of self-esteem among executives, across sex.

Dickstein, E. B. The development of self: theory and measurement. Unpublished dissertation, The Johns Hopkins University, 1972.

> Proposes that with each of five distinct developmental stages of self-concept, there is an appropriate self-esteem type.

Dickstein, E. B. Theory and measurement of self-esteem. *Journal of Multivariate Experimental Personality and Clinical Psychology*, 1973, *1*, No. 1, 23-30.

> A self-esteem measure is developed for children.

Dinardo, T. A. The effects of self-esteem, threat and choseness of sharing a negative impression. Unpublished dissertation, The University of Texas at Austin, 1976.

> Self-esteem has insignificant influence on the situation of sharing a negative impression with a friend.

Dinner, S. H.; Lewkowicz, B. F. & Cooper, F. Anticipatory attitude change as a function of self-esteem and issue familiarity. *Journal of Personality and Social Psychology*, 1972, *24*, No. 3, 407-412.

> Subjects of high manipulated self-esteem showed more anticipatory attitude change toward familiar communication than low self-esteem subjects.

Dion, K. K. & Dion, K. L. Self-esteem and romantic love. *Journal of Personality*, 1975, *3*, N. 1, 39-57.

> In comparison to counterparts, low self-esteem individuals and females expressed: 1) attitudes of greater love, liking, trust, 2) evaluated partners more

favorably, 3) showed less trait congruency between ratings of ideal self and romantic partner.

Dipboye, R. L.; Zultowski, W. H.; Dewhust, D. H. & Arvey, R. D. Self-esteem as a moderator of the relationship between scientific interests and the job satisfaction of physicists and engineers. *Journal of Applied Psychology*, 1978, *63*, No. 3, 289-294.

> Among engineers, self-esteem moderated the relationship in which interest in science was negatively related to intrinsic job satisfaction.

Donahue, P. L. The perception of the autobiographical past as a function of changes in self-esteem. Unpublished dissertation, The Penn State University, 1975.

> There was no support for the hypotheses that manipulated self-esteem influences the subjects autobiographical memories and hence, their present self-perceptions.

Downs, R. A. An analysis of socioeconomic status and self-esteem in relation to minority student academic accomplishments in compensatory programs. Unpublished dissertation, University of Mass., 1975.

> Results support a relationship between socioeconomic status and self-esteem.

Douglas, L. A comparative analysis of the relationship between self-esteem and certain selected variables among youth from diverse racial groups. Unpublished dissertation, University of Michigan, 1969.*

Doyne, S. E. The relationship between self-disclosure and self-esteem in encounter groups. Unpublished dissertation, George Peabody College for Teachers, 1972.

> No relationship was found between the variables, but only females significantly increased in self-esteem during the experience.

Drolet, M. The level of self-esteem and its correlation with certain dimensions on the concept of self in the alcoholic. *Toxicomanies*, 1972, *5*, No. 3, 221-242.

> A synthesis of research on the self-esteem of alcoholics reinforced the hypothesis that alcoholics are characterized by low self-esteem.

Dunbar, S. M. College women's self-esteem and attitudes toward women's roles. Unpublished dissertation, Michigan State University, 1975.

> Tentative support found for the positive relationship between female's self-esteem and the degree of parent communality.

Durley, G. L. A variance analysis of the self-esteem among Black Elementary school children: sex and grade level the determining variables. Unpublished dissertation, University of Massachusetts, 1973.

> Among Black elementary school children, self-esteem rose as education pro-

gressed; males exhibited higher self-esteem than their female counterparts.

Eagly, H. Sex differences in the relationship between self-esteem and susceptibility to social influence. *Journal of Personality*, 1969, *37*, 581-591.

> Among males, self-esteem was found to be non-monotonically related to degree of opinion change, while for females, self-esteem was not a prediction variable.

Edwards, C. D. Stress in the school: A study of anxiety and self-esteem in Black and White elementary children. Unpublished dissertation, The Florida State University, 1972.

> The negative relationship between self-esteem and anxiety was stronger for Black males than White males.

Eisen, M. Characteristic self-esteem, sex and resistance to temptation. *Journal of Personality and Social Psychology*, 1972, *24*, No. 1, 68-72.

> For only males, there exists a strong positive relationship between self-esteem and honesty.

Eisen, R. Birth order, sex, self-esteem and prejudice against the physically disabled. *Journal of Psychology*, 1970, No. 2, 147-155.

> Among females, low self-esteem was associated with prejudice towards the disabled.

Elkins, D. P. (ed.) *Glad to be me: building self-esteem in yourself and others.* Englewood Cliffs, New Jersey: Prentice-Hall, 1976.*

Ellison, C. W. The development of interpersonal trust as a function of self-esteem, status and style. Unpublished dissertation, Wayne State University, 1972.

> A significant interaction between self-esteem and the status of a potential disclosure target was experimentally determined.

Ellison, C. W. & Firestone, I. J. Development of interpersonal trust as a function of self-esteem, target status and target style. *Journal of Personality and Social Psychology*, 1974, *29*, No. 5, 655-663.

> Results indicate that subjects are more willing to disclose information to the reflective style potential disclosure target.

Elton, D.; Stanley, G. U. & Burrows, G. D. Self-esteem and chronic pain. *Journal of Psychosomatic Research*, 1978, *22*, No. 1, 25-30.

> Pain prone subjects had poorer self-esteem than organic and normal groups.

Enwerem, F. O. A study of the effect of selected levels of self-esteem and dogmatism on preference for consonant information. Unpublished dissertation, The University of South Dakota, 1975.

> Manipulated self-esteem was not related to a preference for consonant information.

Epstein, R. & Komorita, S. S. Self-esteem, success-failure and locus of control in Negro children. *Developmental Psychology*, 1970, 4, No. 1, 2-8.

> Among Negro children, failure, rather than success is attributed to external causes and those with high self-esteem were more internal implying that a high self-esteem can cushion the belief in one's powerlessness as a stigmatized minority.

Erickson, G. R. A study of the self-esteem and academic self-concepts of ability and randomly-grouped ninth graders. Unpublished dissertation, University of Minnesota, 1973.

> Differences in self-esteem were related to differences in the group labelling process whereas ability grouped students exhibited negative effects on self-esteem.

Fein, D.; O'Neill, S.; Constance, F. & Velet, K. M. Sex differences in pre-adolescent self-esteem. *Journal of Psychology*, 1975, 90, No. 2, 179-183.

> Individual sex differences in self-esteem were sex-role related.

Fichtler, H.; Zimmerman, R. R. & Moore, R. T. Comparison of self-esteem of prison and non-prison groups. *Perceptual and Motor Skills*, 1973, 36, No. 1, 39-44.

> The more time spent in prison, the lower the self-esteem.

Firnesz, K. M. & Nielse, B. The influence of bibliography on self-esteem. *The Cornell Journal of Social Relations*, 1974, No. 2, 217-224.

> In this bibliotherapy training, lack of self-esteem change was attributed to inadequate levels of the librarian's empathy, respect and genuiness.

Fish, B. & Karabenick, S. Relationship between self-esteem and locus of control. *Psychological Reports*, 1971, 729, 784.

> Higher selfesteem subjects seem to be more internally oriented.

Flannery, R. B. & Baer, D. F. Paradox of experimental failure/experiential success in three models of behaviorally altering self-esteem. *Psychological Reports*, 1975, 35, No. 1, 170.

> No real relationships manifested in comparing the efficacy of hypnosis, suggestions, and coverant control in enhancing student's self-esteem but subjects reported academic gain.

Flippo, F. R. & Levinsohn, P. M. Effects of failure on the self-esteem of depressed and nondepressed subjects. *Journal of Consulting and Clinical Psychology*, 1971, 36, No. 1, 151.

> Under the conditionals, depressed, nondepressed, stabile vs. labile, no significant differences were found concerning the effects of failure in task-solving on self-esteem.

Flippo, F. R. Effects of ambiguity and failure on self-esteem of depressed, nondepressed and quasi-psychiatric control subjects. Unpublished dissertation, University of Oregon, 1972.

> Among depressives, ambiguous feedback was uninfluential concerning self-esteem change.

Franks, D. & Marolla, F. Efficacious actions and social approval as interacting dimensions of self-esteem: a tentative formulation through construct validation. *Sociometry*, 1976, *39*, No. 4, 324-341.

> The concept of self-esteem is operationalixed through the interaction of inner, competence based and outer, approval based dimensions.

Frerichs, M. Relationship of self-esteem and internal-external control to selected characteristics of associate degree nursing students. *Nursing Research*, 1973, *22*, No. 4, 350-352.

> Among nursing students, self-esteem levels and the degree of internal control was positively related to marital status (married) and age.

Friedman, S.; Rogers, P. P. & Gettys, F. Project re-ed: increase in self-esteem as measured by the Coopersmith Inventory. *Perceptual and Motor Skills*, 1975, *40*, No. 1, 165-166.

> Among emotionally disturbed children, positive gains in self-esteem were effected in this high-impact residential treatment center.

Frochle, T. & Zerface, J. Social self-esteem: a further look. *Journal of Consulting and Clinical Psychology*, 1971, *37*, 73-74.

> A followup study using Ziller et al.'s social self-esteem measure indicated that order of presentation of significant persons had no effect on their circle assignment.

Fullerton, W. S. Self-disclosure, self-esteem and risk taking: a study of their convergent and discriminant validity in elementary school children. Unpublished dissertation, University of California at Berkeley, 1972.

> A small correlation was found between students self-ratings of self-esteem and self-disclosure to their mother.

Gardner, R. C. The relationship of self-esteem and variables associated with reading for fourth grade Pima Indian children. Unpublished dissertation, University of Arizona, 1972.

> For boys only, significant relationships were found between self-esteem and language ability, total intelligence, reading achievement expectancy and attitudes toward reading.

Gavin, J. F. Self-esteem as moderator of the relationship between expectancies and job performance. *Journal of Applied Psychology*, 1973, *58*, No. 1, 83-88.

> Among managerial level employees, equivocal support was found indicating that self-esteem is a moderating variable between expectancies and job performance.

Gecas, V. Parental behavior and contextual variations in adolescent self-esteem. *Sociometry*, 1972, *35*, No. 2, 332-345.

> Adolescent self-esteem is highest in a social context (among peers) and lowest in a classroom context.

Gecas, V.; Thomas, D. L. & Weigert, A. Perceived parent child interaction and boy's self-esteem in two cultural contexts. *International Journal of Comparative Sociology*, 1970, *11*, No. 4, 317-324.

> Cross-culturally there is a strong relationship between parental support and a child's self-esteem.

Geisler, J. R. The relationship of self-esteem to face-saving behavior. Unpublished dissertation, California School of Professional Psychology, 1975.

> Results suggest that self-esteem and face-saving behavior are importantly related.

Gendreau, P.; Gibson, M.; Surridge, C. & Hug, J. J. The application of self-esteem measures in corrections; a further report on the *S.E.I. Journal of Community Psychology* 1973, *1*, No. 4, 423-425.

> The self-esteem inventory was found to have adequate validity for a Canadian reformatory sample.

Getsinger, S.; Kunce, J.; Miller, D. & Weinbert, S. Self-esteem measures and cultural disadvantagement. *Journal of Consulting and Clinical Psychology*, 1972, *38*, 149.

> It is concluded that either race and socioeconomic status are minimally related to self-esteem among 6th grade students or that the instruments used are insensitive to the existing differences.

Gilbert, S. J. Effects of unanticipated self-disclosure on recipients of varying levels of self-esteem: A research note. *Human Communication Research*, 1977, *3*, No. 4, 368-371.

> Subjects with intermediate levels of self-esteem were most receptive to a disclosing other.

Gill, M. J. Self-esteem and male's receptiveness to persuasion toward women's liberation ideology. Unpublished dissertation, Washington State University, 1975.

> Individuals with low, manipulated self-esteem tend to view females with traditional attitudes.

Glaser, T. E. Locus of control and self-esteem as a function of sensitivity group participation. Unpublished dissertation, Temple University, 1977.

> There is a small significant correlation between self-esteem and locus of control.

Glick, B. R. Self-esteem, the perception of support during marital conflict and marital satisfaction. Unpublished dissertation, The Ohio State University, 1976.

> Self-esteem influences the perception of remarks as support in disagreeing situations; self-esteem was positively related to marital satisfaction.

Gold, S. R. & Coghlan, A. J. Locus of control and self-esteem among adolescent drug abusers: Effects of residential treatment. *Drug Forum*, 1975-76, No. 5, No. 2, 195-191.*

Golin, S.; Davis, E.; Zuckerman, E. & Nelson, E. & H. Psychology in the community: project self-esteem. *Psychological Reports*, 1970, *26*, No. 3, 735-740.

> Describes a black, urban psychoeducational program in progress.

Graham, D. & Perry, R. P. Limitations in generalizability of the physical attractiveness stereotype: The self-esteem exception. *Canadian Journal of Behavioral Sciences*, 1976, *8*,No. 3, 363-374.

> There is a negative correlation between self-esteem and a subject's tendency to denigrate an attractive other in a socially transgressed role.

Gray, S. S. The relationship of locus of control and self-esteem to the quality and content of daydreams. Unpublished dissertation, University of Tennessee, 1975.

> Self-esteem was negatively related to the dimension of realistic-unrealistic daydreaming.

Greadington, B. G. The affects of Black films on the self-esteem of Black adolescents. Unpublished dissertation, University of Miami, 1977.

> The experimental design of Black children viewing a film once, portraying Black actors and actresses in stereotypic and non-stereotypic roles, is admittedly ineffective as an influence on self-esteem.

Green, R. B. Self-disclosure, self-esteem and perceived similarity. Unpublished dissertation, City University of New York, 1976.

> There is a positive relationship between self-esteem and self-disclosure in a group.

Greenberg, J. S. The masturbatory behavior of college students. *Psychology in the Schools*, 1972, *9*, No. 4, 427-432.

> No relationship was found between self-esteem and masturbatory behavior.

Greenberg, J. S. A study of self-esteem and alienation of male homosexuals. *Journal of Psychology*, 1973, *83*, No. 1, 137-143.

> American homosexuals feel greater alienation than, but have similar levels of self-esteem in comparison to heterosexuals.

Greenberg, J. S. & Archambault, F. X. Masturbation, self-esteem and other variables. *Journal of Sex Research*, 1973, *9*, No. 1, 44-51.

Among students, frequency of masturbation was not related to self-esteem.

Greenhaus, J. H. & Badin, I. J. Self-esteem, performance and satisfaction: some tests of a theory. *Journal of Applied Psychology*, 1974, *59*, No. 6, 722-726.

Only for high self-esteem subjects did performance tend to predict satisfaction on an anagram task.

Heaton, R. C. & Duerfeldt, P. H. The relationship between self-esteem, self-reinforcement and the internal-external personality dimension. *Journal of Genetic Psychology*, 1973, *123*, No. 7, 3-13.

It is suggested that self-esteem, self-reinforcement and the internal-external personality dimension could possibly be aspects of a broader response tendency.

Hecht, H. B. Self-esteem and cognitive dissonance in a naturally occurring situation. Unpublished dissertation, Adelphi University, 1973.

The validity of self-esteem measures are challenged as too general.

Helland, D. J. Sex-role correlates of adolescent self-esteem. Unpublished dissertation, The University of Michigan, 1973.

The self-esteem of adolescent boys was most strongly related to achievement whereas female adolescent's self-esteem was most strongly related to social variables.

Helmreich, R. & Stapp, J. Short forms of the Texas Social Behavior Inventory (TSBI), an objective measure of self-esteem. *Bulletin of the Psychonomic Society*, 1974, *4*, 473-475.*

Hess, K. A & Lindner, R. Dogmatism and self-esteem: A negative relationship confirmed. *Psychological Reports*, 1973, *32*, No. 1, 158.

The findings of K. S. Larsen and G. Schwendiman are confirmed. (See Psych. Abstracts Inter. Vol. 44: 3607.)

Higgins, T. F. The effects of self-help therapeutic community treatment on self-esteem in drug abusers. Unpublished dissertation, Boston University School of Education, 1977.

Over an unspecified length of time, the self-esteem of experimentals improved significantly vs. controls.

Hill, N. C. & Ritchie, J. B. The effect of self-esteem on leadership and achievement: a paradigm and a review. *Group and Organizational Studies*, 1977, *2*, No. 4, 491-503.

A literature review concluded that self-esteem is a significant variable in leader effectiveness; also, he presents a conceptual framework on self-esteem importance in organization contexts.

Hillner, W. M. The effect of self-esteem upon self-evaluation and self-reinforcement. Unpublished dissertation, University of Georgia, 1976.

High self-esteem children set higher goals than low self-esteem children.

Hirschfeld, R. M. et al. Dependency-self-esteem-clinical depression. *Journal of the American Academy of Psychoanalysis*, 1976, *4*, No. 3, 373-388.

> Self-esteem is viewed as an intervening factor in the interaction of interpersonal dependency and depression.

Hoffman, C. E. Empowerment and personality: a study of locus of control, self-esteem and autonomy among members of the united farm workers. Unpublished dissertation, University of Southern California, 1975.

> There were no significant differences found in the self-esteem of union vs. non-union workers.

Hollender, J. W. Self-esteem and parental identification. *Journal of Genetic Psychology*, 1973, *122*, No. 1, 3-7.

> For undergraduate females, self-esteem is positively correlated with parental identification.

Holcomb, L. Role concepts and self-esteem in church women with implications for pastoral counseling. *Journal of Psychology and Theology*, 1975, *3*, No. 2, 119-126.

> There was no significant differences in self-esteem relating to role concepts of church women.

Howard, A. Aspects of self-esteem among Hawaiian-Americans of the parental generation. In W. P. Lebra (Ed.), *Youth, Socialization, and Mental Health: III. Mental Health Research in Asia and the Pacific*. Honolulu, HI: University Press of Hawaii, 1974.*

Howe, M. C. A comparison of the self-esteem body image and movement-concept of adults in different age groups. Unpublished dissertation, Boston University School of Education, 1973.

> From the early to late adult years, self-esteem gradually decreased, reflecting this culture's aging attitudes.

Hoyt, R. Self-identification as lead or character actor as it relates to self-esteem, locus of control and fear of success. Unpublished dissertation, California School of Professional Psychology, Los Angeles, 1977.

> Indications lead to the interrelations of self-esteem and locus of control; self-identification is related to both self-esteem and locus of control.

Husaini, B. A. Achievement motivation and self-esteem: a cross cultural study. *Indian Journal of Psychology*, 1974, *49*, No. 2, 100-108.

> The influence of cultural variability upon self-esteem and the achievement motivation relationship lies within the value system.

Hustak, T. L. The mediating effects of self-esteem and noncontingent feedback in a self-reinforcement paradigm. Unpublished dissertation, University of

Southern Mississippi, 1977.

> Self-esteem modified self-reward behavior toward task performance.

Ickes, W. J.; Wicklurd, R. A. & Ferris, C. B. Objective self-awareness and self-esteem. *Journal of Experimental Social Psychology,* 1973, *9,* No. 3, 202-219.

> Subjects under a condition of self-focused attention exhibited higher self-esteem.

Inkson, J. K. Self-esteem as a moderator of the relationship between job performance and job satisfaction. *Journal of Applied Psychology,* 1978, *63,* No. 2, 243-247.

> Self-esteem served as a moderating variable in the correlations between job performance and intrinsic satisfaction.

Izzeth, R. R. Effects of self-praise and self-esteem on interpersonal attraction. *Representative Research in Social Psychology,* 1976, *7,* No. 1, 1-5.

> Results indicate an interaction between a subject's self-esteem and the positively preevaluated target person.

Johnson, C. D. & Gormly, A. & J. Disagreements and self-esteem: support for the competence-reinforcement model of attraction. *Journal of Research in Personality,* 1973, *1,* No. 2, 165-172.

> Results show that interactions with disagreeing strangers produce decrements in a subject's self-esteem; subjects expressing the greatest dislike for the stranger would experience the greatest decrements.

Johnson, M. The relationship of religious commitment to self-esteem. Unpublished dissertation, Brigham Young University, 1971.*

Johnson, C. Viewer aggression, self-esteem and television character preference as variables influencing social normative judgments of television violence. Unpublished dissertation, University of Maine, 1976.

> The self-esteem level of adolescents cannot serve as a predictor of social judgments on television violence.

Jones, S. C. Self and interpersonal evaluation evaluations: Esteem theories vs. consistency theories. *Psychological Bulletin,* 1973, *79,* No. 3, 185-199.

> He contrasts and derives different predictions from two social-psychological theories on the relation between self and inter-personal evaluation.

Kaplan, H. B. The self-esteem motive and change in self-attitudes. *The Journal of Nervous and Mental Disease,* 1975, *161,* No. 4, 265-275.

> Observations of junior high students supported the postulate of the self-esteem motive.

Kayala, L. M. Internal vs. external self-esteem: a new measure. Unpublished dissertation, The University of Massachusetts, 1977.

> A scale was devised to test the dual process theories of self-esteem (1. social theory and 2) self-opinion that is independent of environmental feedback and social value.)

Karylowski, T. Altruism and interpersonal attraction as function of perceived self-partner similarity and self-esteem. *Polish Psychological Bulletin*, 1975, *6*, No. 2, 63-71.

> Attraction to a similar partner correlated positively with subject's self-esteem. An altruistic motivation is stronger in a relation to a similar partner than to a dissimilar one.

Keller, M. E. Self-disclosure as a function of self-esteem and repression sensitization. Unpublished dissertation, Rutgers University, 1975.

> There is no significant curvilinear or linear relationship between self-esteem and self disclosure for female undergraduates.

Kelly, D. H. Tracking and its impact upon self-esteem: a neglected dimension. *Education*, 1975, *96*, No. 1, 2-9.

> Educational tracking produces a "corroding effect" upon student's self-esteem.

Kelly, G. K. A comparison of male and female levels and components of self-esteem. Unpublished dissertation, Rutgers University, 1976.

> High self-esteem individuals possibly have cross-sex associated characteristics.

Kennedy, M. S. The effect on persuasibility of the client's self-esteem, his or her sex and the sex of the counsellor. Unpublished dissertation, McGill University, 1975.

> A client's self-esteem was found not to be related to client opinion change in counseling.

Kessler, J. J. Self-esteem and inequity dissonance as factors in under-compensation. Unpublished dissertation, Case Western Reserve University, 1972.

> Self-esteem enhancement of a worker increases work quality.

King, L. M. An experimental exploration of the relationship between self-reinforcement, self-esteem and locus of control in 9-11 year old black males. Unpublished dissertation, University of California at Los Angeles, 1972.

> Self-esteem is significantly related to social reinforcement.

King, M. R. & Manaster, G. J. Body image, self-esteem, expectations, self-assessments and actual success in a simulated job interview. *Journal of Applied Psychology*, 1977, *62*, No. 5, 589-594.

> In a simulated job interview, a significant relationship was found between a subject's success expectations and self-esteem.

King, V. M. Active discipline: an exploration of parental power and its effects on the child's self-esteem. Unpublished dissertation, California School of

Professional Psychology, Los Angeles, 1973.

> Discipline which fosters self-esteem has three components: acceptance, control and training.

Klein, J. W. Jewish identity and self-esteem. Unpublished dissertation, The Wright Institute, 1977.

> A positive relationship exists between a positive Jewish identity and self-esteem.

Klemer, R. H. Self-esteem and college dating experiences as factors in mate selection and marital happiness: A longitudinal study. *Journal of Marriage and the Family*, 1971, *33*, No. 1, 183-187.

> Women with high self-esteem went steady less, dated more and got married earlier.

Knox, N. B. Sex-role orientation and self-esteem in career-committed and home oriented women. Unpublished dissertation, California School of Professional Psychology, San Francisco, 1977.

> Women with an androgynous sex-role orientation had the highest levels of self-esteem.

Koepsel, E. A. The effectiveness of individually guided education on the development of self-esteem in middle school students. Unpublished dissertation, Marquette University, 1975.

> The self-esteem of students in an individually guided learning climate is comparable to those in a traditional school system.

Kokenes, B. Grade level differences in factors of self-esteem. *Developmental Psychology*, 1974, *10*, No. 6, 954-958.

> He investigated the construct validity of the Coopersmith Self-esteem Inventory.

Korman, A. K. Self-esteem, social influence and task performance: some tests of a theory. Proceedings of the 76th Annual Convention of the American Psychological Association, 1968, 567-568.*

Krauss, H. H. & Critchfield, L. L. Contrasting self-esteem theory and consistency theory in predicting interpersonal attraction. *Sociometry*, 1975, *38*, No. 2, 247-260.

> In predicting interpersonal attraction, self-esteem theory alone accounted for data adequately.

Kunce, J. T.; Gestinger, S. H. & Miller, D. E. Educational implications of self-esteem. *Psychology in the Schools*, 1972, *9*, No. 3, 314-316.

> The study reveals nominal relationship between self-esteem and academic achievement and home environment.

Laitman, R. J. Family relations as an intervening variable in the relationship of birth order and self-esteem. Unpublished dissertation, Case Western Reserve University, 1975.

>Family relations were found to be a powerful influence on self-esteem.

Lampl, M. Defensiveness, dogmatism and self-esteem. Unpublished dissertation, Yeshiva University, 1968.

>There is a positive relationship between self-esteem and defensiveness.

Lanza, E. R. An investigation of various antecedents of self-esteem as related to race and sex. Unpublished dissertation, Ball State University, 1969.

>Students with high self-esteem are more likely to have mothers with high self-esteem; fathers with stable jobs value education in the family and basically, like themselves.

Larsen, K. & Schwendiman, G. Authoritarianism, self-esteem and insecurity. *Psychological Reports*, 1969, *25*, 229-230.

>Subjects exhibiting a high level of authoritarianism were low in self-esteem.

League, B. & Jackson, D. Conformity, veridicality and self-esteem. *Journal of Abnormal and Social Psychology*, 1964, *68*, 113-115.

>In a nonsocial condition of the Blake-Brehin procedure, low self-esteem subjects were found to be less accurate than subjects high in self-esteem.

Leake, D. The measurement of self-esteem. Unpublished master's thesis, Ohio State University, 1970.*

Leonard, R. L.; Walsh, W. B. & Osipow, S. H. Self-esteem, self-consistency and second vocational choice. *Journal of Counseling Psychology*, 1973, 20, No. 1, 91-93.

>Self-esteem is positively related to a second vocational choice which is consistent with personality style.

Littell, W. J. An investigation of possible moderating effects of self-esteem on vocational choice and classification. Unpublished dissertation, University of Kansas, 1973.

>Self-esteem did not act as a moderator of vocational choice.

Llewellyn, R. C. Do praise and criticism have different effects on low and high self-esteem children? Unpublished dissertation, Fuller Theological Seminary Graduate School of Psychology, 1973.

>For low self-esteem subjects there is a positive relationship between praise and accuracy in task performance.

Logiudice, J. F. The relationship of self-esteem, testing anxiety and sixth grade student's arithmetical problem solving efficiency under variant test instructions. Unpublished dissertation, St. Johns University, 1970.

>A relationship exists between self-esteem and the level of test anxiety. Satisfactory self-esteem was related to academic success.

London, M. & Klimoski, R. J. Self-esteem and job complexity as moderators of attitudes toward work and effectiveness as seen by self, supervisors and peers. Proceedings of the 81st Annual Convention of the American Psychological Association, 1973, *8*, 559-600.

Self-esteem did not act as a moderator of the relationship.

London, M. & Klimoski, R. J. Self-esteem and job complexity as moderators of performance and satisfaction. *Journal of Vocational Behavior*, 1975, *6*, No. 3, 293-304.

Self-esteem did act as a moderator of the performance/satisfaction relationship among registered nurses.

Loney, J. The relationship between impulse control and self-esteem in school children. *Psychology in the Schools*, 1974, *11*, No. 4, 462-466.

A strong association was found between impulse control and self-esteem.

Love, B. B. Self-esteem in women related to occupational status: a biracial study. Unpublished dissertation, Northwestern University, 1974.

There were significant self-esteem differences between Black and White women across all occupations and self-esteem was related to reasons for working.

Lowry, R. J. (ed.) *Dominance, self-esteem, self-actualization: germinal papers of A. H. Maslow.* Monterey, California, Brooks/Cole, 1973.*

Loxley, J. C. Sex-role androgyny and its effects on self-esteem, adjustment and performance on sex-appropriate and sex-inappropriate tasks. Unpublished dissertation, Southern Illinois University at Carbondale, 1976.

More androgynous traited women had higher self-esteem than less androgynous.

Luck, P. N. & Heiss, J. Social determinants of self-esteem in adult males. *Sociology and Social Research*, 1972, *57*, No. 1, 69-84.

The self-esteem of adult males is influenced by their occupational success, whether utilizing objective indicators, (prestige level, income, etc.) or subjective indicators (personal satisfaction, lack of stress).

Lyons, M. Cognition and affect in social psychology: the case of self-esteem. Paper presnted at the 40th Meeting of the Southern Sociological Society.*

Mahoney, E. R. Body cathexis and self-esteem: the importance of subjective importance. *Journal of Psychology*, 1974, *88*, No. 1, 27-30.

There is no relationship between a subject's stated importance of body aspects and the statistical correlations between body cathexis and self-esteem.

Mahoney, E. R. & Finch, M. D. Body cathexis and self-esteem: a re-analysis of the differential contribution of specific body parts. *Journal of Social Psychology*, 1976, *99*, No. 2, 251-158.

> Due to methodological flaws, earlier statements that certain body parts are important to self-esteem is refuted.

Maier, D. & Herman, A. The relationship of vocational decidedness and satisfaction with dogmatism and self-esteem. *Journal of Vocational Behavior*, 1974, *5*, No. 1, 95-101.

> There are distinct differences in self-esteem and dogmatism between vocationally decided and undecided subjects.

Maile, C. A. Self-esteem and source credibility as determinants of attitude change. Unpublished dissertation, University of Georgia, 1975.

> Dissonance theory is extended to explain the 1) negative linear, 2) inverted U-shape and 3) positive linear relationship between self-esteem and persuasability.

Manganiello, J. A. A psychological investigation of heroin addiction: the self-esteem future time perspective and locus of control of contemporary heroin addicts. Unpublished dissertation, Boston University School of Education, 1974.

> Heroin addicts are characterized by low self-esteem, external locus of control and lack of future goals.

Mann, D. W. When delinquency is defensive: self-esteem is defensive: self-esteem in deviant behavior. Unpublished dissertation, University of Michigan, 1976.

> A model is presented which proposes the presence of conscious self-esteem and unconscious self-esteem within individuals.

Mansfield, R. Self-esteem, self-perceived abilities and vocational choice. *Journal of Vocational Behavior*, 1973, *3*, No. 4, 433-441.

> High self-esteem persons are more likely to perceive themselves as possessing the necessary vocational abilities in their chosen occupation.

Many, M. A. & Many, W. A. The relationship between self-esteem and anxiety in grades four through eight. *Educational and Psychological Measurement*, 1975, *35*, No. 4, 1017-1021.

> There is a negative relationship between self-esteem and anxiety among elementary and junior high school children.

Marolla, J. A. A study of self-esteem as a two dimensional construct. Unpublished dissertation, University of Denver, 1974.

> Self-esteem is presented as differentiated into structural individualistic dimensions.

Martin, J. R. Self-esteem, reciprocity of liking and perceived social acceptance. Unpublished dissertation, University of California at Berkeley, 1975.

A subject's perceived acceptance by both primary and secondary groups interact in their effects on self-esteem.

Maslow, A. H. A test for dominance feeling (self-esteem) in college women. *Journal of Social Psychology*, 1940, *12*, 255-170.

Dominance feeling is a construct determined by several factors (e.g. self-esteem, self-confidence) and is one aspect of a more socially sensitive construct called dominant behavior.

Mason, E. J. The relationship between perceived success and failure on the learner's level of self-esteem. Unpublished dissertation, University of Wisconsin, 1972.

Perceived success or failure did not significantly affect self-esteem.

Mathes, E. W. & Kahn, A. Physical attractiveness, happiness, neuroticism, and self-esteem. *Journal of Psychology*, 1975, *90*, No. 1, 27-30.

For women only, physical attractiveness was found to correlate positively with self-esteem.

Matteson, R. Adolescent self-esteem, family communication, and marital satisfaction. *Journal of Psychology*, 1974, *86*, No. 1, 35-47.

A positive relationship exists between adolescent self-esteem and their view of facilitative communication with parents.

Meltzer, M. L. & Levy, B. I. Self-esteem in a public school. *7Psychology in the School*, 1970, *7*, No. 1, 14-20.

Anecdotal observations made at an inner city junior high school on those aspects of school life that lead to dissatisfaction, low achievement and school dropout in students and faculty.

McCarthy, J. D. & Yancey, W. L. Uncle Tom and Mr. Charlie: Metaphysical pathos in the study of racism and personal disorganization. *American Journal of Sociology*, 1971, *76*, No. 4, 648-672.

Exploratory research which questions, as being based on a stereotype, the hypothesis that U.S. Negroes have low self-esteem and experience identity crises.

McCormick, C. H. & Karalinus, R. A. Relationship of ethnic groups' self-esteem and anxiety to school success. *Educational and Psychological Measurement*, 1976, *36*, No. 4, 1093-1100.

Among Blacks, no differences in self-esteem between high and low achievement reading groups.

McElroy, D. & Bernstein, H. The role of parents in the developing self-esteem in a hearing impaired child. *Volta Review*, 1976, *78*, No. 5, 209-223.

Parents must view hearing-impaired children in a larger, social context by allowing the child a sense of control in the home environment.

McKinney, T. T. Self-esteem in a competitive environment: Does success matter? Paper presented at 1971 Annual Meeting of the Georgia Sociological and Anthropological Association.

> There is no significant correlation between self-esteem and success as measured in relation to individual achievement, group achievement and group evaluation of individual achievement.

McNulty, T. G. The effects of the human development program on the self-esteem, self-esteem behavior, social acceptance and academic achievement of children. Unpublished dissertation, Lehigh University, 1975.

> The human development progrm had no effect on the self-esteem level of 3rd graders.

McReynolds, P. The motives to attain success and to avoid failure; historical note. *Journal of Individual Psychology*, 1968, *24*, No. 2, 157-161.

> From an Adlerian perspective, the relative nature of failure-avoidance motivation and success-attainment motivation is explored historically, beginning with William James.

McQuaide, M. M. & Walsh, E. J. Occupation, age and self-esteem: A comparison of older and younger White workers in seven occupations. Paper presented at 1977 meeting of Pennsylvania Sociological Society.

> The experimental data challenge the hypothesis that age and self-esteem are negatively related.

Meacham, J. A. A dialectical approach to moral judgment and self-esteem. *Human Development*, 1975, *18*, No. 3, 159-170.

> Moral judgments and self-esteem are interdependent.

Miller, T. W. Communicative dimensions of mother-child interactions as they affect the self-esteem of the child. *Proceedings from the Annual Convention of the American Psychological Association*, 1971, Vol. 6, 241-242.

> There was a positive correlation between the effects of verbal and nonverbal parental behavior and the child's self-esteem.

Miller, T. W. Male self-esteem and attitudes toward women's roles. *Journal of College Student Personnel*, 1973, *14*, No. 5, 302-406.

> In non-college subjects and male subjects from small, private, predominantly male educational institutions, low self-esteem was related to negative attitudes towards women's liberation.

Miller, T. W. Effects of maternal age, education and employment status on the self-esteem of the child. *Journal of Social Psychology*, 1975, *95*, No. 1, 141-142.

> There is a positive relationship between maternal educational level and a child's self-esteem.

Micucci, J. A. Self-esteem and preference for consonant information. *Cornell Journal of Social Relations,* 1972, 7, No. 2, 63-74.

> In a task solving group, members with low self-esteem preferred consonant rather than dissonant information.

Mishken, M. A. Self-esteem as a moderator in the relationship between job ability and job performance. Unpublished dissertation, University of Tennessee, 1973.

> Self-esteem acts as a moderator in the relationship between job ability and job performance.

Modell, E. A. An investigation of children's self-esteem and incidence of behavior problems as correlates of parental permissiveness.

> Among female children, high self-esteem was related to moderate maternal permissiveness.

Montijo, J. A. The relationships among self-esteem, group pride and cultural group identification. Unpublished dissertation, Adelphi University, 1974.

> Among urban Puerto-Ricans, self-esteem was negatively correlated with group pride and with identification as an American.

Morrison, T. L. & Thomas, M. D. Self-esteem and classroom participation. *Journal of Educational Research,* 1975, *68,* No. 10, 374-377.

> Results were inconclusive due to the inconsistency of the measures employed.

Morrison, T. L. Thomas, M. D. & Weaver, S. J. Self-esteem and self-estimates of academic performance. *Journal of Consulting and Clinical Psychology,* 1973, *41,* No. 3, 412-415.

> There were disagreements between the 3 self-esteem measures used, leading to obvious implications of validity.

Morval, M. & Morval, J. Concerning the concept of self-esteem and some possibilities of its measurement. *Bulletin de Psychologie* 1971- 1972, *25,* 145-150.

> Examines self-esteem from psychoanalytic, social psychological, and existential phenomenological viewpoints.

Morval, M. & Morval, J. Self-esteem and interpersonal needs in girls between 15 and 18. *Revue de Psychologie Appliquee,* 1972, *22,* No. 2, 67-75.

> There is a positive correlation between self-esteem and the need for inclusion in social groups and a negative correlation between self-esteem and the need to control others.

Moser, K. Preventative psychotherapy: implementation of an intervention strategy to raise self-esteem. Unpublished dissertation, Indiana University, 1973.

The data do not allow for conclusive statements about the merits of this intervention strategy.

Moyal, B. R. Locus of control, self-esteem, stimulus appraisal and depressive symptoms in children. *Journal of Consulting and Clinical Psychology*, 1977, No. 5, 951-952.

In children, self-esteem was significantly correlated with depressive symptoms.

Myers, L. W. Black women and self-esteem. *Sociological Inquiry*, 1975, *45*, 240-249.

In exploring the effects of the matriarchally structured family on American Black women's self-esteem, it was concluded that the reference group used is other Black women; the family structure does not lower self-esteem and the maintenance of self-esteem is a reference group process.

Neistein, S. & Katkovsky, W. The effects of inconsistent reinforcement on the negative self-reinforcing behavior of high and low self-esteem individuals. *Journal of Personality*, 1974, *42*, No. 1, 78-92.

There is a negative, direct relationship between self-esteem and the rate of negative self-reinforcement as the percentage of inconsistent reinforcement increases.

Nemoto, K. Effects of self-esteem on person perception: I. *Japanese Journal of Experimental Social Psychological*, 1973, 13, No. 1, 31-39.

Self-esteem and the congruency between one's feeling toward others and perception of others' feelings toward oneself were positively related when others were positively perceived.

Nemoto, K. Effects of self-esteem on person perception: II. *Japanese Journal of Experimental Social Psychology*, 1973, 13, No. 1, 31-39.

Self-esteem was positively correlated with perceptual accuracy of others' feelings and negatively with others' negative feelings.

Newman, D. E. The personality of violence: conversations with protagonists. *Mental Health and Society*, 1974, 1, 328-344.

It was observed that among men living violent lives, the importance of self-esteem was central.

Nocks, J. J. & Bradley, D. L. Self-esteem in an alcoholic population. *Diseases of the Nervous System*, 1969, *30*, No. 9, 611-617.

Among acute, male alcoholics, self-esteem was found to be positively related with smoking (cigarettes); negatively with the increasing duration of the awareness of a drinking problem, whereas subjects who denied any problem had higher self-esteem.

Norem-Hebeisn, A. A. Differentiated aspects of the self-esteeming process among suburban adolescents and dysfunctional youth. Unpublished dissertaton, University of Minnesota, 1974.

>The lower self-esteem of dysfunctional adolescents manifests in differentiated personalities unique to each category of dysfunction studied.

Norem-Hebeisen, A. A. A multidimensional construct of self-esteem. *Journal of Educational Psychology*, 1976, *68*, No. 5, 559-565.

>A conceptualization of self-esteem is presented which concluded that among adolescents, stress and unwillingness to cooperate were negatively related to self-esteem.

Oaklander, H. Self-esteem diversity of backgrounds and clarity of communication in engaged couples. Unpublished dissertation, Michigan State University, 1972.

>A married couple with similar levels of self-esteem exhibited more dysfunctional communication and tended to have a more conflictual type of relationship as compared to a couple with differing levels of self-esteem who complemented each other.

O'Brien, E. F. & Epstein, S. Naturally occurring changes in self-esteem. *Personality and Social Psychology Bulletin*, 1974, *1*, No. 1, 384-386.*

O'Donnell, W. J. Test anxiety related to self-esteem in neutral and examination conditions. *Bulletin of the North Carolina Psychological Association*, 1976, 18-20.

>Among college students, a strong inverse relationship exists between the direction of change in anxiety and the direction of change in self-esteem, under neutral and examination conditions.

O'Donnell, W. J. Adolescent self-esteem related to feelings toward parents and friends. *Journal of Youth and Adolescence*, 1976, *5*, No. 2, 178-185.

>Self-esteem in adolescents appeared as significantly related to the primary group as to the secondary group.

Ohlenkamp, E. A. The relationship among test anxiety, self-esteem and achievement for cooperative career education students in grades eleven and twelve. Unpublished dissertation, Northern Illinois University, 1976.

>Among 11th and 12th graders there was a negative relationship between self-esteem and anxiety and between test anxiety and academic achievement; there was a positive relationship between self-esteem and academic achievement.

Orpen, C. & Lisus, G. Self-esteem and the relationship between need fulfillment and job satisfaction. *Journal of Psychology*, 1974, 93, No. 2, 307-308.

>For high self-esteem subjects, a lower correlation was obtained between self-rated need fulfillment and job satisfaction than for low self-esteem subjects.

Page, J. P. Relationship between sex role conformity and self-esteem, anxiety and motive to avoid success. Unpublished dissertation, The City University of New York, 1973.

Self-esteem was found to be unrelated to sex role conformity status among female undergraduates.

Page, R. A. The effects of self-esteem and sex on attributions by actors and observers regarding the causes of success and failure. Unpublished dissertation, University of Rochester, 1973.

High self-esteem individuals exhibit a more internal locus of control.

Page, W. F. Self-esteem and internal versus external control among Black youth in a summer aviation program. *Journal of Psychology*, 1975, *89*, No. 2, 307-311.

Significant gains were made in self-esteem by subjects under 16 years old and those from middle income families.

Patterson, A. H. The effects of a season of high school football upon the aggressiveness, self-esteem and innovativeness of the student-athlete. Unpublished dissertation, Northwestern University, 1973.

There is strong *inferential* evidence that self-esteem is reciprocally related to athletic performance.

Paulos, A. J. Acute self-esteem effects on racial attitudes measured by rating scale and bogus pipeline. Proceedings of the 81st Annual Convention of the American Psychological Association, 1973, *8*, 165-166.

There is a negative relationship between self-esteem and prejudice toward Blacks.

Pawelkiewicz, W. M. & McIntire, W. G. Field dependence-independence and self-esteem in pre-adolescent children. *Perceptual and Motor Skills*, 1975, *41*, No. 1, 41-42.

For boys, there is a correlation between field independence and self-esteem.

Penney, R. Self-esteem and the search for self-awareness. Unpublished dissertation, Michigan State University, 1973.

There is a negative relationship between self-esteem and awareness-seeking behavior.

Perlman, D. Self-esteem and sexual permissiveness. *Journal of Marriage and the Family*, 1974, *36*, No. 3, 470-473.

The sexual permissiveness self-esteem relationship is dependent on cultural norms.

Piers, E. V. Children's self-esteem, level of esteem certainty, and responsibility for success and failure. *Journal of Genetic Psychology*, 1977, *130*, No. 2, 295-304.

A self-esteem model is suggested involving a modification of attribution theory.

Plante, J. A. A study of future time perspective and its relationship to self-esteem and social responsibility of high school students. Unpublished dissertation, University of Massachusetts, 1977.

> A positive correlation was found between self-esteem and an active future orientation.

Platt, J.; Eisenman, R. & Darbes, A. Self-esteem and internal-external control: a validation study. *Psychological Reports*, 1970, *26*, 162.

> There was no correlation found between Ziller, et al.'s self-esteem measure and Rotter's Internal-External Control scale.

Pollack, L. J. The differential effects of ego threat on the tactical self-presentation of low, moderate and high self-esteem children. Unpublished dissertation, Syracuse University, 1978.

> Results led to the speculation that high self-esteem individuals react to failure by increasing self-esteem and low self-esteem individuals react to failure by self-punishment.

Pollard, R. J. The differential effects of initial and induced self-esteem on changes in interpersonal perception following the performance of a harmful act. Unpublished dissertation, University of Washington, 1974.

> All the subjects were uninfluenced by the attempted self-esteem manipulation.

Pope, M. G. Construction of a self-esteem scale. *Sociological Focus*, 1971, *4*, No. 3, 83-89.

> In developing a scale to measure the self-esteem of undergraduate students, the most common referent was other college students.

Prieto, A. G. & Robbins, M. C. Perceptions of height and self-esteem. *Perceptual and Motor Skills*, 1975, *40*, No. 2, 395-398.

> A positive correlation exists between self-esteem and a subject's own perception, and his peers and teachers' perceptions of his height.

Primavera, L. H.; Simon, W. E. and Primavera, A. M. The relationship between self-esteem and academic achievement: An investigation of sex differences. *Psychology in the Schools*, 1974, *11*, No. 2, 213-216.

> There is a positive relationship between self-esteem and performance on academic exams.

Prytula, R. E. & Thompson, N. D. Analysis of emotional indicators in human figure drawings as related to self-esteem. *Perceptual and Motor Skills*, 1973, *37*, No. 3, 795-802.

> There was no statistical support for the body-image hypothesis as it relates to self-esteem.

Qadri, A. J. & Kaleem, G. A. Effects of parental attitudes on personality adjustment and self-esteem of children. *Behaviorometric*, 1971, *1*, No. 1, 19-24.

A positive relationship was found between children's self-esteem and parental permissiveness and self-esteem and parental acceptance.

Raben, C. S. & Klimoski, R. J. The effects of expectations upon task performance as moderated by levels of self-esteem. *Journal of Vocational Behavior*, 1973, *3*, No. 4, 475-483.

Only high self-esteem individuals differed significantly in their response to manipulated expectations of a task performance.

Rathus, S. A. & Siegal, L. J. Delinquent attitudes and self-esteem. *Adolescence*, 1973, *8*, 265-276.

Small correlations allowed an inference to be made that an inverse relationship existed between delinquent's self-esteem and their attitudes toward the criminal justice system.

Recely, N. L. Level of self-esteem and conformity to sex role stereotypes. Unpublished dissertation, University of Colorado, 1973.

There is a positive correlation between self-esteem and the amount of conformity to the male sex-role in both females and males.

Regan, J. W.; Gosselink, H.; Huback J. & Ulsh, E. Do people have inflated views of their own ability? *Journal of Personality and Social Psychology*, 1975, *31*, No. 2, 295-301.

It was found that subjects, when faced with the possibility of losing self-esteem, engaged in self derogation.

Reschly, D. J. & Mittleman, A. The relationship of self-esteem status and task ambiguity to the self-reinforcement behavior of children. *Developmental Psychology*, 1973, *9*, No. 1, 16-19.

A direct, positive relationship between self-esteem status and self-reinforcement rates was observed.

Rice, J. H. The relationship of male sex-role identification and self-esteem to aggressive behavior. Unpublished dissertation, United States International University, 1975.

There is a negative relationship between self-esteem and aggressive tendencies in males.

Rickson, S. T. Self-esteem, reference group orientation and academic achievement. Unpublished dissertation, University of Washington, 1977.

A positive relationship was found between a student's self-esteem and his academic achievement.

Rios-Garcia, L. R. Self-esteem, defense styles and conformity. Unpublished dissertation, Florida State University, 1975.

This is a critical review of the literature which shows self-esteem to be negatively related to conformity behavior.

Riskind, J. H. Controllability and behavioral compliance with the counselor's recommendations: Effects of time perspective and self-esteem on weight loss. Unpublished dissertation, Yale University, 1977.

> Subjects with chronic self-esteem enhanced their feelings of personal control by exhibiting a short-range, realistic goal orientation.

Robbins, G. L. The effects of leader styles on self-esteem, attitudes and interpersonal coping style of T-group participants. Unpublished dissertation, University of Iowa, 1974.

> There was no relationship supported between leader style and group member outcome or between group member goal choice and member outcome in a T-group.

Rosenthal, J. H. Self-esteem in dyslexic children. *Academic Therapy*, 1973, *9*, No. 1, 27-39.

> Dyslexic children have lower self-esteem (than non-dyslexic) and dyslexic from an aware and understanding family have higher self-esteem than those from an unaware family.

Rothfarb, H. I. A study of the psychological needs and self-esteem of college men who exercise regularly. Unpublished dissertation, Boston College, 1970.

> There is a positive relationship between self-esteem and the amount of intentional exercise.

Russell, P. R. The effects of a psychological education class on self-esteem, locus of control and vocational choice of community college students. Unpublished dissertation, Cornell University, 1975.

> In a structured small group, positive feedback, value clarification and stressing participant's strengths proved effective in improving self-esteem.

Ryckman, R. M. & Cannon, D. W. Relationship between self-esteem and internal external control for men and women. *Psychological Reports*, 1973, *32*, No. 3, 1106.

> As a correlate of locus of control self-esteem was not affected by sex differences.

Ryckman, R. M. & Cannon, D. W. Multidimensionality of locus of control and self-esteem. *Psychological Reports*, 1975, *37*, No. 3, 786.

> Among female undergraduates, there is a positive relationship between self-esteem and 1) personal locus of control 2) freedom from other's control.

Rynersom, B. C. Need for self-esteem in the aged: A literature review *Journal of Psychiatric Nursing and Mental Health Services*, 1972, *10*, No. 1, 22-26.*

Sachs, D. H. The effects of similarity, evaluation and self-esteem on interpersonal attraction. *Representative Research in Social Psychology.* 1976, 7, No. 1, 44-50.

> The predicted interaction of self-esteem and similarity variables was evident only for the subject's perceived intelligence of the stranger.

Sachs, D. L. The impact of group counseling on self-esteem and other personality characteristics. Unpublished dissertation, University of Michigan, 1974.

> This group counseling experience tended to effect large changes in individual self-esteem, both positively and negatively.

Saito, I. & Inoue, K. (Cooperation competition and self-esteem.) *Japanese Journal of Psychology,* 1971, 42, No. 3, 147-152.*

Samuels, D. D. A study of the relationship between maternal anxiety and self-esteem of Head Start children. Unpublished dissertation, Michigan State University, 1977.

> Highly anxious mothers tend to have children with low self-esteem.

Schaeffer, G. M.; Schuckit, M. A. & Morrissey, E. R. Correlation between two measures of self-esteem and drug use in a college sample. *Psychological Reports,* 1976, *39*, No. 3, 915-991.

> Concerning drug use and self-esteem, only heavy alcohol use was related to low self-esteem.

Schiff, E. The relationship of women's sex-role identity to self-esteem and ego development. Unpublished dissertation, University of Maryland, 1977.

> Androgynous women have higher self-esteem than feminine or undifferentiated women.

Schlenker, B. R.; Soraci, S. & McCarthy, B. Self-esteem and group performance as determinants of egocentric perceptions in cooperative groups. *Human Relations,* 1976, *29*, No. 12, 1163-1176.

> Self-esteem was not related to perceptions of responsiblity (personal or environmental) for group performance, but high self-esteem subjects shifted credit for group success toward themselves and group failure away from themselves.

Schneider, D. J. & Turkat, D. Self-presentation following success or failure: defensive self-esteem models. *Journal of Personality,* 1975, *13*, No. 1, 127-135.

> Those subjects with high defensive self-esteem presented themselves more positively after failure (versus success), than did genuine high self-esteem subjects.

Schonbar, R. Group co-therapists and sex-role identification. *American Journal of Psychotherapy,* 1973, 27, No. 4, 539-547.

> Low self-esteem is proposed as being related to the type of neurosis associated with sex-role identity.

Schwab, J. A. The effects of self-esteem and vocational maturity on the level of occupational choice. Unpublished dissertation, University of Notre Dame, 1974.

There is a significant relationship between one's self-esteem on his occupational goals and aspirations.

Schwartz, A. N. Volunteers help build patient's self-esteem. *Hospital and Community Psychiatry*, 1970, *21*, No. 3, 87-89.

Report of a project in which attractive women volunteers attended group gatherings of institutionalized males to help patients build self-esteem.

Schwartz, A. N. An observation of self-esteem as the linchpin of quality of life for the aged; an essay. *Gerontologist*, 1975, *15*, No. 5, 470-472.

Self-esteem is the most crucial factor is successful aging.

Schwendiman, G.; Larsen, K. & Dunn, F. Social position, social desirability and self-esteem. *Psychological Reports*, 1970, *27*, No. 1, 117-118.

There is a positive correlation between a person's self-esteem and the desirability of his social position.

Scott, S. Self-esteem in women as a function of participation in groups. Unpublished dissertation, United States International University, 1975.

Group participation insignificantly enhances self-esteem.

Sell, J. M. Effects of subject self-esteem test performance feedback and counselor attractiveness of influence in counseling. *Journal of Counseling Psychology*, 1974, *21*, No. 4, 342-344.

The self-esteem of an experimental subject is not related to the development of counselor attractiveness.

Shainwald, R. G. The effect of self-esteem on opinion leadership. Unpublished dissertation, University of Georgia, 1973.

There is a positive relationship between self-esteem and a subject's interpersonal influence in communication.

Sheehan, C. & Walsh, E. J. Sex, work satisfaction and self-esteem: the effects of cross-sex incumbency in sex-typed occupations. Paper presented at the 1977 meeting of the Pennsylvania Sociological Society.

There was no effect on self-esteem in the sample.

Shelibow, B. An investigation into the relationship between self-esteem and skin color among Hispanic children. *Graduate Research in Education and Related Disciplines*, 1973, *1*, No. 1, 64-82.

Black Hispanic children have lower self-esteem than White Hispanic children.

Shrauger, J. S. Self-esteem and reactions to being observed by others. *Journal* of Personality and Social Psychology, 1972, 23, No. 2, 192-200.

> High self-esteem subjects had a more positive performance assessment of themselves than low self-esteem subjects.

Shrauger, J. S. & Rosenberg, S. E. Self-esteem and the effects of success and failure feedback on performance. *Journal of Personality*, 1970, *38*, No. 3, 404-417.

> Task performance following failure feedback was poorer than that following success, with high self-esteem subjects improving performance after success and low-self esteem subjects performing worse after failure.

Silber, E. & Tippett, J. Self-esteem: clinical assessment and measurement validation. *Psychological Reports*, 1965, *16*, 1017-1071.

> Utilizing several testing methods, self-esteem was proposed to be the degree of congruence between a person's self-image and his ideal self-image.

Silverman, A. F.; Pressman, M. E. & Bartel, H. W. Self-esteem and tactile communication. *Journal of Humanistic Psychology*, 1973, *13*, No. 2, 73-77.

> Higher self-esteem persons were more intimate on tactile communication, found the task easier and perceived the communication more clearly. Results support the idea that *touch* can be used as a means of self-disclosure.

Silverman, A. I. The effects of preferred-perceived environmental compatibility and self-esteem on managerial in-basket behavior. Unpublished dissertation, Temple University, 1972.*

Simon, W. E. Note on smoking and self-esteem. *Psychological Reports*, 1972, *31*, No. 2, 666.

> No relation between the variables was found.

Simon, W. E. & Simon, M. G. Self-esteem, intelligence and standardized academic achievement. *Psychology in the Schools*, 1975, *12*, No. 1, 97-100.

> Significant relationships exist between self-esteem and standardized academic achievement; self-esteem and verbal I.Q.

Simpson, K. C. & Boyle, D. Esteem construct generality and academic performance. *Educational and Psychological Measurement*, 1975, *35*, No. 4, 897-904.

> Among undergraduates, the relationship between esteem measures and actual examination performance was strongest for the task measures of self-esteem.

Singh, U. P. & Tapeshwar, P. Self-esteem, social-esteem and conformity behavior. *Psychologia: An International Journal of Psychology in the Orient*, 1973, *16*, No. 2, 61-68.

> Conformity and low self-esteem were found to be significantly related among male postgraduate students.

Sjoberg, L. Self-esteem and information processing. *Goteborg Psychological Reports*, 1976, *6*, No. 14.

> A theory develops in which the preservation of self-esteem is postulated as a central force in goal oriented belief systems.

Slavson, S. R. Because I live here, NY:NY, International Universities Press, 1971.

> Describes a long-term research project outlining "Vita-Erg" therapy used in two closed wards for psychotic women.

Smart, M. S. & Smart, R. C. Self-esteem and social-personal orientation of Indian 12- and 18-year-olds. *Psychological Reports*, 1970, *27*, No. 1, 107-115.

> Among preadolescents the average self-ideal congruence scores were highest for Indian girls, than Indian boys followed by American girls and boys, respectively.

Smerd, S. J. The relationship between inner-city high school girls' perception of academic competence and self-esteem. Unpublished dissertation, University of Pittsburgh, 1977.

> Researcher concludes that it *seems* academic achievements by Blacks builds self-esteem, which *inherently* leads to openness toward others.

Smith, A. D. Effects of self-esteem enhancement on teacher's acceptance of innovation in a classroom setting. Unpublished dissertation, Yale University, 1973.

> Positive feedback on performance enhances self-esteem and increases acceptance of innovations.

Smith, R. B.; Tedeschi, J. T.; Brown, R. C. & Lindskold, S. Correlations between trust, self-esteem, sociometric choice and internal-external control. *Psychological Reports*, 1973, *32*, No. 3, 739-743.

> Among 4th and 5th graders, self-esteem was not correlated with any of the other variables.

Smith, R. C. Self-esteem as moderator variable in the relationship between manifest need of nurturance and satisfaction. *Journal of Clinical Psychology*, 1972, *28*, No. 3, 347-348.

> Self-esteem acts as a moderator variable in the relationship between nurturance and satisfaction.

Smith W. P. & Bordonaro, F. Self-esteem and satisfaction as affected by unexpected social status placement. Sociometry, 1975, *38*, No. 2, 223-246.

> Unexpected status manipulation to a position above peer group resulted in personal satisfaction and lower self-esteem.

Smokler, C. B. The development of self-esteem and femininity in early adolescence, Unpublished dissertation, the University of Michigan, 1974.

The self-esteem of females was positively related to having feminine comptencies, but negatively related to traditional feminine personality characteristics.

Sparling, J. J. The etiology of self-esteem in childhood and adolescence. Unpublished dissertation, the University of Michigan, 1968.

The researcher generates a broad hypothesis suggesting that a multi-factor interaction, over time, produces patterns of self-esteem.

Spillman, B. M. Cognitive dissonance, self-esteem and the process of self-persuasion. Unpublished dissertation, University of Utah, 1974.

The process of protecting self-esteem produces more cognitive reorganization than the motivation to reduce value inconsistency.

Stang, D. J. Conformity, ability and self-esteem. *Representative Research in Social Psychology*, 1972, *3*, No. 2, 97-103.

Self-esteem measures had small positive correlations with task ability and small negative correlations with conformity.

Stebbins, R. A. Modesty, pride and conceit: variations in the expression of self-esteem. 1972, paper presented at the 67th Annual Meeting of American Sociological Association.

The verbal expressions of self-esteem and explored, utilizing hypotheses about the concepts of modesty, pride and conceit in relation to structural and situaional conditions.

Steffenhagen, R. A. Toward a self-esteem theory of drug dependence: a position paper. *Journal of Alcohol and Drug Education*, 1977, *22*, No. 2, 1-3.

Placing self-esteem at the apex of the personality, a self-esteem theory of drug dependence is posited, based on Adler's Individual Psychology.

Stein, S. L. The interrelationships among self-esteem, personal values and interpersonal values. Unpublished dissertation, Northern Illinois University, 1969.

Self-esteem correlated significantly with academic achievement.

Stephan, W. G. School desegregation: An evaluation of predictions made in Brown vs. Board of Education. *Psychological Bulletin*, *85*, No. 2, 217-238.

A tentative conclusion drawn from social scientists' testimony in Brown vs. Board of Education is that the self-esteem of Blacks rarely increases in desegregated schools.

Stericker, A. B. Fear of success in male and female college students: sex-role identification and self-esteem as factors. Unpublished dissertation, Loyola University of Chicago. 1976.

Self-esteem was found not to be related to fear of success in undergraduates.

Sternberg, W. C. Self-esteem as a mediating variable of attributions. Unpublished dissertation, City University of New York, 1976.

> This study, using behavioral measures and questionnaires, supports the proposition that self-esteem acts as a mediator variable concerning the types of attributions an individual makes.

Sterner, G. A. Birth order and self-esteem as determinants of affiliative behavior under ego-threatening conditions Unpublished dissertation, Wayne State University, 1972.

> A model was developed to explain affiliative behavior under threatening conditions which assumed there is an interaction effect between birth order position and self-esteem.

Stevens, W. D. The effects of didactic group therapy on the self-esteem of potential school dropouts. Unpublished dissertation, Southern Illinois University, 1974.

> Didactic group therapy is effective in changing self-esteem under proper social conditions.

Stewart, R. A. Integration of tolerance of ambiguity and persuasibility studies of self-esteem. *Psychological Reports*, 1968, *23*, No. 3, 1104.

> Describes a curvilinear relationship between self-esteem and persuasibility.

Stone, V. A. Individual differences and innoculation against persuasion, *Journalism Quarterly*, 1969, *46*, No. 2, 267-273.

> Subjects with low self-esteem are more reliant on sources (v. content) for determining the correctness of ideas; hence how a subject with low self-esteem views a source will make a greater difference in his response (than a high self-esteem subject).

Stotland, E. Self-esteem and violence by guards and state troopers of Attica. *Criminal Justice and Behavior*, 1973, *3*, No. 1, 85-96.*

Stotland, E. & Dunn, R. Identification, oppositeness, authoritarianism, self-esteem and birth order, *Psychological Monographs*, 1962, *76*, No. 9, 21.

> Persons with low self-esteem identified more with a similar-poor model than high self-esteem individuals.

Street, C. P. Changes in self-esteem, dependency and depression as a result of participation in a self-esteem building workshop. Unpublished dissertation, United States International University, 1976.

> Significant correlations were found between self-esteem and dependency; self-esteem and depression, and between dependency and depression.

Stroebe, W.; Eagly, A. H. & Stroebe, M. S. Self-esteem and the perceived course of friendly and unfriendly acts. *Personality and Social Psychology Bulletin*, 1974, *1*, No. 1, 387-389.

> There is a positive correlation between a subject's self-esteem and the attributing of a positive self-evaluation by others to personal feelings of that evaluator.

Stroebe, W.; Eagly, A. H. & Stroebe, M. S. Friendly or just polite? The effect of self-esteem on attributions. *European Journal of Social Psychology*, 1977, 7, No. 3, 265-274.

There is a significant interaction between self-esteem and evaluation positivity.

Suga, Sawako. The relation between the self-esteem and the human relations of the adolescent. *Japanese Journal of Educational Psychology*, 1975, 23, No. 4, 224-229.

Results support the positive correlation between adolescent self-esteem and acceptance by others.

Sutherland, S. H. A study of the effects of a marathon and a traditional encounter group experience on self-esteem, defensive behavior and mood. Unpublished dissertation, Texas Tech. University, 1972.

There was no differnce in self-esteem found between the experimental and control group.

Taylor, J. B. & Reitz, W. E. The three faces of self-esteem. *Research Bulletin* #80, Department of Psychology, University of Western Ontario.*

Taylor, L.M. A comparison of self-esteem and self-concept of academic ability in three groups of black adolescents. Unpublished dissertation, University of Minnesota, 1974.

A significant positive relationship exists between self-esteem and self-perceived academic ability.

Teahan J. E. & Hug, J. Some effects of audio-visual techniques on the aspirational level of self-concept of Negro students. *Journal of Human Relations*, 1969, 17, No. 2, 291-310.

The U.S. Negro, due to his absence of cultural models and lack of history is forced to look to contemporary models for identification and enhancement of their self-esteem.

Timm, S. A. The behavioral correlates of mothers of low and high self-esteem. Unpublished dissertation, University of Nebraska-Lincoln, 1974.

Mothers with high self-esteem tended to give more rewards and make fewer negative remarks to their children.

Tittle, C. R. Institutionalized living and self-esteem. *Social Problems*, 1972, 20, No. 1, 65-77.

The data show that total institutions affect self-esteem negatively, but not pervasively.

Trautner, H. M. & Schuster, B. On the significance of the self-image and the perceived parent image for the problem of delinquency. (German) *—rchiv fur Psychologie*, 1975, 127, No. 1-2, 116-130.

Delinquents showed no less self-esteem than non-delinquents of the same socioeconomic status.

Trenkel, A. Pleasure and self-esteem (German) *Zeitschrift fur Klinische Psychologie and Psychotherapie*, 1975, 23, No. 3, 224-231.

> The experience of pleasure and self-esteem was positively correlated among neurotic patients.

Turrall, G. M. Differential effects of sensitivity training and Adlerian parent training upon the self-esteem of academic underachievers. Unpublished dissertation, Boston University School of Education, 1975.

> The self-esteem of underachieveing child benefits over time from sensitivity training an Adlerian parent training.

Uhl, G. B. The effects of perceived helper status and recipient self-esteem on help-seeking. Unpublished dissertation, Ohio State University, 1974.

> There is a positive relationship between a subject's self-esteem and his willingness to seek help.

Upshaw, H. S. & Yates, L. W. Self-persuasion, social approval, and task success as determinants of self-esteem following impression management. *Journal of Experimental Social Psychology*, 1972, 24, 209-210.

Vance, J. & Richmond, B. O. Cooperative and competitive behavior as a function of self-esteem. *Psychology in the Schools*, 1975, 12, No. 2, 225-229.

> There is a negative relationship among children between cooperative behavior and self-esteem.

Van Gorder, E. J. Self-esteem as a variable in response to frustration. Unpublished dissertation, California School of Professional Psychology, San Francisco, 1975.

> Subjects with high self-esteem exhibited no aggressive behavior in response to frustration and were less anxious than low self-esteem subjects following attack.

Vaughan, S. T. Raising self-esteem through cognitive counseling. Unpublished dissertation, University of California, Los Angeles, 1974.

> The total counseling mode produced significant changes in self-esteem.

Volpe, R. Feedback facilitated relaxation training as primary prevention of drug abuse in early adolescence. *Journal of Drug Education*, 1977, 7, No. 2, 179-194.

> Relaxation training is suggested as a form of primary prevention of anxiety and for developing the self-esteem involving individuals who are drug abusers.

Wallston, B. S. The effects of sex-role, self-esteem and expected future integration with an audience for help-seeking. Unpublished dissertation, University of Wisconsin, 1972.

> Among males, self-esteem was negatively related to help-seeking behavior.

Ward, S. H. & Braun, J. Self-esteem and racial preferences in black children. *American Journal of Orthopsychiatry*, 1972, *42*, No. 4, 644-647.

> Among Black children, a significant, positive relationship was found between self-esteem scores and preference of a black puppet over a white one.

Warren, N. T. Self-esteem and sources of cognitive bias in the evaluation of past performance. *Journal of Consulting and Clinical Psychology*, 1976, *44*, No. 6, 966-975.

> Among male subjects a negative correlation exists between self-esteem and the size of the discrepancy between successful goal criteria and perceived performance.

Washburne, N. F. Postnote. *Sociological Focus*, 1971, *4*, No. 3, 90-101.

> The researcher claims Pope's scale is crude and insufficiently tested, though Washburne originally proposed the scale's creation.

Washington, C. S. A method for developing self-esteem and authenticity in para-counselors and counselors. Unpublished dissertation, University of Massachusetts, 1976.

> This counselor training program for Blacks enhanced self-esteem.

Waters, L. K. & Roach, D. Self-esteem as a moderator of the relationship between task success and task-liking. *Psychological Reports*, 1972, *31*, No. 1, 69-70.

> The relationship between task success and task liking was stronger for high self-esteem subjects.

Watkins, D. Self-esteem as a moderator in vocational choice: a test of Korman's hypothesis. *Australian Psychologist* 1975, *10*, No. 1, 75-80.

> There is no relationship between self-esteem and teacher's perceptions of personal abilities and satisfaction concerning vocational choice.

Watkins, D. The development and evaluation of self-esteem measuring instruments. *Journal of Personality Assessment*, 1978, *42*, No. 2, 171-182.

> He proposes a self-esteem measure that takes into account the subject's value system.

Weinberger, D. M. Frequency of group counseling as a variable affecting student self-esteem and classroom behavior with male students at the seventh grade level. Unpublished dissertation, The American University, 1975.

> Self-esteem was not significantly influenced by group counseling for adolescent males.

Wells, L. E. Self-esteem: its conceptualization and measurement. Unpublished dissertation, University of Wisconsin-Madison, 1975.

> This study tries to delimit as well as analyze the self-esteem concept as a social scientific construct subsumed under a broader theoretical topic of self-conception.

Wetzel, B. C. The effects of assertive training on the self-esteem of counselors in training. Unpublished dissertation, University of Pittsburgh, 1977.

> There was no significant effect on the self-esteem of individuals who participated in group assertive training.

Weiner, Y. Task ego involvement and self-esteem as moderators of situationally devalued self-esteem. *Journal of Applied Psychology*, 1973, *58*, No. 2, 225-232.

> High task involvement and high self-esteem lead to a production increase.

Wilcox, A. H. Effects of self-esteem, motive to avoid failure and order of presentation on the consideration of discrepant and nondiscrepant vocational interest inventory results. Unpublished dissertation, University of Maryland, 1973.

> It is statistically indicated that relationships exist between the three variables, but in a way more complex than determined.

Williams, R. L. & Byars, H. Negro self-esteem in a transitional society. *Personnel and Guidance Journal*, 1968, *47*, No. 2, 120-125.

> General finding concerning Negro adolescent students indicate low self-confidence, defensive in their self-descriptions and confused, concerning their self-identity.

Williams R. L. & Byars, H. The effect of academic integration on the self-esteem of southern Negro students. *Social Psychology*, 1970, *80*, No. 2, 183-188.

> Black students in segregated schools with Caucasian instructors made significantly greater gains in self-evaluation than students in totally segregated or newly desegregated schools.

Wilson, J. P. & Wilson, S. B. Sources of self-esteem and the person X situation controversy. *Psychological Reports*, 1976, *38*, No. 2, 355-358.

> Sex differences were found for the major sources of self-esteem.

Wilson, S. R. & Benner, L. A. The effects of self-esteem and situation upon comparison choices during ability evaluation. *Sociometry*, 1971, *34*, No. 3, 381-397.

> Males, in a public competitive situation show a positive correlation between self-esteem and their choice, by ranked ability of a comparison other.

Wingard, G. L. The effects of marital adjustment and self-esteem of parents on children's perceptions of parental behavior. Unpublished dissertation, University of Notre Dame, 1977.

> A strong relationship exists between parental self-esteem and marital adjustment; and the child's perception of parents as accepting.

Wober, M. Explorations on the concept of self-esteem. *International Journal of*

Psychology, 1971, *6*, No. 2, 147-155.

> This cross-cultural study clearly indicates that vast differences in criteria and level of self-esteem exists between both cultural and occupational groups.

Wortitz, J. G. A study of self-esteem in children of alcoholics. Unpublished dissertation, Rutgers University, 1976.

> Children living in alcoholic homes have lower self-esteem than those from non-alcoholic homes.

Wood, F. H. & Johnson, A. Coopersmith Self-Esteem Inventory scores of boys with severe behavior problems. *Exceptional Children*, 1972, *38*, No. 9, 739-740.

> These subjects scored significantly lower than the norm in mean self-esteem.

Woodward, C. Self-esteem: a self-presentation interpretation. Unpublished dissertation, University of Southern California, 1977.

> Proposes personality to be an interpersonal phenomenon and that self-esteem expression has normative limitations which constantly change with the social situation.

Wright, R. J.; Fox, M. & Noppe, L. The interrelationship of creativity self-esteem and creative self-concept. *Psychology*, 1975, *12*, No. 5, 1115.*

Youngleson, M. L. The need to affiliate and self-esteem in institutionalized children. *Journal of Personality and Social Psychology*, 1973, *26*, No. 2, 280-286.

> The poor socializing environment inherent in institutions leads to reduced self-esteem.

Zak, I. Jewish background, self-esteem, Jewish-American identity, and attitudes toward Israel. Unpublished dissertation, New York University, 1973.

> Self-esteem had an inverse effect on the behavioral tendencies in Jews and no direct influence on the affective tendencies.

Zeitner, R. M. The pupillometric response as an index of self-esteem. Unpublished dissertation, Brigham Young University, 1975.

> For only females, in self-portrait, observation, the greater the pupillometric response, the poorer the self-esteem.

Zellner, M. Self-esteem reception and influencibility. *Journal of Personality and Social Psychology*, 1970, *15*, No. 1, 87-93.

> Among male high school students, their acute (manipulated) self-esteem point of maximum influenceability increased as the situational messages became more complex.

Ziller, R. C.; Hagey, J.; Smith, M. & Long, B. H. Self-esteem: a self-social construct. *Journal of Consulting and Clinical Psychology*, 1969, 33V, No. 1, 84-95.

Research results emanating from an evolving theory of social self-esteem, suggest that self-acceptance and social acceptance are interdependent concepts.

Zivelonghi, V. O. The relationship between self-esteem and the primary emotions. Unpublished dissertation, Claremont Graduate School, 1976.

Self-esteem is positively related to joy and acceptance and is negatively related to sorrow and disgust.

SUBJECT INDEX